Man's body

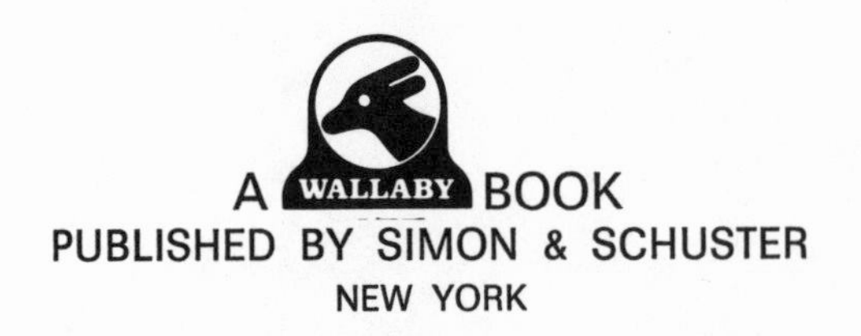

An Owner's Manual

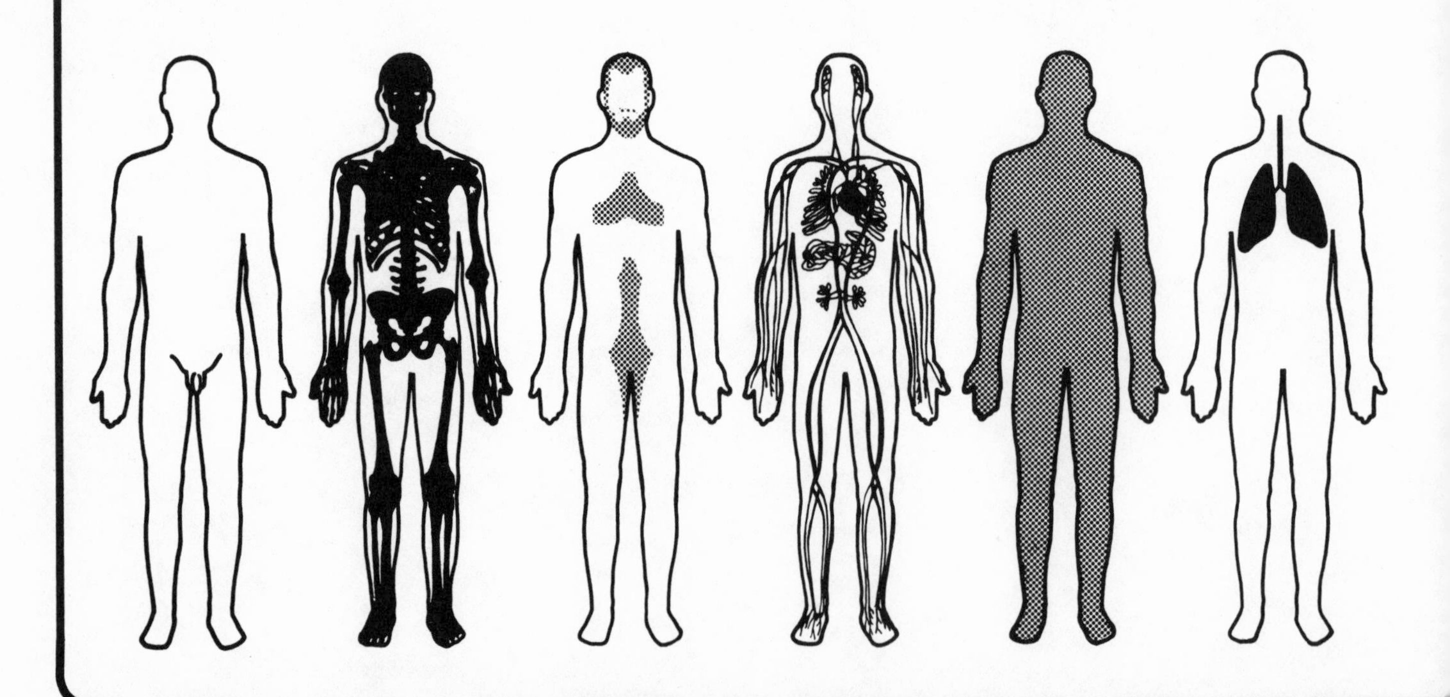

MAN'S BODY

by the Diagram Group

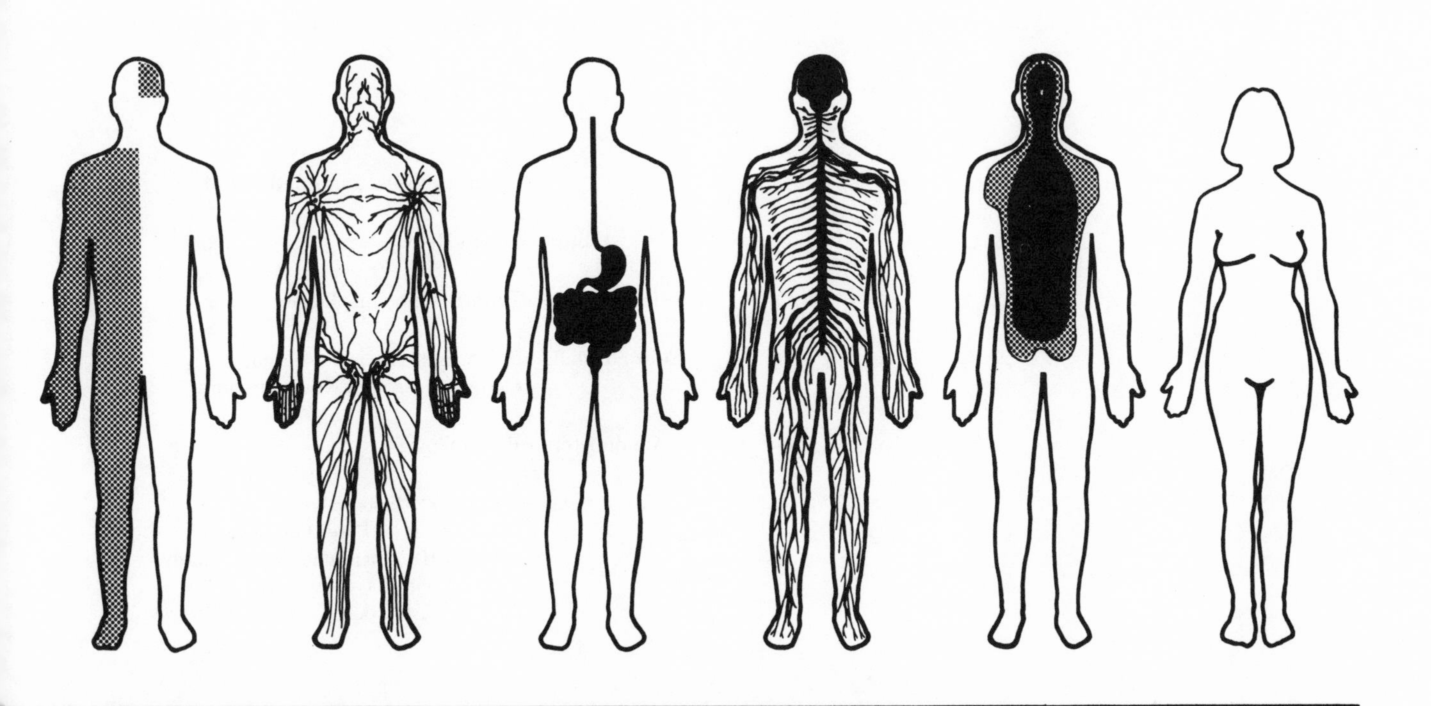

Revised Edition published 1981.

Published by Wallaby Books
A Simon & Schuster Division of
Gulf & Western Corporation
Simon & Schuster Building
1230 Avenue of the Americas
New York, New York 10020

10 9 8 7 6 5 4 3 2 1
Manufactured in the United States of America

Library of Congress Cataloging in Publication Data

Diagram Group.
Man's body.

Reprint of the 1976 ed. published by Paddington
Press, New York.
Includes index.
1. Men—Health and hygiene. 2. Men—Physiology.
I. Title.
RA777.8.D5 1980 613'.04234 80-24674

ISBN 0-671-41619-7

Revisions Joseph Ballinger, Barbara B. Buchholz

Diagram Visual Information Ltd.

Editor David Heidenstam

Associate editors Ruth Berenbaum, Jefferson Cann

Editorial staff Susan Leith, Julie Vosburgh,
Catherine Groom, Kathryn Dunn

Art director Robin Crane

Artists Jeff Alger, Allison Blythe,
Robert Galvin, Peter Golding,
Richard Hummerstone, Susan Kinsey,
Roger Kohn, Pavel Kostal,
Kathleen McDougall, Graham Rosewarne

FOREWORD

The male body is usually a mystery to its owner. The purpose of this book is to unravel some of that mystery.

Its standpoint is that of the ordinary man. Medical science and its language are complex; and so are the functions and malfunctions of the male body. MAN'S BODY sets out to make a wide range of information and practical guidance clear and concise.

The editors have brought together both international statistical evidence and the insights of recognized specialists; and all this material has been presented to a panel of practicing physicians for their review and commentary.

The problem of clear presentation resulted in a special solution. Illustrations and charts help make the array of information readily comprehensible. Individual panels, numbered for cross-reference, lead the reader through the issues that his questions raise.

Since MAN'S BODY's publication in 1977, however, medical science has made new discoveries, conquered old problems, gained new insights. We now know more about the risks associated with smoking, drinking, and combining drugs. We know more about infertility; for example, that the woman may have an antibody reaction to the man's sperm. We have also learned more about treatments for these and other problems, and new diagnostic procedures and medicines are being developed constantly. Every day our understanding of the workings of the human body is being modified and expanded.

MAN'S BODY has been revised to focus on the new developments in medical science since 1977. The revised edition is just as simple to use as the original; its diagrams are just as precise.

This book is intended to provide helpful everyday information in one volume, to dispel many myths, and to give the reader a sound understanding and fuller enjoyment of man's body.

CONTENTS

BODY CARE

DRUGS

WOMAN'S BODY: A NON-OWNER'S GUIDE

An asterisk in the text refers to an index entry.

CONCEPTION

A01 SEX DETERMINATION

WHY SEXUAL REPRODUCTION?
Some creatures - such as the amoeba - reproduce by just splitting in two. That may be convenient! But the resulting offspring are very predictable. One amoeba can father endless generations: but the youngest will still be identical with the first. Sexual reproduction, in contrast, gives almost infinite variety, for the offsprings' characteristics are a jumbled mixture from both parents' family trees. Some have some talents, and some have others - and some manage to combine many talents: all of which helps a species as complex as man to survive, in a complex and demanding world.
SEXUAL INHERITANCE
Every cell in the human body contains a "blueprint" of information, on the basis of which it was constructed. This information is contained in 23 pairs of chromosomes, which lie in the nucleus of the cell. The chromosomes determine the output of protein, the basic building unit: which proteins the cell manufactures, when, and how. This in turn determines the cell's characteristics and activities.
When a cell divides to make the body grow, the pairs of chromosomes double up before the division. This means both new cells still get 23 pairs, and still get every piece of information that the old cell had. But when the body produces cells for sexual reproduction, it divides cells without doubling their chromosomes first. The pairs separate and each sexual cell gets only 23 single chromosomes, one of each pair. So each of these cells has only half the information that goes into a normal cell.
The sperm is the male example of such a cell, and the ovum is the female example. When the two unite, the new fertilized cell, from which the offspring grows, contains 23 pairs of chromosomes again - each parent having contributed half.
BOY OR GIRL?
Of the 23 pairs of chromosomes in a body cell, 22 are always matching pairs - each chromosome in the pair is similar. Women also have their 23rd pair identical: they are both called X chromosomes. But men, instead, have two chromosomes that do not match. One is an X, as in women; the other is different, and is called a Y chromosome. It is these final chromosomes that contain the code that determines sex. The XX combination occurs in, and produces, a female; the XY combination, a male.
When the female cell splits, for sexual reproduction, the sexual cell that results contains one chromosome from each of the 23 pairs - including one X chromosome. When the male cell splits, for sexual reproduction, the sexual cell contains one chromosome from each of the 22 identical pairs, plus either the X or the Y - but not both. Which it is determines the offspring's sex. If it is an X it forms a pair with the female's X - a female child occurs. If it is a Y, it gives the XY non-pair that is typical of, and forms, a man.
More males are conceived than females- but males die off at a faster rate, even in the womb. There are more male stillbirths than female stillbirths, and the sooner the stillbirth occurs in the term of pregnancy, the more likely it is to be male. At four months there are about two male stillbirths for every female; at full term it is more like 1.5 to 1. As a result, the the ratio of fetus males to females declines, until at full term, in advanced societies, it is about 105 or 106 males for every 100 females.

A02 BOY OR GIRL?

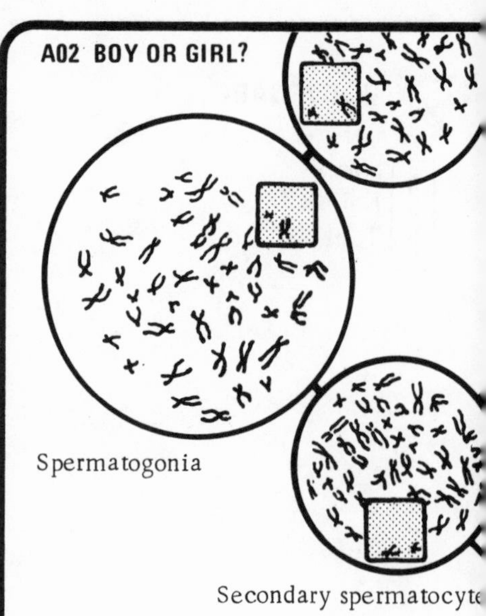

Male cell division (above) results in two spermatozoa, one with an X chromosome (a), the other with a Y chromosome (b). (See shaded boxes.)
Female cell division (below) results in one ovum, with an X chromosome (c) (the other cells degenerate).
The ovum is fertilized (d) by the sperm with the Y chromosome, so the child is male.

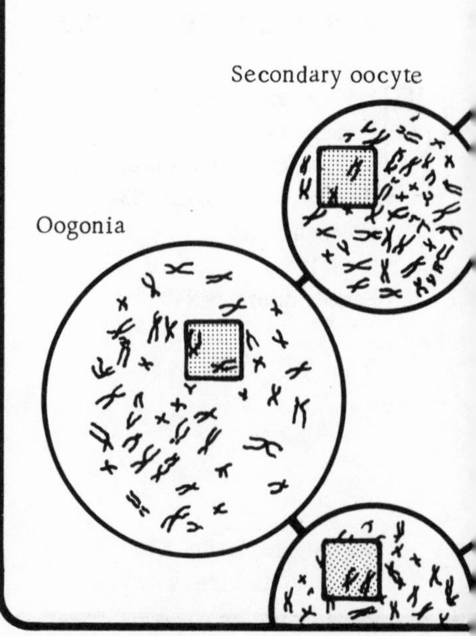

A03 MOMENT OF FERTILIZATION

On the right we show the edge of a female ovum - magnified about 50,000 times. (The ovum varies a great deal in size; but despite its minuteness, it is always by far the largest cell that the body produces.) Below we show three spermatazoa, magnified by the same amount. The ovum has just been fertilized by the topmost spermatozoon. Immediately the ovum's outer wall hardens, to prevent any more from entering.

For a description of the processes of conception, see M05.

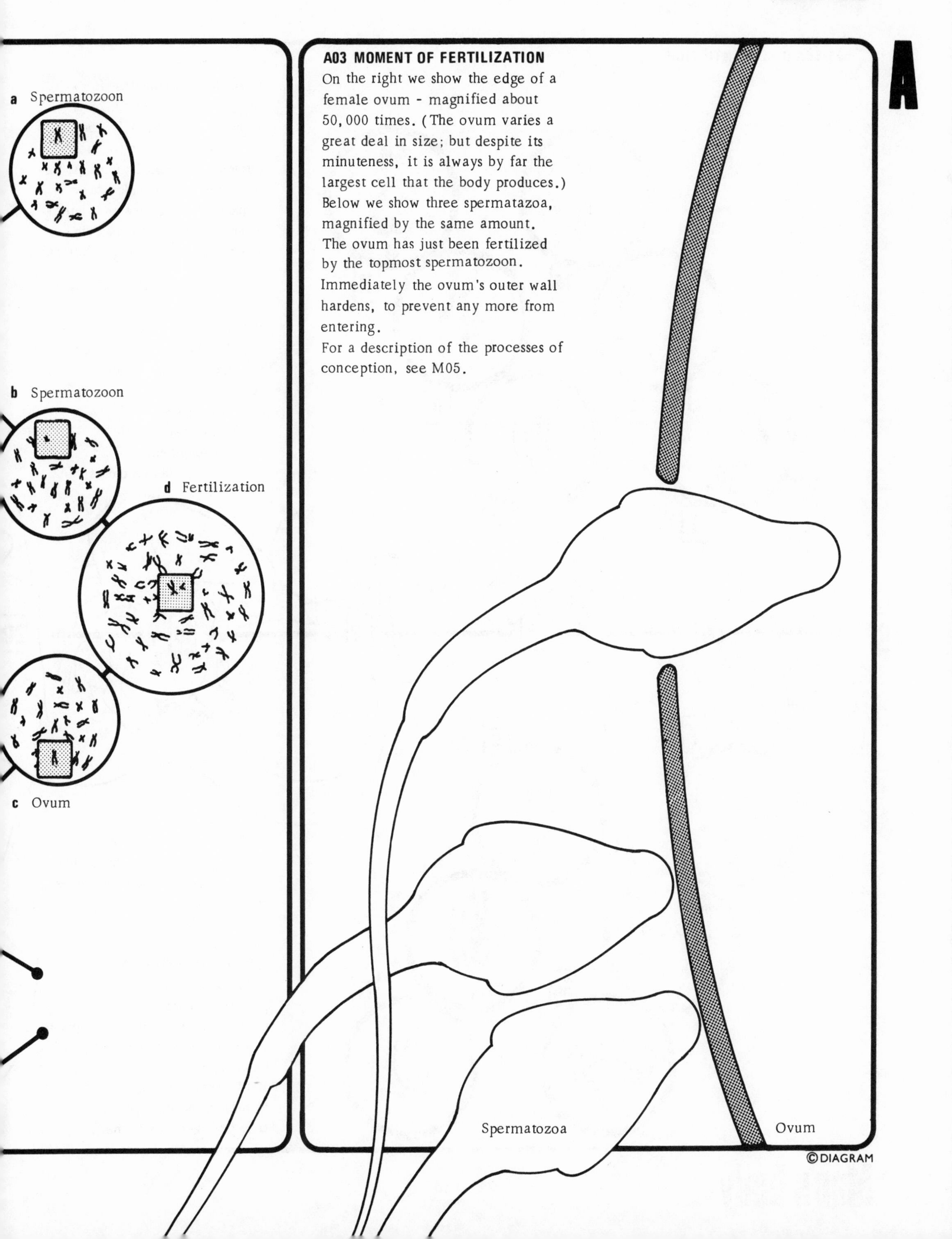

A04 SEX DIFFERENTIATION

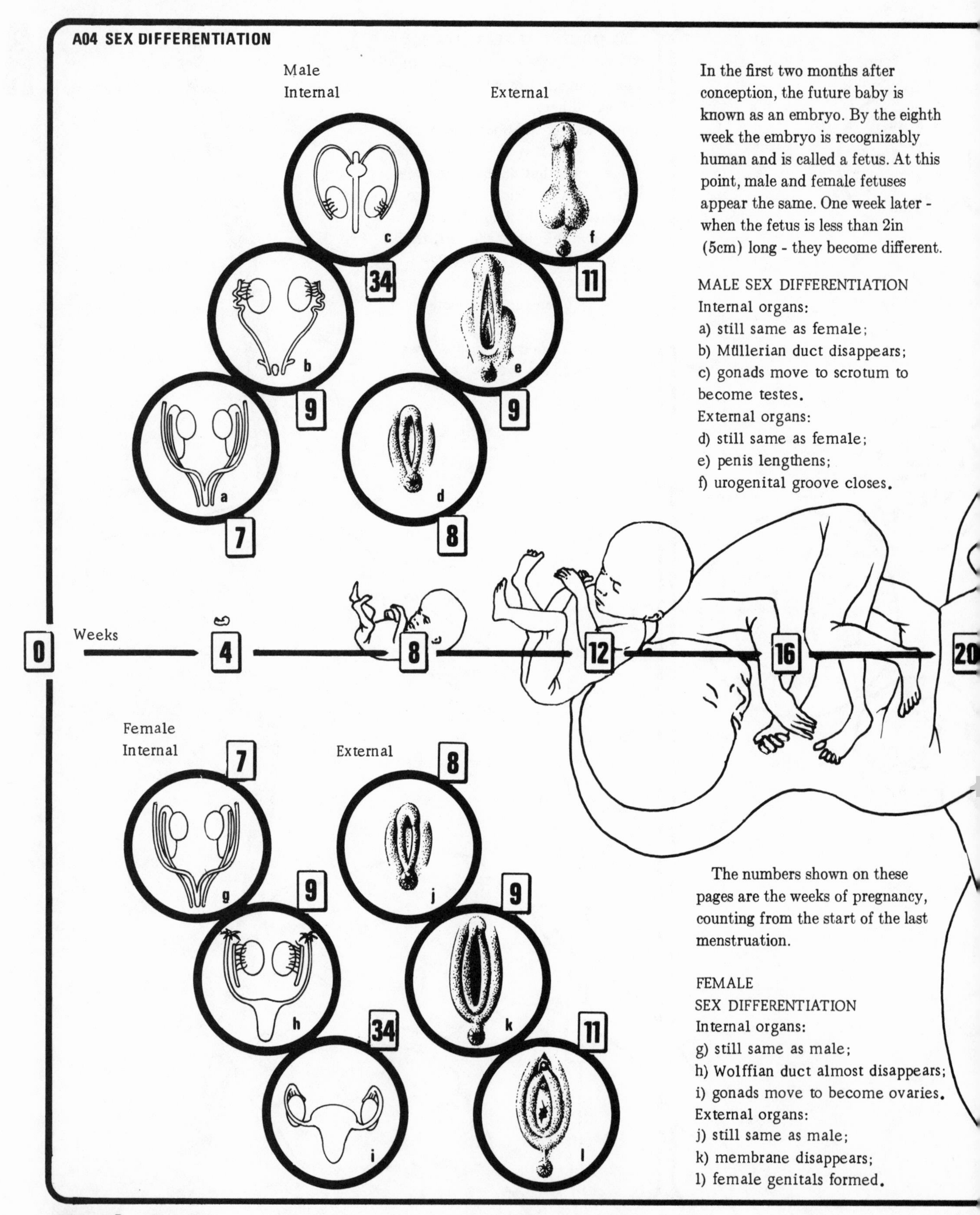

In the first two months after conception, the future baby is known as an embryo. By the eighth week the embryo is recognizably human and is called a fetus. At this point, male and female fetuses appear the same. One week later - when the fetus is less than 2in (5cm) long - they become different.

MALE SEX DIFFERENTIATION
Internal organs:
a) still same as female;
b) Müllerian duct disappears;
c) gonads move to scrotum to become testes.
External organs:
d) still same as female;
e) penis lengthens;
f) urogenital groove closes.

The numbers shown on these pages are the weeks of pregnancy, counting from the start of the last menstruation.

FEMALE
SEX DIFFERENTIATION
Internal organs:
g) still same as male;
h) Wolffian duct almost disappears;
i) gonads move to become ovaries.
External organs:
j) still same as male;
k) membrane disappears;
l) female genitals formed.

The centerline drawings show the average actual size of the fetus, at four-week intervals.

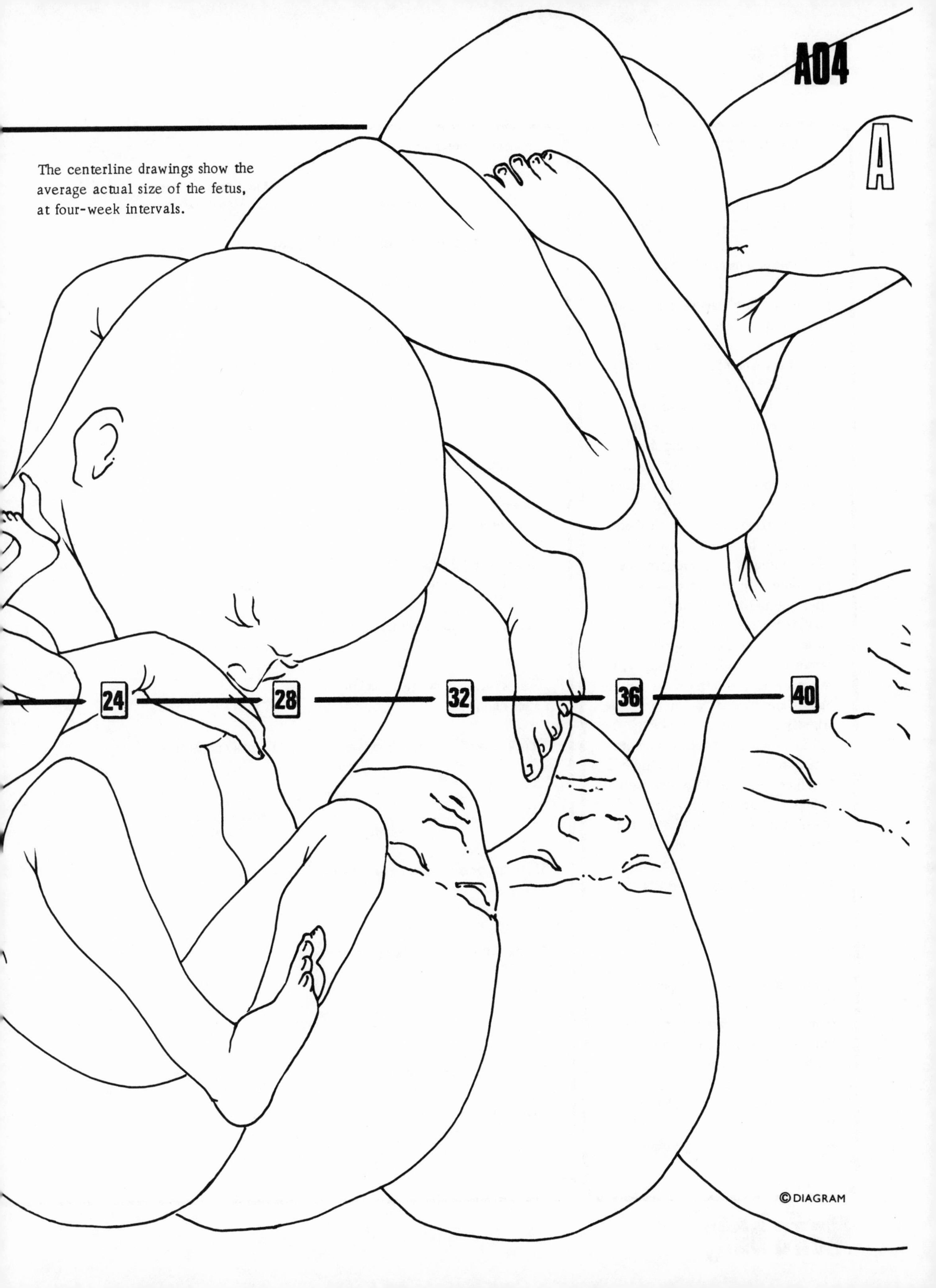

A05 BIRTHWEIGHT

The 6ft kangaroo has a less than 1gm baby; the blue whale a nearly 10 ton one. Human babies that have survived have ranged from under 2lb to over 29lb - but it is far healthier just to be an average 7lb 4oz.
In fact the boys' average is slightly higher (7½lb), and the girls' (just over 7lb) correspondingly lower. Boys' hearts and lungs are already marginally bigger at birth too (though their livers are lighter). All this is not because boys are later than girls in leaving the womb (in which case boys would have more time to develop before birth). In fact, if anything, there is a very slight tendency for there to be more boys among babies born after unusually short pregnancies, and more girls among those born after unusually long ones.
However, "premature babies" are quite often defined by birthweight, rather than length of pregnancy. On this criterion, slightly more female babies are termed "premature", as slightly more are under 5½ lb (2.5 kg) in weight. But really they are often "full-term low birthweight". Whether underweight or overweight, babies that are far from the average have less likelihood of survival. Average-weight babies have under a 2% death rate; 6 or 9 lb babies a 3% one; 4½ or 10½ pounders a 10% rate. Those that do survive are also more likely to be handicapped.
Perfectly normal babies vary greatly in rate of development. Sitting up for a few moments without support can start any time between 5 months and a year - walking without help any time between 8 months and 4 years. Parents should not think that delay is always very serious, or that it is likely to have a lasting effect.

A06 DEVELOPMENT

Characteristic	Most Babies First Do This Between
How he or she uses hands and eyes:	
Follows an object with his eyes for a short distance	Birth and 6 wks
Follows with his eyes from one side all the way to the other side of his head	2 mos and 4 mos
Brings his hands together in front of him	6 wks and 3½ mos
Grasps a rattle placed in his fingers	2½ mos and 4½ mos
Passes a toy from one hand to the other	5 mos and 7½ mos
Grasps a small object (like a raisin) off a flat surface	5 mos and 8 mos
Picks up a small object using thumb and finger	7 mos and 10 mos
Brings together two toys held in his hands	7 mos and 12 mos
Scribbles with a pencil or crayon	12 mos and 24 mos

Characteristic	Most Babies First Do This Between
How he or she uses ears and voice:	
Pays attention to sounds	Birth and 6 wks
Makes vocal sounds other than crying	Birth and 6 wks
Laughs	6 wks and 3½ mos
Squeals	6 wks and 4½ mos
Turns toward your voice	4 mos and 8 mos
Says "Dada" or "Mama"	6 mos and 10 mos

Characteristic	Most Babies First Do This Between
Uses Dada or Mama to mean one specific person	10 mos and 14 mos
Imitates the speech sounds you make	6 mos and 11 mos

Characteristic	Most Babies First Do This Between
How he or she handles whole body:	
Holds head off of bed for a few moments while lying on stomach	Birth and 4 wks
Holds head upright lying on stomach	5 wks and 3 mos
Holds head steady when you hold him in sitting position	6 wks and 4 mos
Rolls over from front to back, or from back to front	2 mos and 5 mos
Sits without support when placed in a sitting position	5 mos and 8 mos
Gets himself into sitting position in crib or on floor	6 mos and 11 mos
Takes part of his weight on his own legs when held steady	3 mos and 8 mos
Stands holding on	5 mos and 10 mos
Stands for a moment alone	9 mos and 13 mos
Stands alone well	10 mos and 14 mos
Walks holding onto furniture	7½ mos and 13 mos
Walks alone across a room	11 mos and 15 mos

Characteristic	Most Babies First Do This Between
How he or she behaves with other people:	
Looks at your face	Birth and 1 mo
Smiles when you smile or play with him	Birth and 2 mos
Smiles on his own	6 wks and 5 mos
Pulls back when you pull a toy in his hand	4 mos and 10 mos
Tries to get a toy that is out of reach	5 mos and 9 mos
Feeds himself crackers	5 mos and 8 mos
Drinks from a cup by himself	10 mos and 16 mos
Uses a spoon, spills little	13 mos and 24 mos
Plays peek-a-boo	6 mos and 10 mos
Plays pat-a-cake	7 mos and 13 mos
Plays with a ball on the floor	10 mos and 16 mos

NOTE: A baby who was born before he was expected—who was "premature"—will normally be later in development. If your baby was early by a month, add one month to the above ages to find out when to expect him to do things. If he was two months early, add two months, etc.

Information from U.S. Department of Health and Human Services, Office of Child Development.

A07 GROWTH, HEIGHT, AND WEIGHT

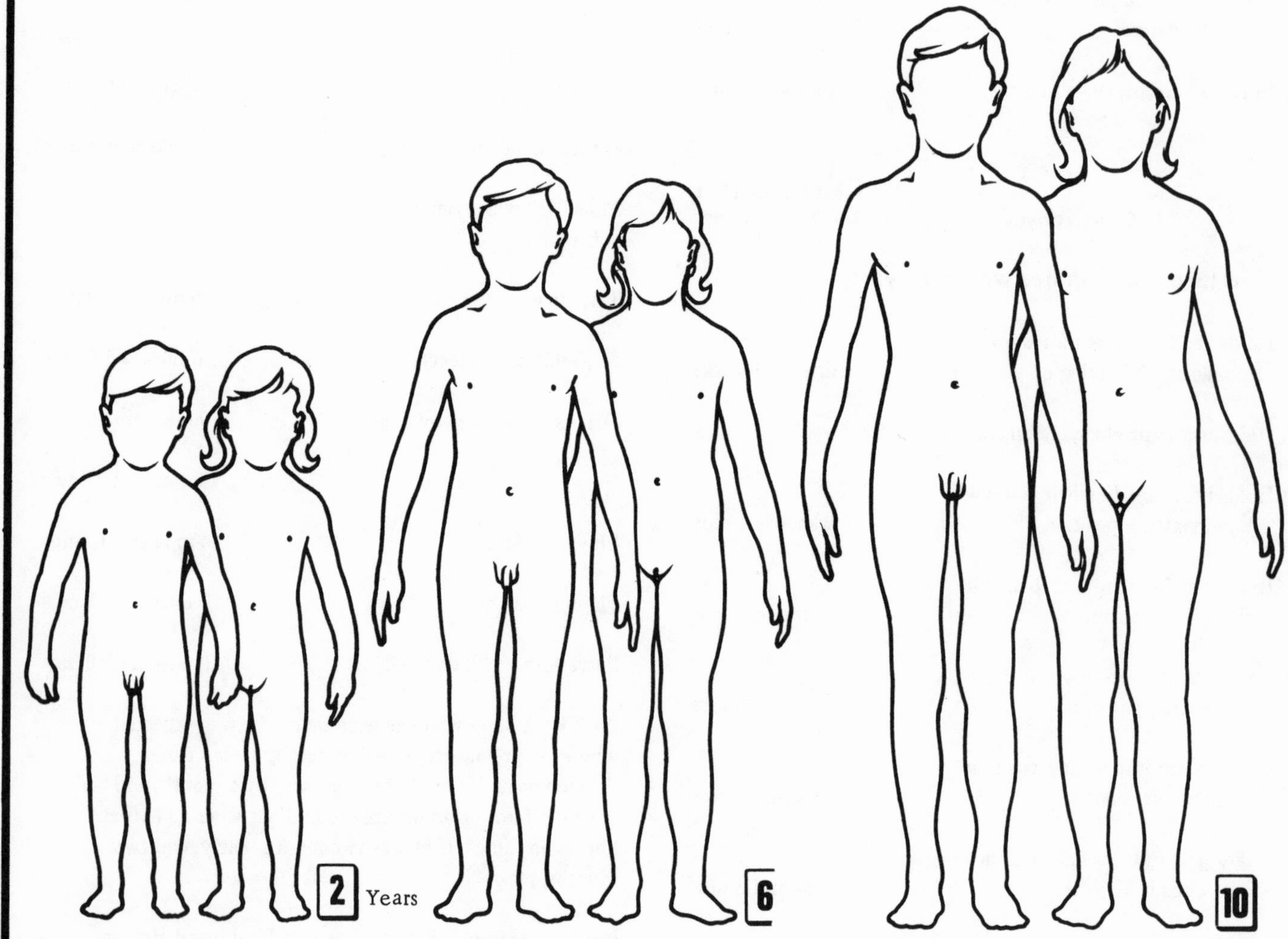

	2	6	10
1	2ft 10in, 27lb (2ft 10in, 25lb)	3ft 9in, 46lb (3ft 8in, 42lb)	4ft 6in, 70lb (4ft 5in, 68lb)
2	49.5%	65.2%	78.0%
3	51.3%; 47.0%	67.8%; 63.8%	79.7%; 76.4%

The first figures give typical heights and weights for each age (figures for girls in brackets). The next figures tell you how much of his final adult height a boy is likely to have achieved at each age, eg 78% at age 10. So you can calculate, from his actual height, how tall a boy will be as an adult; eg a boy 4ft 8in at 10 is likely to be almost 6ft.
Of course, such predictions are averages only. In fact there are two reasons why a child may be taller than average at a given age. He may be going to be a tall person; or he may just be further along in his development than most others - so he will stop sooner and they will catch up.
This is the reason for the final set of figures. They give the percentage of final height that a child has reached if his skeletal development

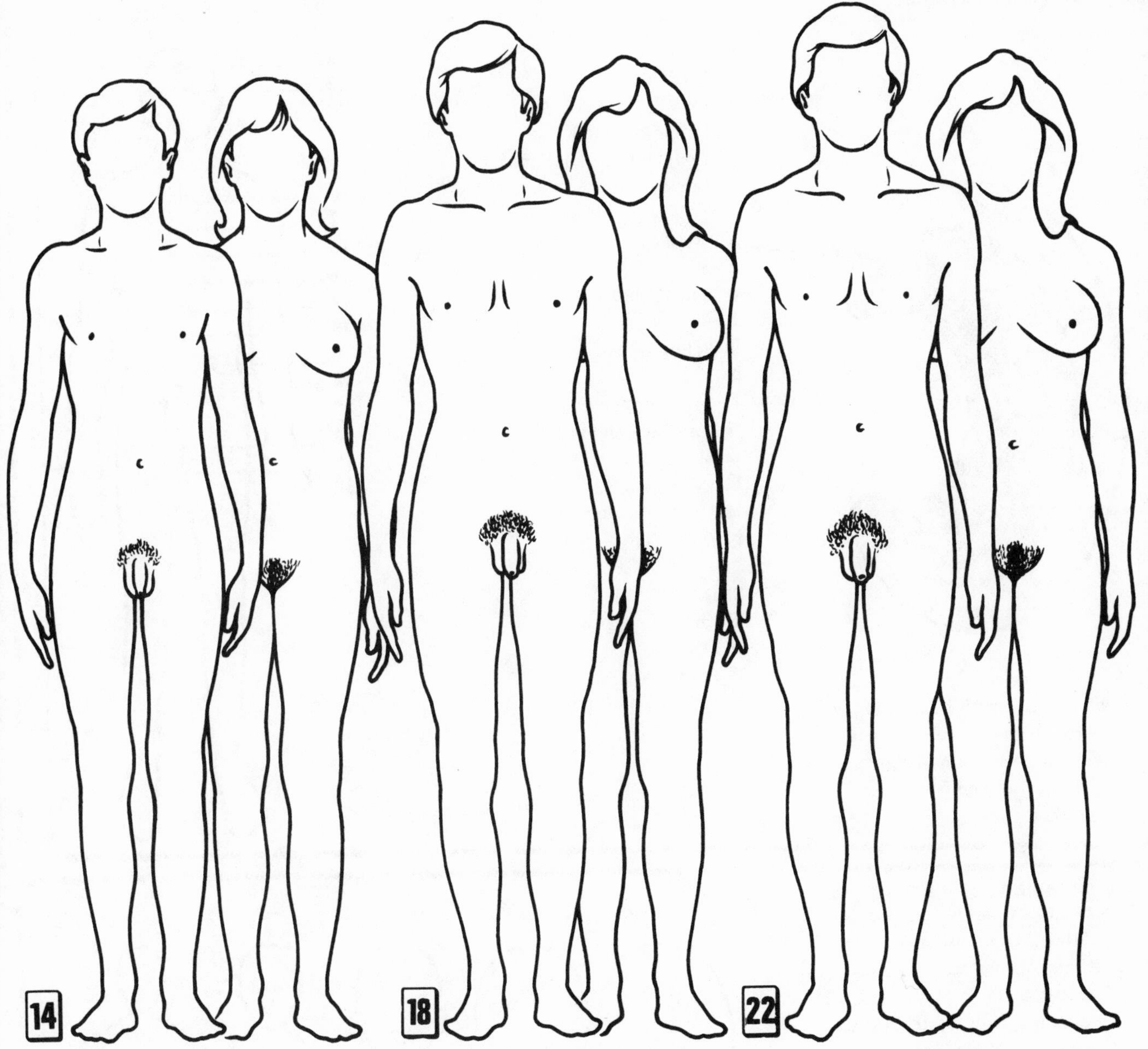

5ft 3in, 108lb (5ft 2in, 109lb)
91.5%
95.8%; 87.6%

5ft 8in, 143lb (5ft 3in, 120lb)
99.8%
100.0%; 99.2%

5ft 9in, 155lb (5ft 3in, 125lb)
100%

is a year ahead of (first figure), or a year behind (second figure), the average. For example, a 10 year old boy of advanced development may have grown 79.7% of his final height - he has not so much further to go. A same age boy with slow development may only have grown 76.4% of his final height. So such figures give a more accurate prediction if a child's physical development is not average. Scientists use X rays of bone formation to determine skeleton age - but you can get a rough idea by noting a child's development of permanent teeth. Compare the ages at which his teeth appear with those in D41. If the teeth appear at the earlier ages shown, his development is advanced; if at the later ages, slow; if between, average.

A08 EMBRYO AND ADULT

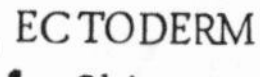

ECTODERM
1 Skin
2 Lining of mouth
3 Conjunctiva and cornea
4 Lens

MESODERM
5 Brain
6 Spinal cord
7 Eye
8 Sclera of eye
9 Kidney
10 Reproductive organs
11 Cartilage and bone
12 Skeletal muscle
13 Heart
14 Uterus (in woman)
15 Outer wall of gut

ENDODERM
16 Thyroid
17 Liver
18 Pancreas
19 Inner wall of gut

Only a few days old, the growing embryo of a human being already has three distinct layers of cells, which will go to form different parts of the finished body.

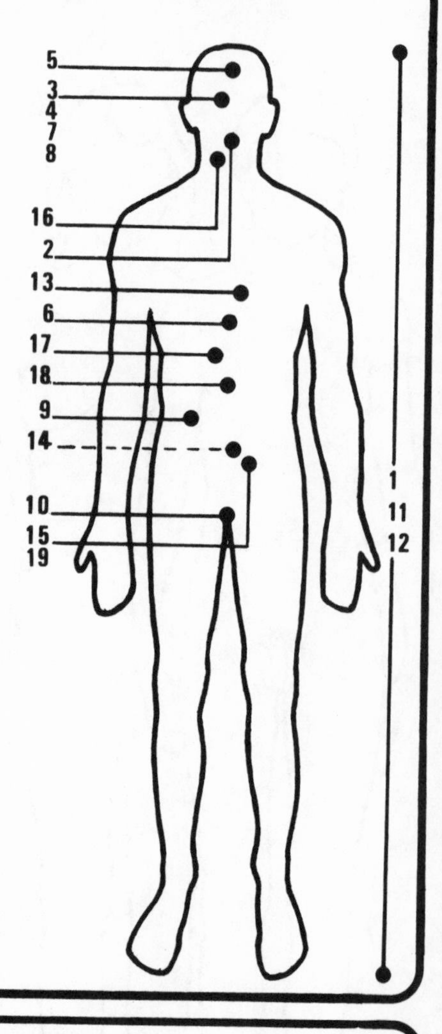

A09 CHANGING PROPORTIONS

In a two month fetus, the body's main divisions are already formed. But its proportions are very different from those of an adult, or even a baby. Only the trunk will stay constant, at three-eighths of body length. The head, instead of forming half the body length will be just a quarter at birth, and a seventh at 25. And the legs will shoot up, from an eighth of body length, to three-eighths, and then half in the adult. Compare too how long the trunk is, and how wide the shoulders are, against the head's dimensions.

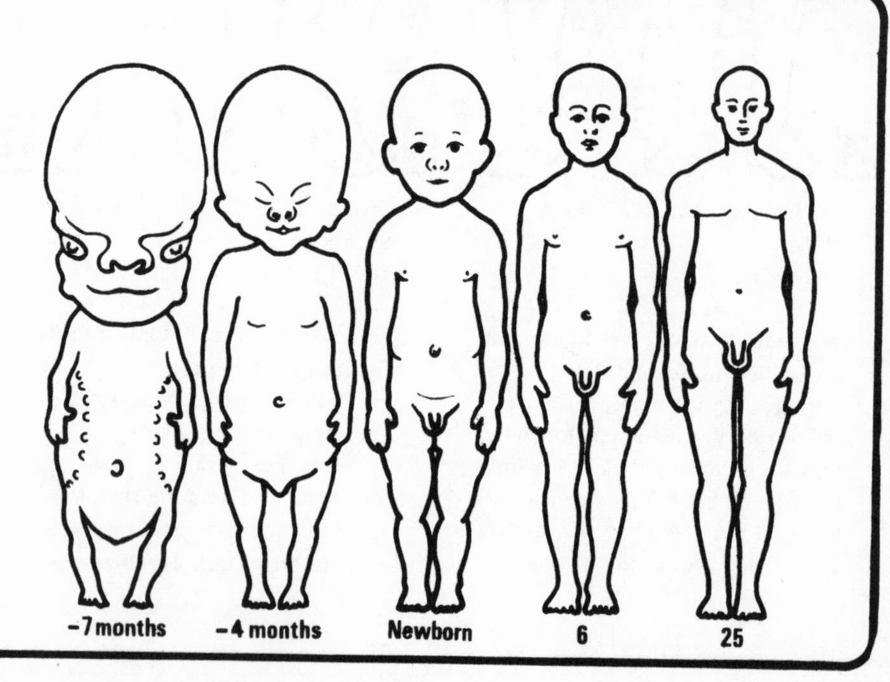

A

A10 GROWTH OF PARTS

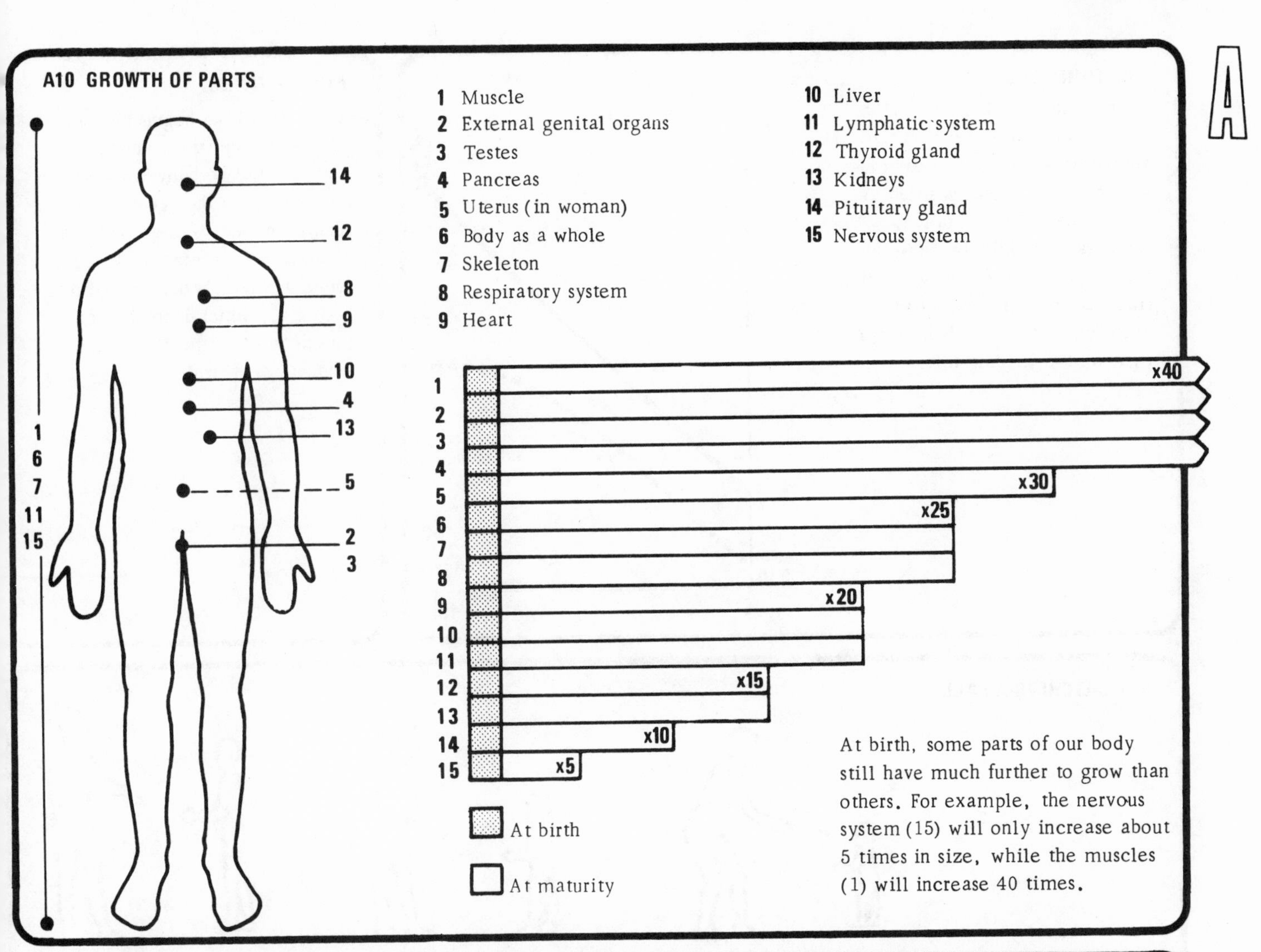

At birth, some parts of our body still have much further to grow than others. For example, the nervous system (15) will only increase about 5 times in size, while the muscles (1) will increase 40 times.

A11 RATE OF GROWTH OF PARTS

This graph shows how fast the different parts of the body grow. Slowest are the genitals: testes, epididymides, seminal vesicles prostate, etc. Next in speed is the body as a whole - its skeleton, muscles, external dimensions, blood volume; also many of its internal organs. Fastest - at first - are the central nervous system (brain and spinal cord) and many of the head's dimensions. And fastest of all, for a while, is the lymphatic system - only to shrink back down again. This is the only part of the body to blow up to much larger than its final size.

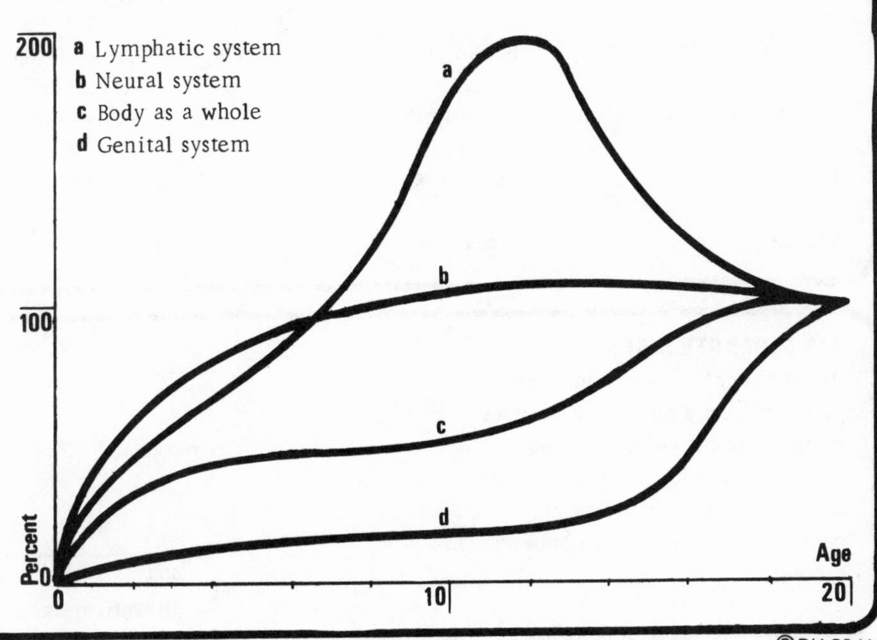

A12 THROWING

Increase in throwing distance is mainly marked by development of an overarm throw. This coincides with changes in feet position to allow greater body rotation. A right-handed child uses a weight shift from rear left foot to leading right foot on delivery. In an adolescent, the shift is from rear right foot to leading left.

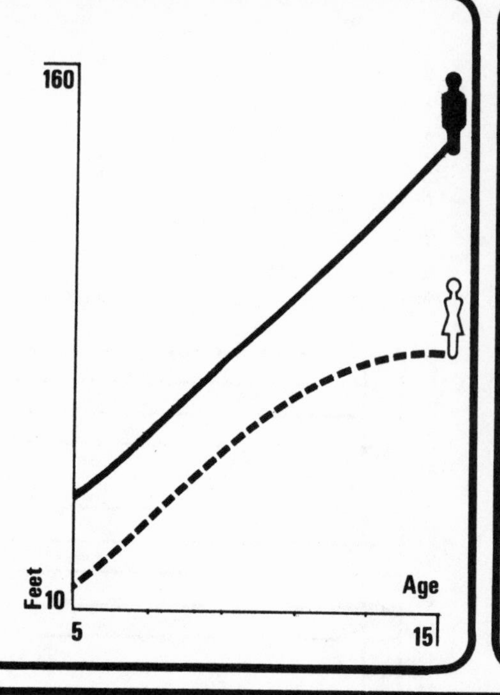

A13 SPRINTING

A simplified run begins by about 18 months, but true running (with a moment of no body support) does not appear till the age of 3. Adult running pattern is established by about 5 or 6. Thereafter speed of running is largely determined by body size, which increases the length and the strength (and so frequency) of stride.

A15 CATCHING A BALL

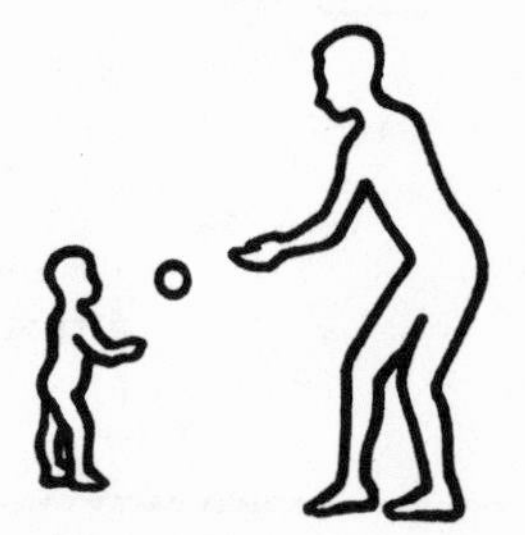

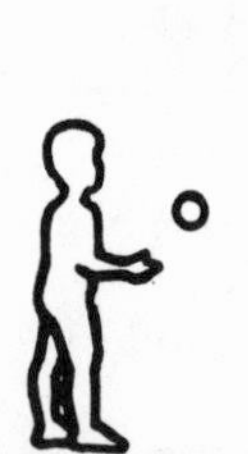

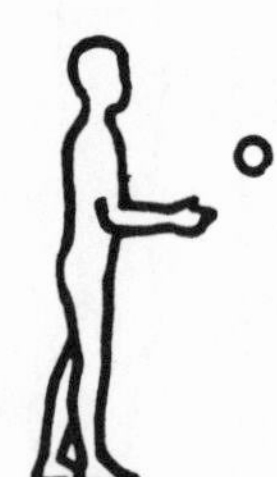

	2 years	5 years	15 years
General strategy	Almost nil	Half formed	Complete
Hand movements	Static	Intentional and appropriate, but excessive	Directed, smooth, and effective
Timing and co-ordination	Almost nil	Effective but slow	Co-ordinated, and unhurried
Eye gaze	On thrower	On thrower, ball, and hands	On ball
Stance	Rigid	Jerky	Adaptive

A16 STRENGTH INDEX

These strength scores summarize grip, pull, and push. The strongest child is almost twice as strong as the weakest. Most boys are stronger than most girls - but there is considerable variation within each group.

Girls

Boys

100 150 200

Strength index

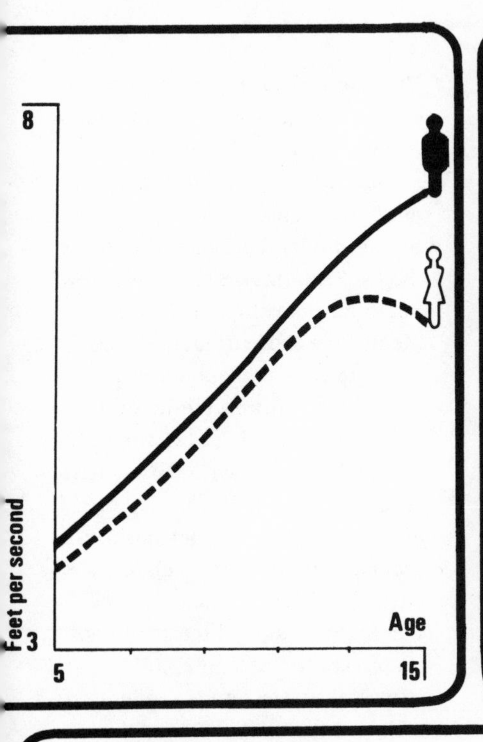

A14 STANDING JUMP

This shows development of the standing broad jump - taking off and landing on both feet. (The running jump confuses the situation by adding in running abilities.) Achievement in boys continues at an almost steady rate throughout childhood and adolescence.

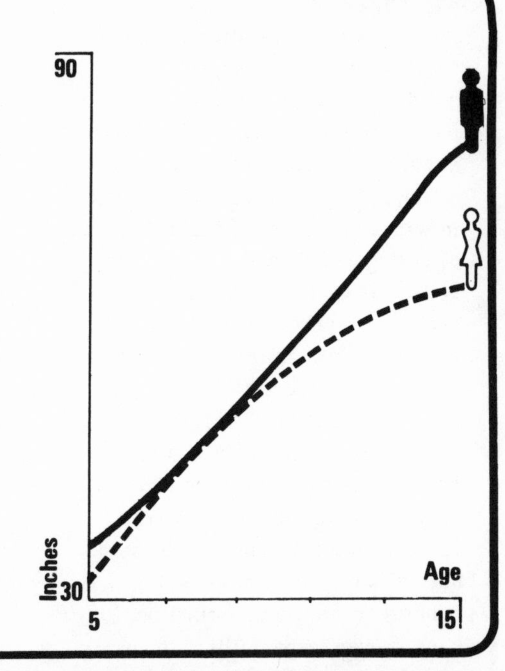

A17 MUSCULAR STRENGTH

Here we show how different aspects of strength develop with age. The main determinant of strength is body size. This is not surprising, since muscle is 40% of body weight. But body weight only accounts for 30 to 35% of strength variation, and height for only another 10%. Age in itself (independent of growth) also shows some effect - perhaps because of developments in the centers of motor control. But strength also varies with constitutional factors such as somatotype*: mesomorphs are stronger for size than ectomorphs, and ectomorphs than endomorphs.

Hand grip

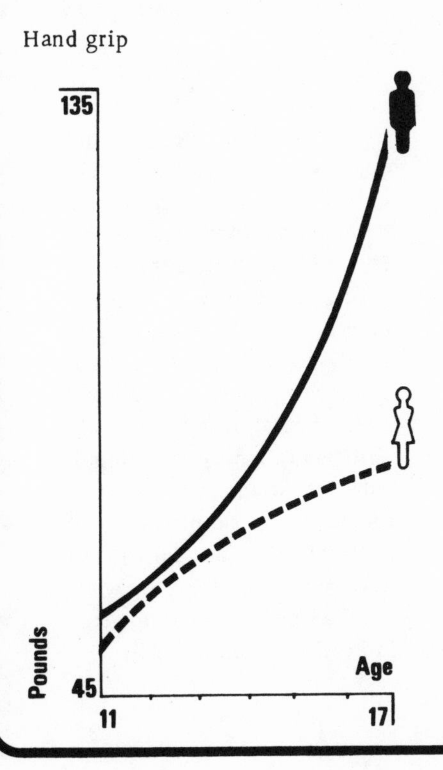

Arm pull

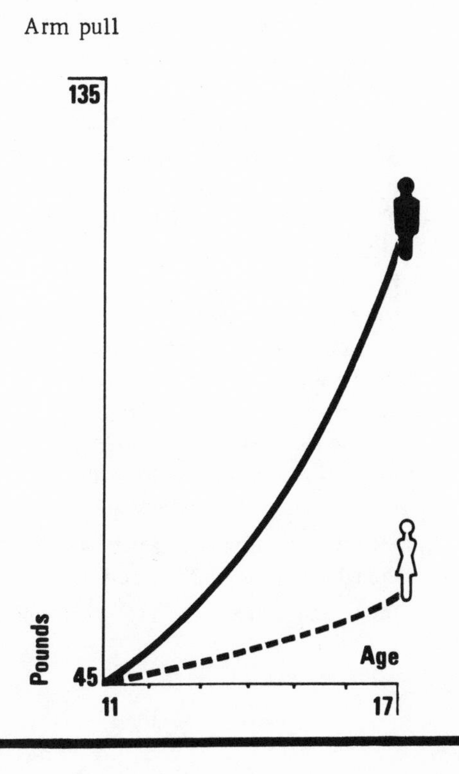

Arm push

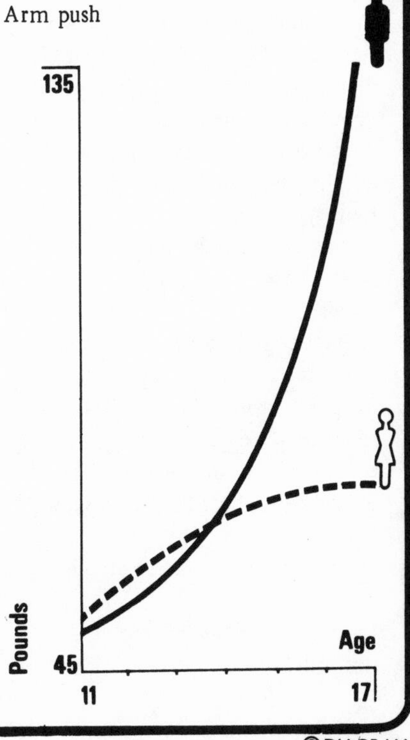

A18 PUBERTY

Puberty is the time when a human being starts being able to have a child. In a boy, the testes start producing sperm. (In a girl, ova begin to mature, and menstruation* occurs.) But this sexual fact is tied in with many other changes, affecting almost every part of the body - as well as with the long period of psychological change, leading up to adulthood, that we call adolescence.

PHYSICAL DEVELOPMENT

The changes of puberty in a boy can start at any time from about 10 years of age to about 15, and finish between 14 and 18. So some normal boys have completed puberty before other normal ones have started (especially as those who do start earlier also tend to take less time over it). But on average the changes start at about 12, and reach a peak between 13 and 14.

The sequence of events can also vary, but a typical sequence would be:

1) the testes and scrotum begin to enlarge;
2) the first pubic hair appears at the base of the penis;
3) the penis begins to enlarge; and, about the same time
4) there is a sudden rapid gain in height (the "adolescent growth spurt");
5) the shoulders broaden;
6) the voice deepens as the larynx grows;
7) hair begins to appear in the armpits and on the upper lips;
8) sperm production reaches a level at which semen may well be ejaculated during sleep;
9) the pubic hair begins to show color;
10) the prostate gland enlarges; and
11) there is a sudden increase in strength.

Other particular changes of puberty include: increased oiliness and coarseness of the skin; and development of body odor for the first time from the armpits and genitals (other areas such as the feet also smell stronger than before).

At the same time, more generally, many other tissues of the body increase in size; blood pressure, blood volume, and the number of red blood corpuscles, all rise; the heart slows down; body temperature falls; breathing slows down - but the lungs' capabilities increase; and bones grow harder, and more brittle, and change in proportion. Typically, by about 17¾, the bulk of growth is over. Height, for example, usually only gains another 2% after that. (In other cases, of course, puberty and growth may still be under way.)

THE HORMONES INVOLVED

The changes of puberty are produced by "hormones" - chemicals manufactured in certain organs of the body called "glands". Hormones travel round the body in the bloodstream, and affect how cells in other parts of the body work and develop.

The signal to produce the hormones of puberty comes from the hypothalamus, a part of the brain. The signal apparently has to wait until the hypothalamus has matured to a certain point. But when it appears, it acts on the pituitary, an important gland at the base of the brain, and this begins to produce two hormones called FSH* and LH*. (Their full names refer to their role in the female body, where they are also the trigger hormones of puberty - though more LH is produced in men.)

The two hormones act, in a boy, on the testes. After about a year, while their level builds up, LH stimulation results in the testes producing testosterone, the main masculinizing hormone of puberty. Testosterone makes the penis grow, pubic hair develop, and so on. Meanwhile FSH stimulates the testes to start producing sperm.

To keep a limit on the level of sexual activity, both LH and FSH are under what is called "negative feedback control". That is, the effects they have hinder their own production, so their level falls, until their very absence creates the conditions in which they can reappear. For example, LH stimulates testosterone production, which reacts back on the hypothalamus. As a result, the hypothalamus sends out a message cutting back LH production. As LH is then no longer stimulating testosterone production, the testosterone level falls - allowing LH to start to be made again. (With FSH, the control mechanism is probably not the testosterone level.)

INFLUENCES ON TIMING

In this century, puberty in the western world has been starting younger and younger. No one is quite sure why, though it may be due to rising living standards. But, between different children, the age of puberty varies with inherited family traits, nutrition level, general living conditions, and physical and psychological state (mental disturbance and long childhood illness can each delay puberty). It also varies with somatotype*. Children who will be mesomorphs as adults tend to have puberty early; those who will be ectomorphs have puberty late; while those who will be

A

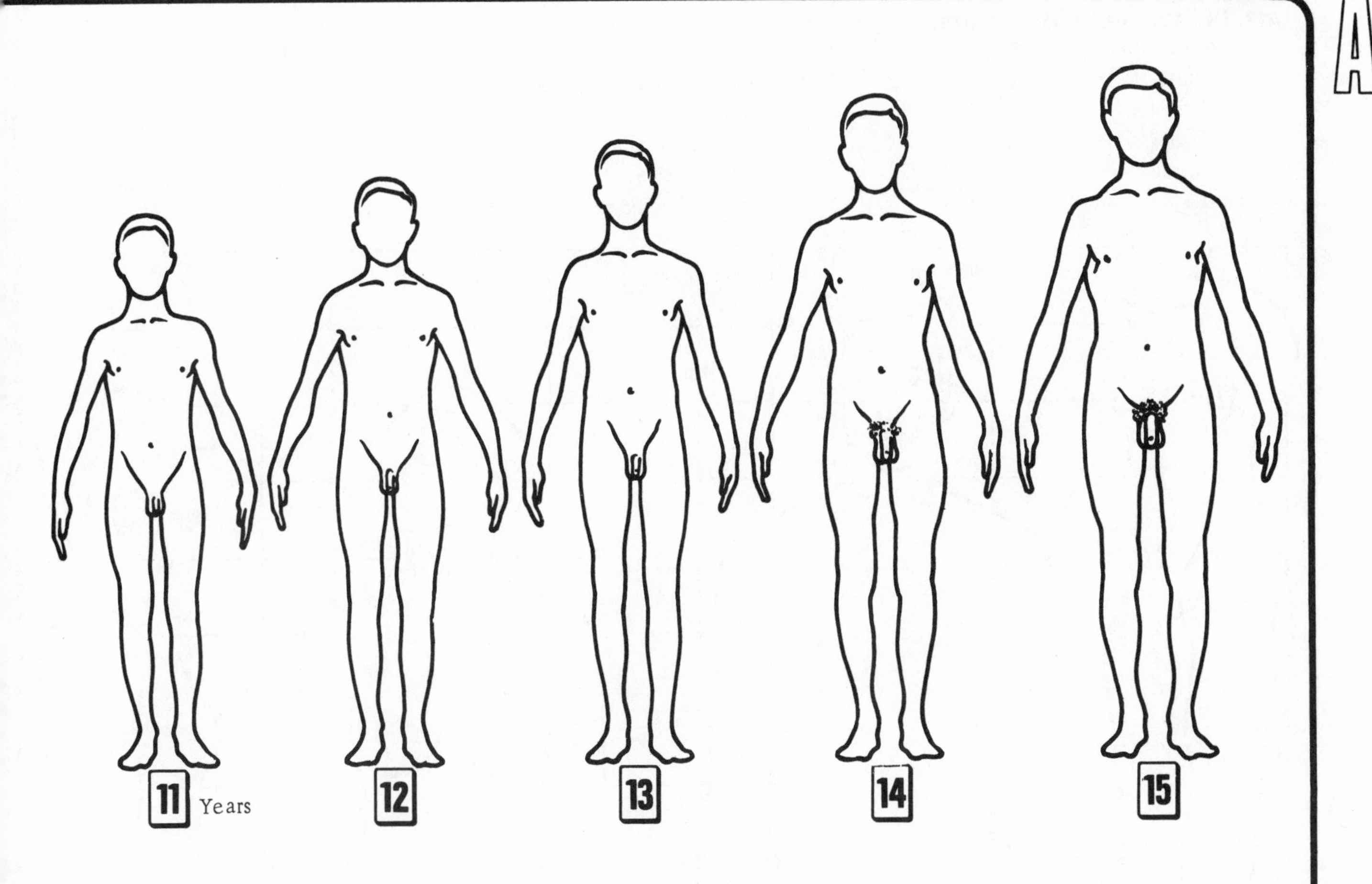

endomorphs seem perhaps to start early but finish late. All these are more important than any effect - if there is one - of race or climate. However, the rate of puberty does vary with the season of the year. Growth in height is usually fastest in spring, growth in weight in autumn. In fact, this is true for all ages - not just adolescence.

PHYSICAL PROBLEMS

Puberty can fail to occur, in rare cases, because of hormonal imbalance. Also certain disorders become more common after puberty: acute myeloid leukemia, bone cancer - and, less seriously, short-sightedness. But many of the so-called physical problems ot puberty are really only psychologically significant. Very early or late development, skin troubles, and increased body odor, are all more embarrassments than anything else.

A common but temporary problem can be extreme lethargy - which is both physical and psychological in cause and effects. Psychologically, it can be due to the great psychic changes going on at this time, which can result in anxiety, self-consciousness, and boredom with old pastimes and roles. Physically, it can be due to the effects of the hormones, or the growth spurt, or just too many late nights.

It is worth mentioning some normal physical events of puberty which can be misconstrued as abnormal.

a) The thyroid gland often enlarges, but should go down again when puberty is completed.

b) Fat may develop due to faulty appetite control in the brain (not to glands or gluttony). It may disappear later, but it is best to begin the practice of diet control.

c) Almost a third of boys develop a slight swelling beneath the breast nipple. This vanishes within 1 to $1\frac{1}{2}$ years.

A19 THE AVERAGE HUMAN BEING

The average man is just over 5ft 9in tall. He weighs almost 162lb, his chest is 38¾in round, his waist 31¾in, his hips 37¾in. The maximum weight he reaches is about 172lb, and that is between the ages of 35 and 54.

The average woman is almost 5ft 3¼in tall. She weighs almost 135lb, her bust is 35½in, her waist 29¼in, her hips 38in. The maximum weight she reaches is about 152 lb, and that is between the ages of 55 and 64.

These figures are for people in the USA.

The average man and woman do not exist.

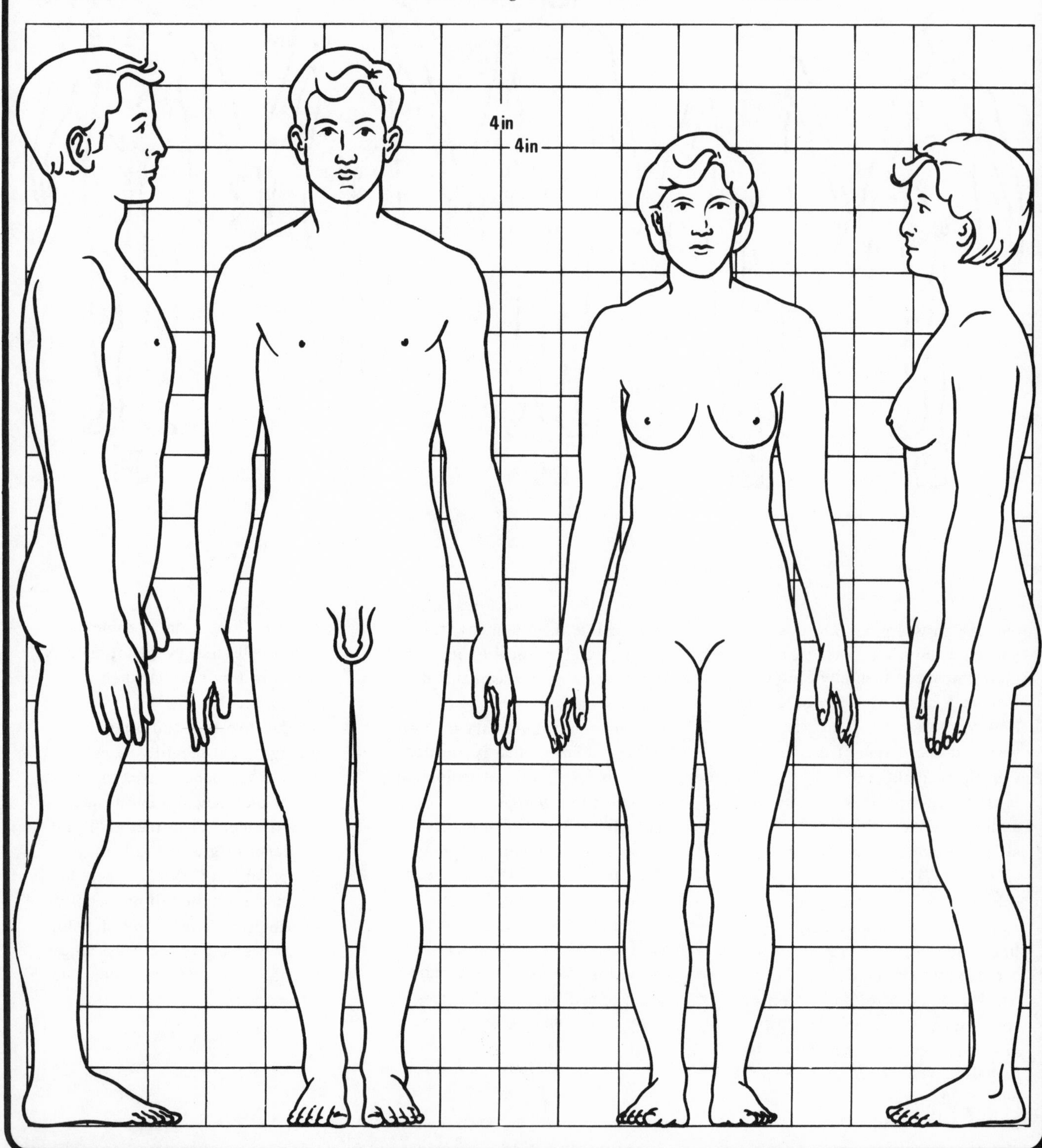

A

A20 NORMAL AND ABNORMAL

The range of the normal is fairly small; the range of the possible is fairly wide. A convenient example is height. In every 100 men, 95 are between 5ft 4in and 6ft 2in. But the tallest man that has ever lived (whose height has been verified) was 8ft 11in tall at death (age 22), and the shortest 26½in (age 21).
In fact, the distribution of many physical characteristics in a population can be summed up in a curve called the "normal distribution" curve, shown below. The range of the characteristic goes all the way from a to z, and there are people at every point in between. But there are very few people at either of the extremes - and very many in the central area.

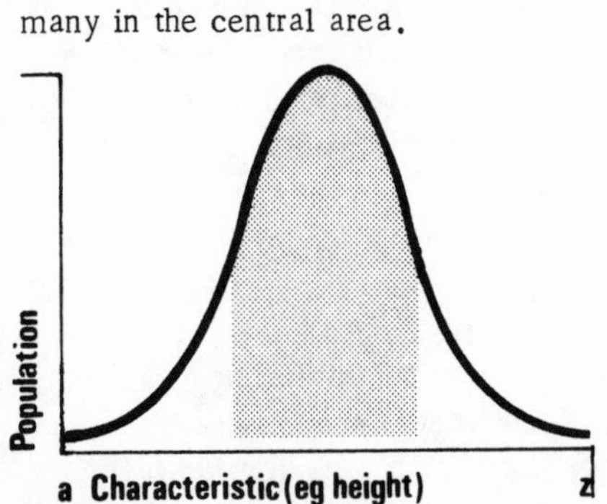

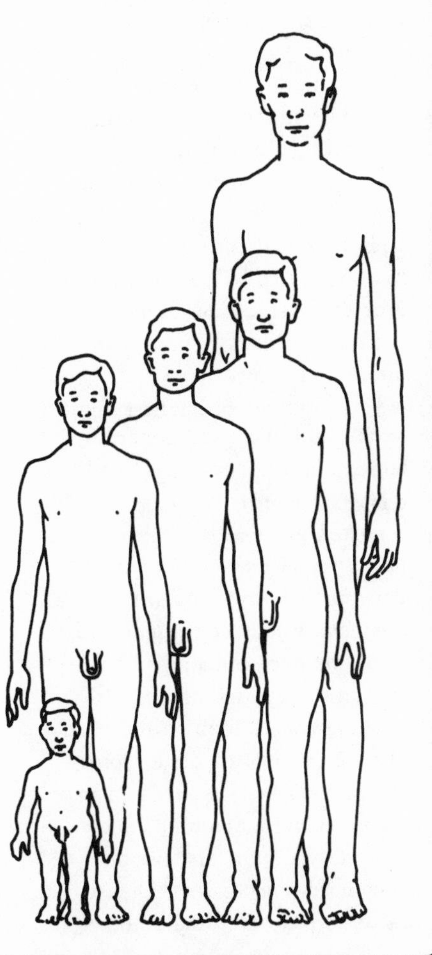

A21 OUR MAKE-UP

In every 100 men, 95 weight between 127 and 209 lb (for women it is 95 and 195lb). In the average 162lb man, about 43% of the weight is muscle, 14% is fat, 14% bone and marrow, 12% internal organs, 9% connective tissue and skin, and 8% blood. The weight distributes: 47% in the trunk and neck, 34% in the legs, 12% in the arms, and 7% in the head. Broken down into his elements, man is 65% oxygen, 18.5% carbon, 9.5% hydrogen, 3.3% nitrogen, 1.5% calcium, 1% phosphorous, 0.35% or less each of potassium, sulfur, chlorine, sodium, and magnesium, with traces of iron, iodine, zinc, fluorine, and other elements. This gives him enough water to fill a 10 gallon barrel, enough fat for 7 bars of soap, enough phosphorus for 2,200 match heads, and enough iron for a 3in nail.

A22 MAN AND WOMAN

This shows how some characteristics of the typical man and woman compare.

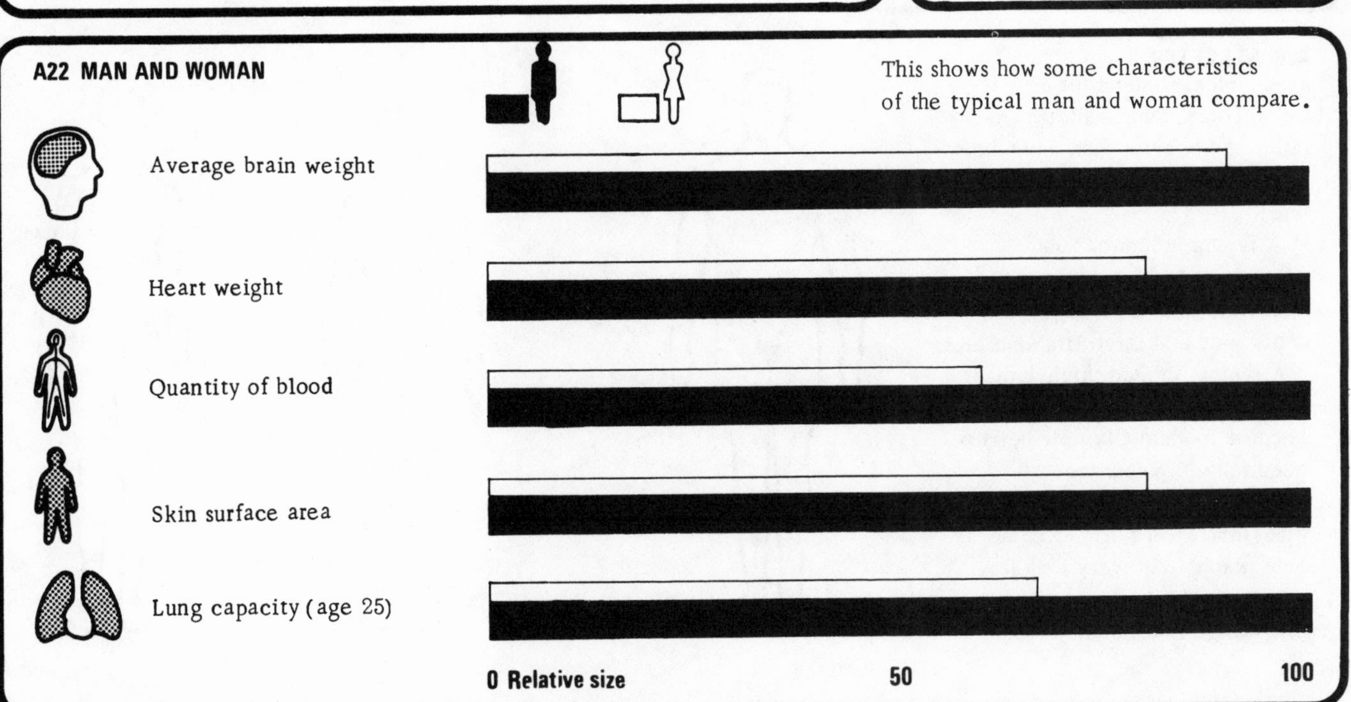

A23 SOMATOTYPES

There have been attempts to classify human body types ever since Hippocrates. In the 1940s the American psychologist W H Sheldon put forward a new approach, called somatotyping. He did not suggest that there was any set number of body types, to one of which everyone had to belong. Instead, he felt that all the infinite variety of forms could be analyzed in terms of just three tendencies. Any individual body could be described, by judging how far each of these three variables was represented in it.

The three variables he called endomorphy, mesomorphy, and ectomorphy. Endomorphy is the tendency to soft roundness in the body, mesomorphy the tendency to muscularity, and ectomorphy the tendency to "linearity". A very endomorphic person would be stocky, with a large, round body, a short, thick neck, and short arms and legs with fat upper arms and thighs. (An endomorph also normally has considerable body fat - though he would still be an endomorph without it.)

A very mesomorphic person would be strongly built, with broad muscular shoulders and chest, very muscular arms and legs, and little body fat. (Other body types can also put on muscle, by body building. But the type they can put on cannot - at least after puberty - turn them into a mesomorph.)

A very ectomorphic person would be tall and thin, with a narrow body, thin arms and legs, little body fat, and stringy muscles.

Recognizing these body types was not especially new. But Sheldon drew up a scale for each variable. Someone's body could score from 1 to 7 on each tendency - but if it scored very high on one, it could not score high on the others also. By listing all three scores, the person's body type was then recorded and pinpointed. Such "somatotype numbers" list the endomorphy score first, then the mesomorphy, then the ectomorphy.

So a really extreme endomorph would be 711, an extreme mesomorph 171, an extreme ectomorph 117.

In practice, such extremes seldom occur - but nor are most people an "average" 444. A typical population dots itself over a somatotype chart like the shots of an unsuccessful marksman.

Sheldon's system assumes that our somatotype never changes - with age, or diet, or exercise.

In reality, some experts believe that somatotype can be altered a little by exercise during puberty. But all agree that, by the time we are sixteen or seventeen, we are basically stuck with what we are.

So, for example, a knowledge of which sports events favor which somatotype can guide a young athlete in deciding his ambitions.

Somatotyping is carried out in practice by assessment from three photographs using carefully standardized postures. The scoring is a matter of judgement, but experienced assessors rate the same body very similarly.

A26 ATHLETES

a) A typical shot-putter or weightlifter. Such athletes are taller and heavier than any others, with large arms relative to their legs.

b) A typical 100m or 200m sprinter - relatively short and muscular, with short legs relative to his body and large limb muscles.

c) A typical modern high-jumper - less ectomorph than in the past, because modern Olympic heights need muscle power too.

d) A typical traditional high-jumper: a fairly extreme ectomorph, with very long legs relative to his body.

e) Average man.

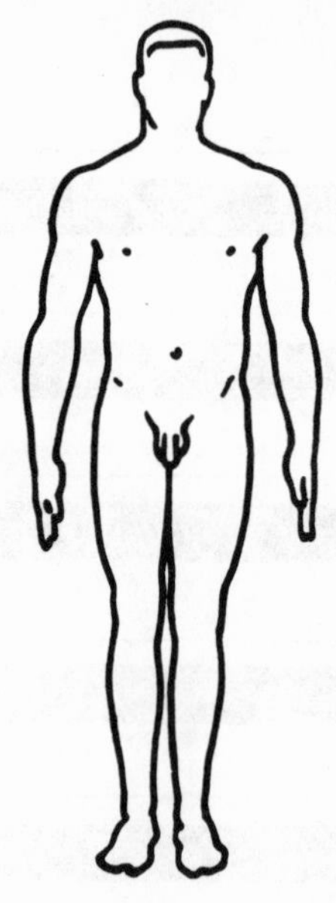

a Shotputter

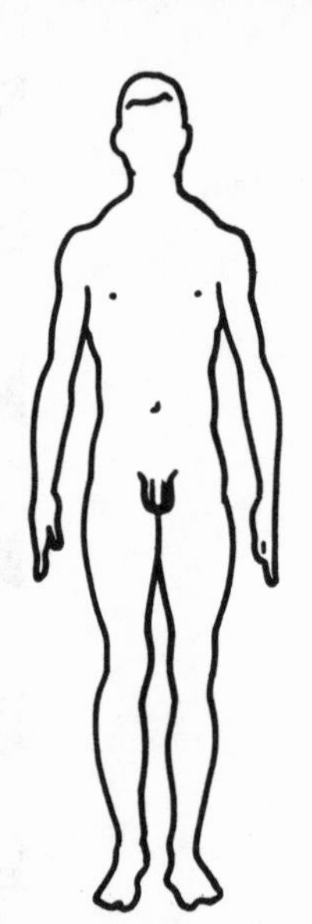

b Sprinter

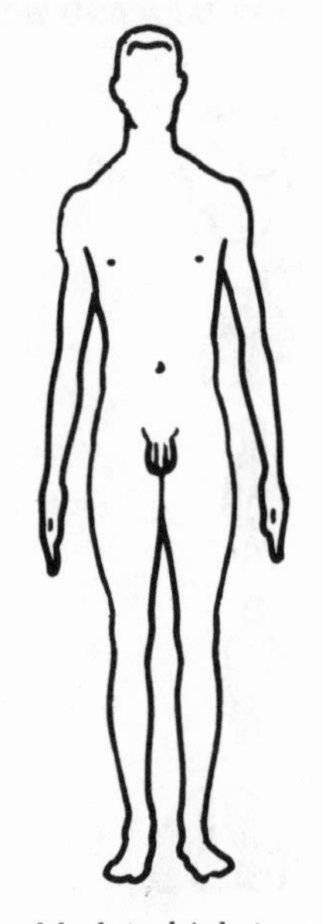

c Modern high jumper

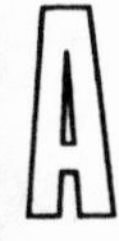

A24 TAKE THREE MEN

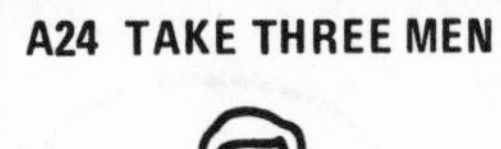

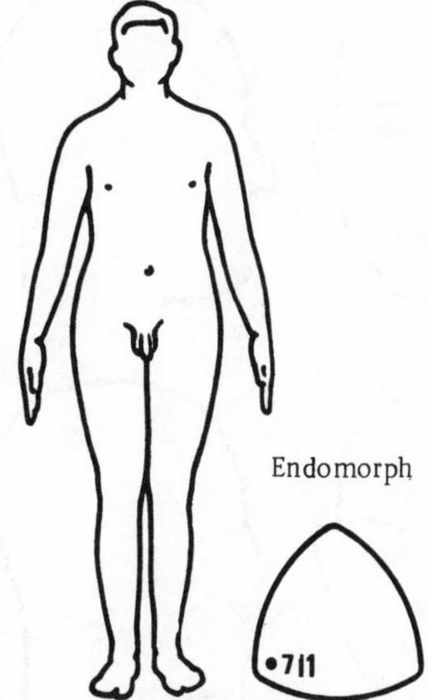

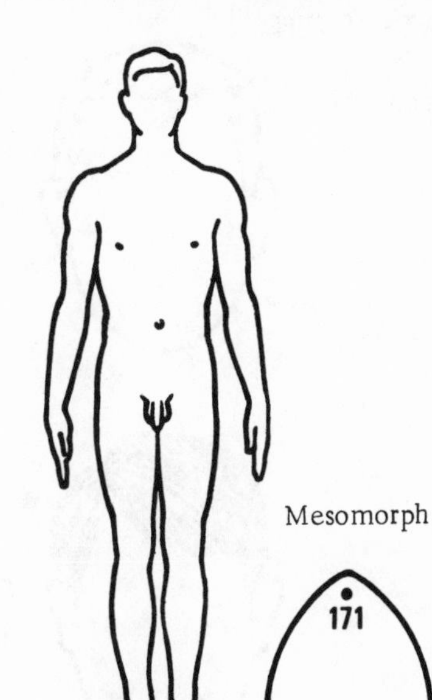

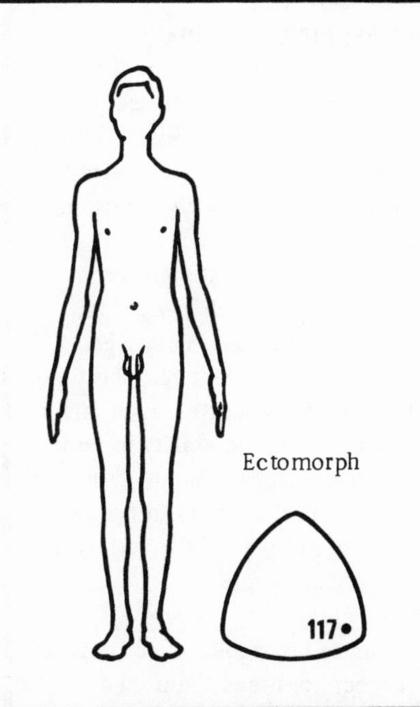

A25 SCATTER PATTERN

The somatotypes of 4000 US college students show a wide distribution over the chart, with some concentration around the center. In contrast, a sample of Olympic track and field athletes shows a great bias towards mesomorphy and ectomorphy.

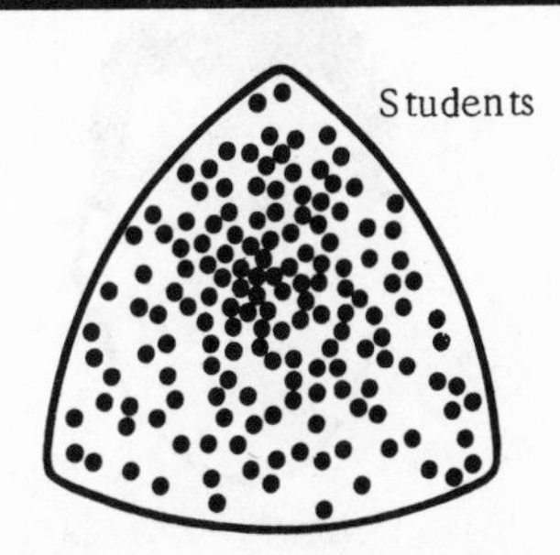

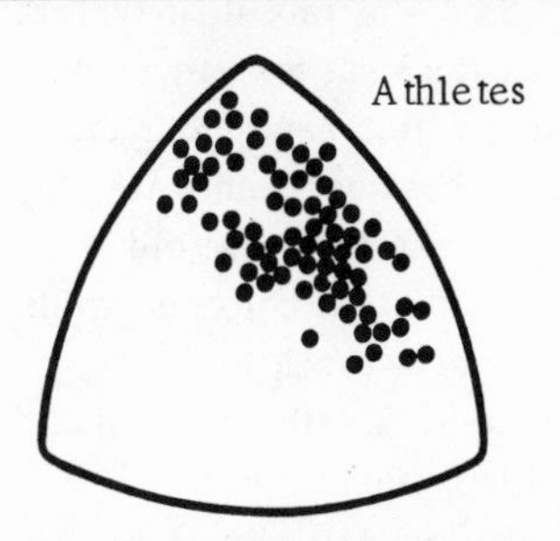

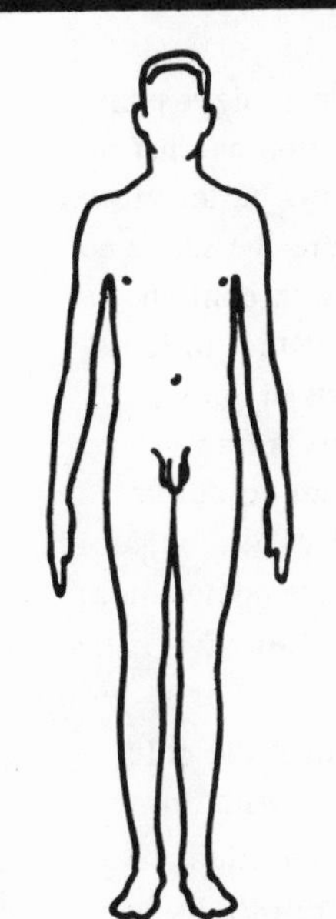

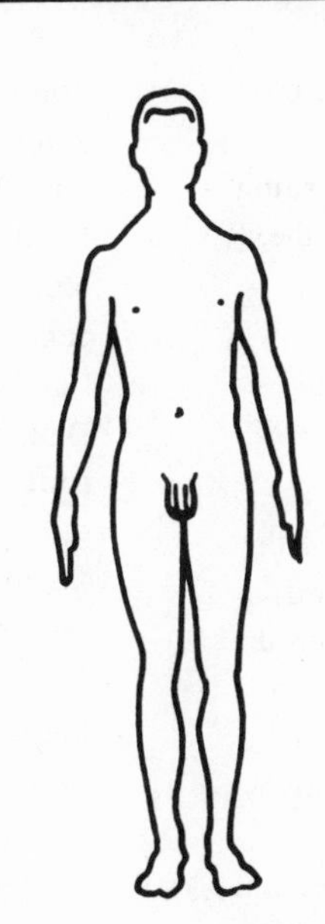

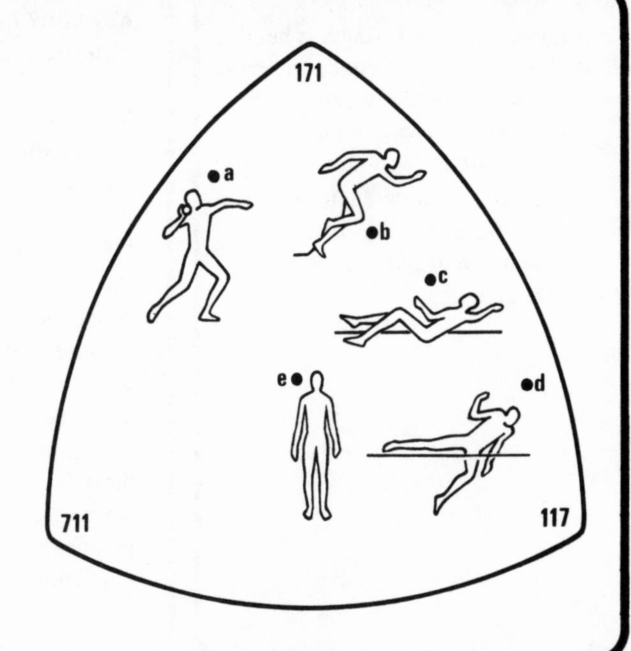

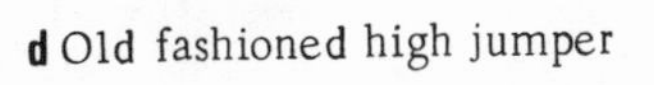

d Old fashioned high jumper

e Average man

ETHNIC VARIATIONS

A27 ETHNIC VARIATIONS

No one now is very happy with the word "race": it has been too much a part of man's inhumanity to man. But patterns of ethnic variation do, of course, exist - fairly consistent differences in the physical characteristics of different peoples. We are all aware of how people vary in stature, skin color, hair type, and facial features. But the ethnologist also notices such things as blood type, the ability to taste certain substances, and even the type of wax that forms in the ear. All these are part of the variety of human inheritance.

Three great ethnic groups - caucasoid, mongoloid, and negroid - account between them for almost all of the world's population. We have tried to illustrate their typical characteristics. But sometimes the differences within each group are as large as those between them. Taking, for example, the old preoccupation, skin color: negroids range from near black to sallow; mongoloids from yellowish to flat white to deep bronze; and caucasoids from fair pinkish in northern Europe, to the dark brown people of southern India.

Another extreme variable is height. It is less totally inherited, and more immediately determined by environment, than other ethnic criteria. But not only does it vary widely among individuals of a given people, but also between different peoples of the same ethnic group.

A28 ETHNIC TYPES

Basic facial characteristics

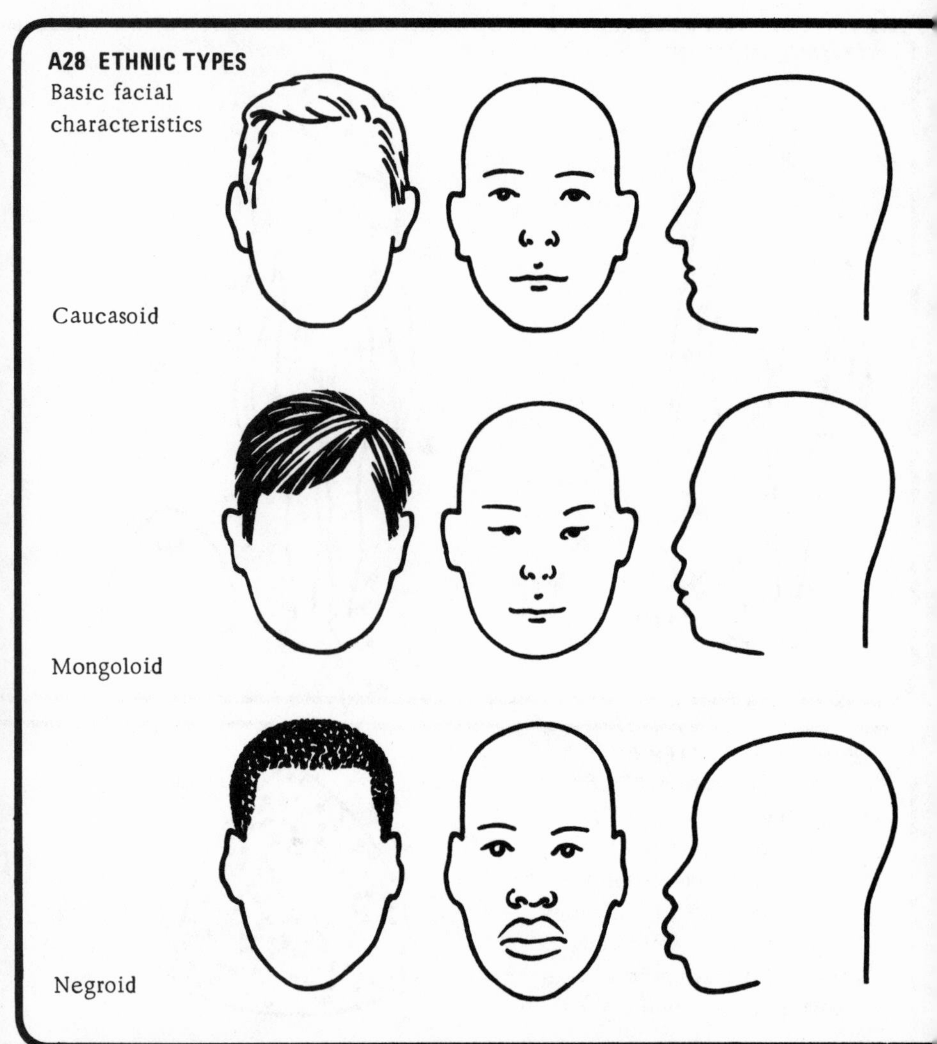

A30 BODY AND CLIMATE

Animals of a species differ in coat color, size, limb length, and location of fat deposits, according to climatic conditions where they live. Some of man's variations are also related to climate.

ETHNIC FEATURES

The environment did not make people acquire inheritable characteristics - but it did decide which characteristics flourished. Those people who flourished bred among themselves, and passed on these features (which are not, of course, lost if the inheritor moves to a new environment).

Skin color is a well-known example. The extra melanin* in dark skins gives added protection against the sun. Pale skin allows better vitamin D* formation, where the sun is no problem. Yellow skin contains a dense keratin* layer that reflects light well in deserts or snow.

Dark eye color also protects against sunlight; and so do the thick, folded eyelids of mongoloids.

Negroid hair protects against heat on the scalp, but allows sweat loss from the neck. Straight hair, grown long, protects against the cold.

Noses typically vary with air humidity. In dry conditions they are longer and narrower, so

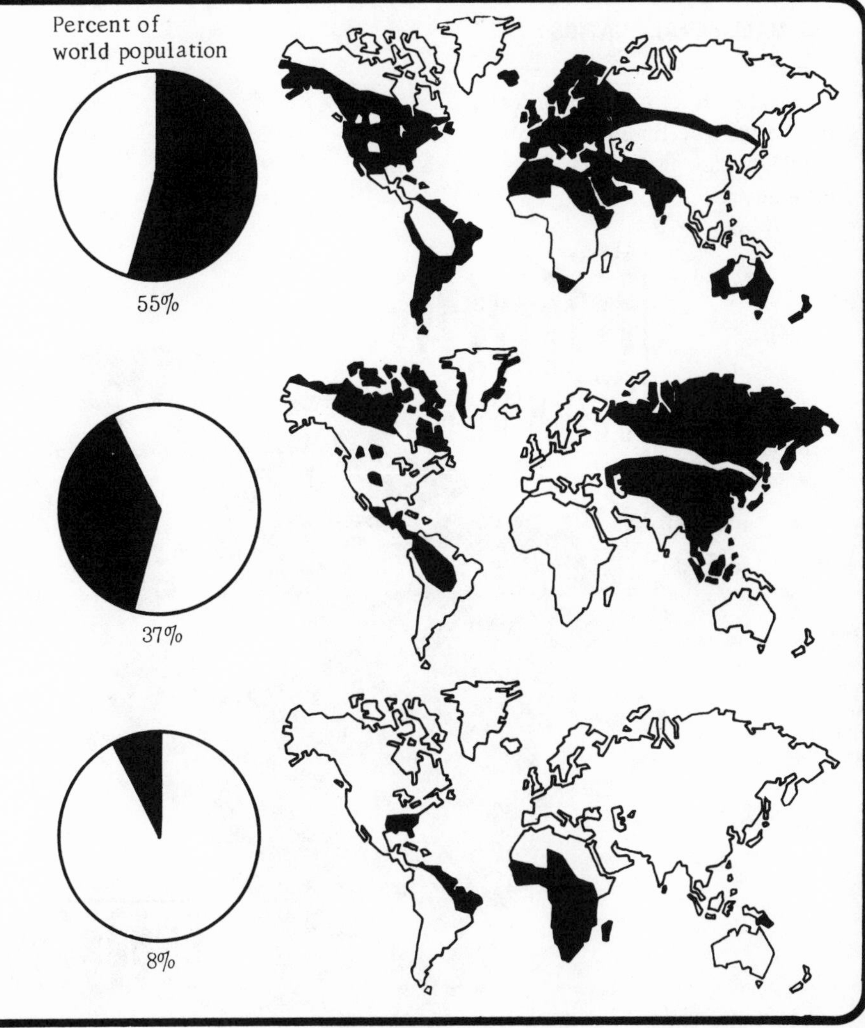

A29 ETHNIC VARIETY

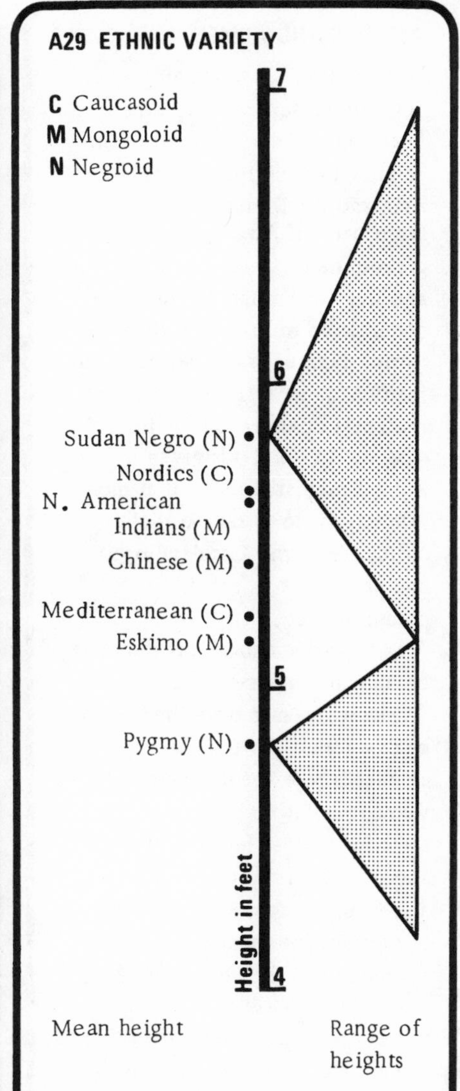

inhaled air is moistened. But the flat mongoloid face developed as protection against the cold, and here the nose is not prominent and exposed. The Eskimo have taken this further, by developing facial fat.

OTHER VARIABLES

Other features, not entirely inherited, also vary with climate. Average weight is greater the colder it is. The Eskimo averages 170lb, the Irishman 157lb, the Spaniard 132lb, the Algerian Berber 125lb. Body shape also varies: two bodies that weigh the same can have very different surface areas. Body area is larger, for weight, the hotter it is, for a large area gives more skin from which to sweat and to radiate heat. Metabolic rate varies in the same way. A typical European has a "thermal equilibrium" of 77°F; i.e. with that temperature around him, naked, standing still, he shows no tendency to get hotter or colder. The Eskimo's metabolic rate is 15 to 30% higher than the European's, giving him a lower thermal equilibrium, while an Indian's, Brazilian's, or Australian's rate is 10% lower than the European's.

Height relates partly to ethnic factors - but little to overall ethnic group. Above, left, average heights, for a sample selection of peoples, reveal a jumbled sequence of negroids, caucasoids, and mongoloids (eg negroid peoples are both shortest and tallest). Also, even within a people, other genetic and environmental variations prevent too much consistency. Above, right, for example, the height range shows the tallest pygmy as tall as the shortest Sudan Negro.

MEN AND WOMEN

A31 MEN AND WOMEN

World-wide, there are just over 100 women for every 100 men. But this ratio varies greatly from country to country. In most of Asia and the Middle East, and large parts of Africa, men predominate; in the United States and western Europe, women. In general, in primitive parts of the world, lack of contraception and medical facilities increases the maternal death rate in childbirth. Also the lower status given to women may still mean that more effort is made to save a male child. Yet some less developed countries show a female predominance.

A male predominance can also arise because of immigration, as in Alaska where men were the first to go in search of fortune. As standards rose, the numbers of women caught up. But Canada still has fewer women per 100 men than the United States; and in the United States itself, female predominance was not reached until the census of 1950.

THE AGE PATTERN

In most societies, more men than women are born. The ratio is generally about 105 male babies for every 100 female. But, in modern American and western European society, more males than females die at each age before old age is reached (except perhaps for a brief period during childhood). In other words, female life expectancy is longer. So the older one is, the more women of that age group there are for every 100 men. Parity between the sexes is usually reached between the ages of 30 and 40. After this, female predominance grows steadily, until at 95 a man is outnumbered 4 to 1.

A32 MALE-FEMALE RATIOS

The map tints show the male-female ratios for most countries in the world. The lines of symbols pinpoint a few places that have very different ratios.

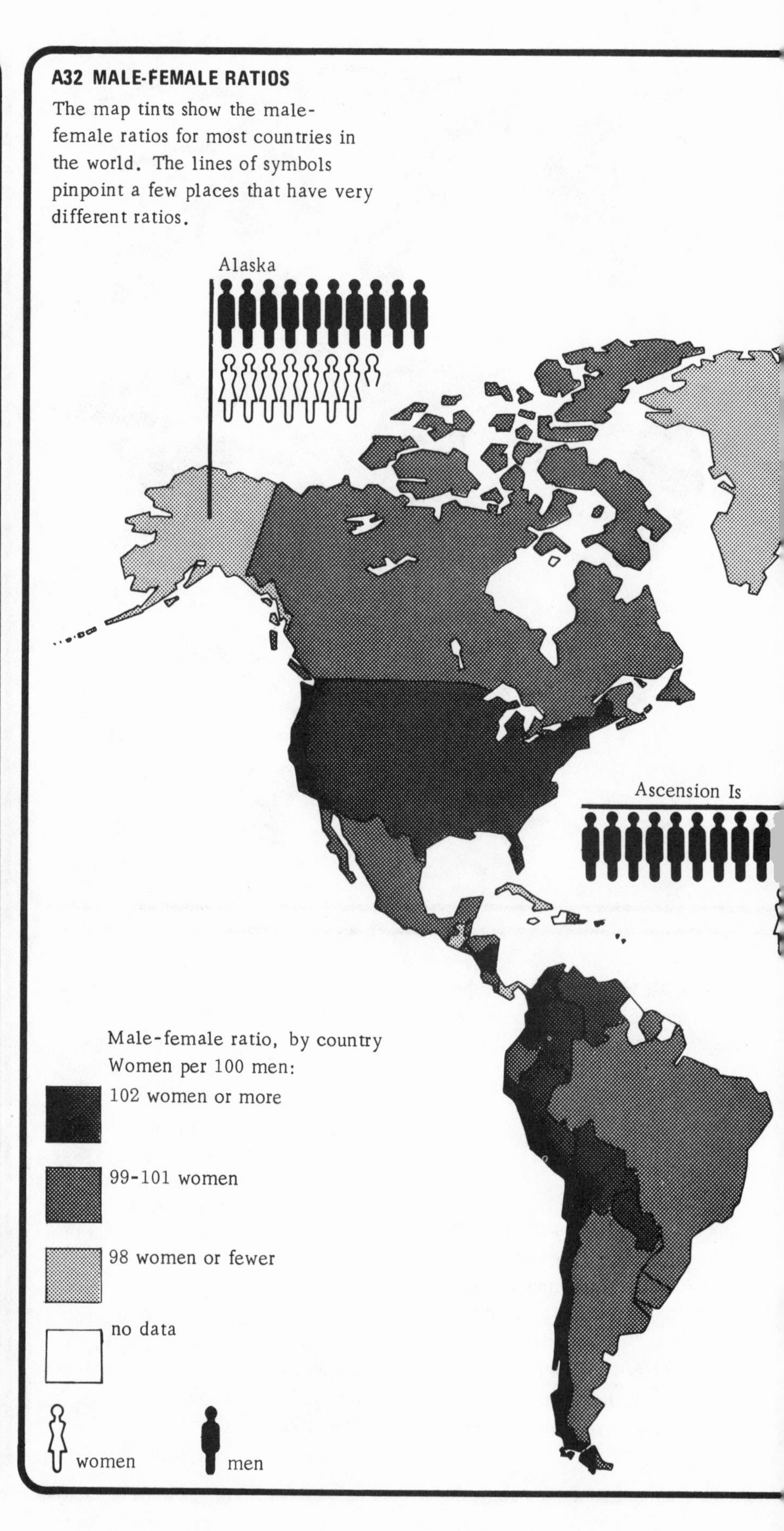

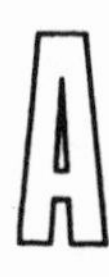
A

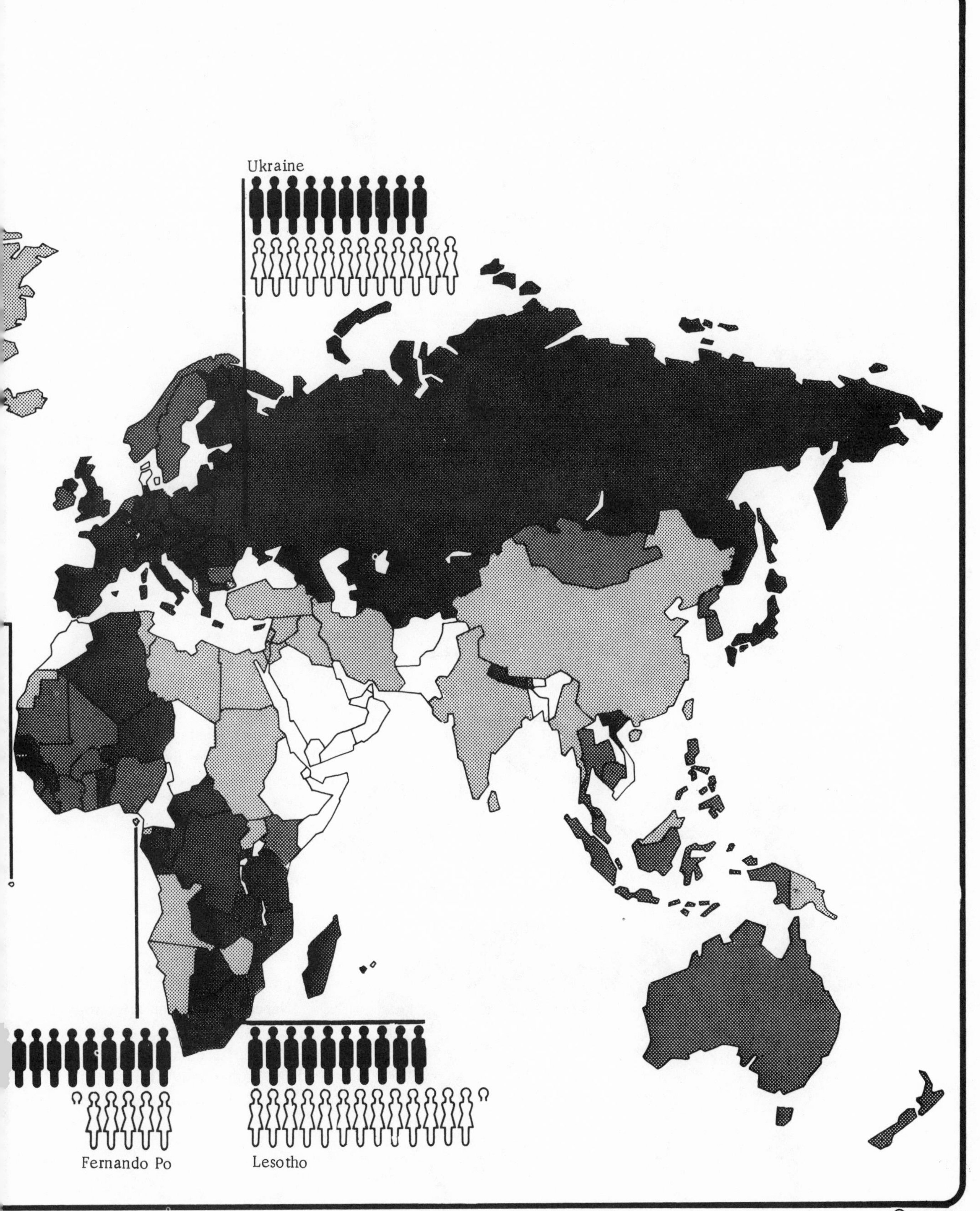
Ukraine
Fernando Po
Lesotho

LIFE EXPECTANCY 1

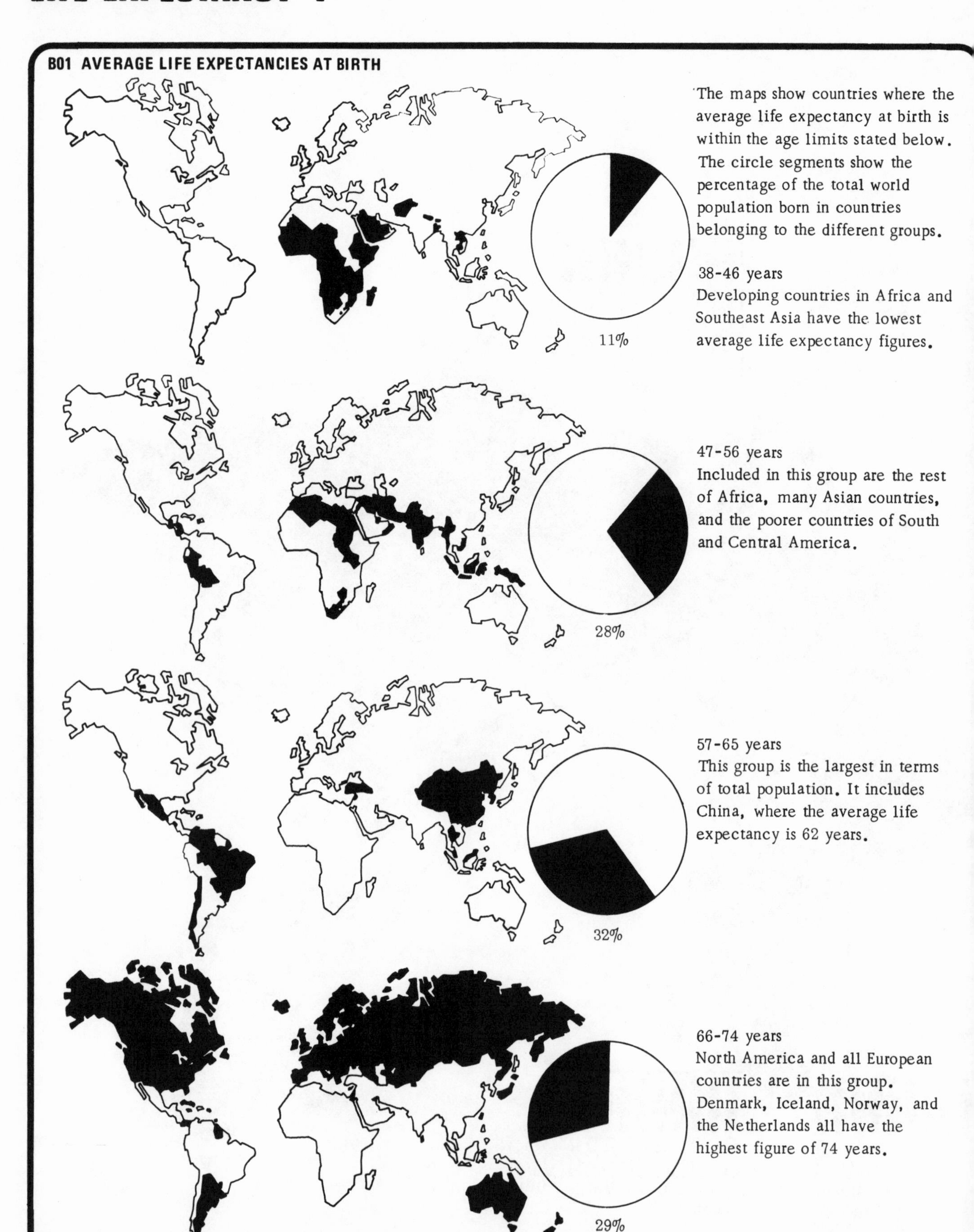

The maps show countries where the average life expectancy at birth is within the age limits stated below. The circle segments show the percentage of the total world population born in countries belonging to the different groups.

38-46 years
Developing countries in Africa and Southeast Asia have the lowest average life expectancy figures.

47-56 years
Included in this group are the rest of Africa, many Asian countries, and the poorer countries of South and Central America.

57-65 years
This group is the largest in terms of total population. It includes China, where the average life expectancy is 62 years.

66-74 years
North America and all European countries are in this group. Denmark, Iceland, Norway, and the Netherlands all have the highest figure of 74 years.

B02 A LONG LIFE

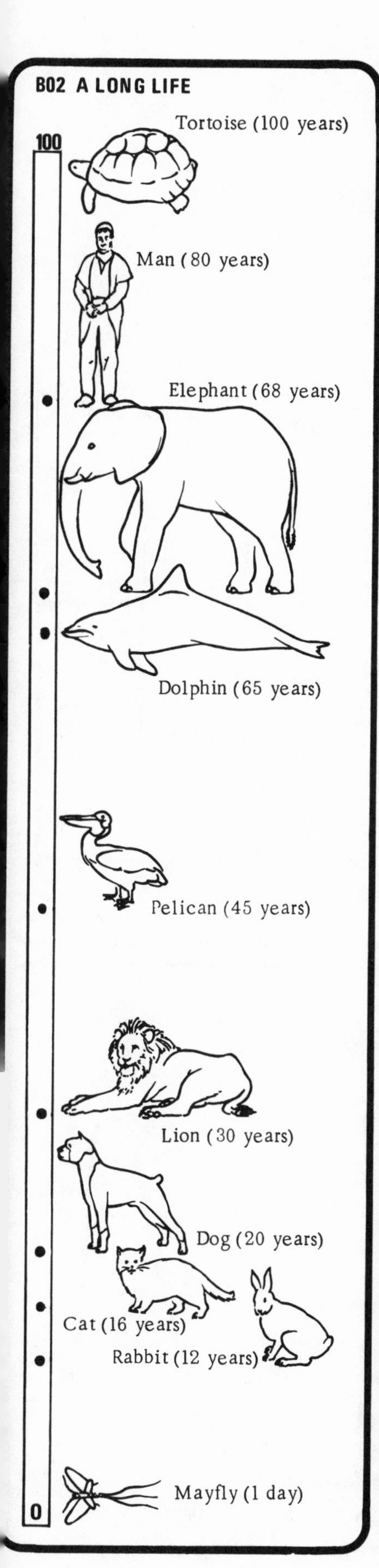

B03 PAST LIFE EXPECTANCIES

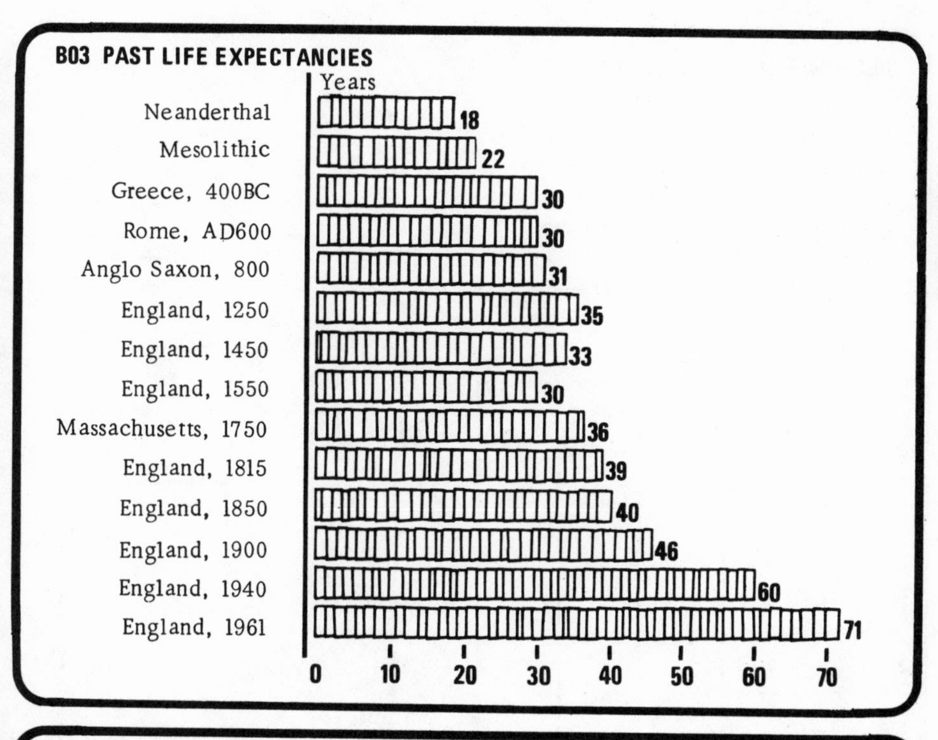

B04 MEN AND WOMEN

On average, women live longer than men in most countries of the world. (In the selection below, for example, only India is the exception.) But no one is quite sure why women live longer. It may be some factor in their physical constitution. Alternatively, it may be the consequence of the different types of work that men and women, at present, tend to do.

Average male age at death

Average female age at death

Years

Chile

Colombia

Gabon

India

Japan

Mexico

Sweden

United States

Zaire

0 10 20 30 40 50 60 70

LIFE EXPECTANCY 2

B05 HOW LONG WILL I LIVE?
Look at the bottom of this first table, and find your age now. Then look up the column - the number at the top is the age you can expect to live to. But you are likely to live longer if your father also lived to an old age - as the second table shows.

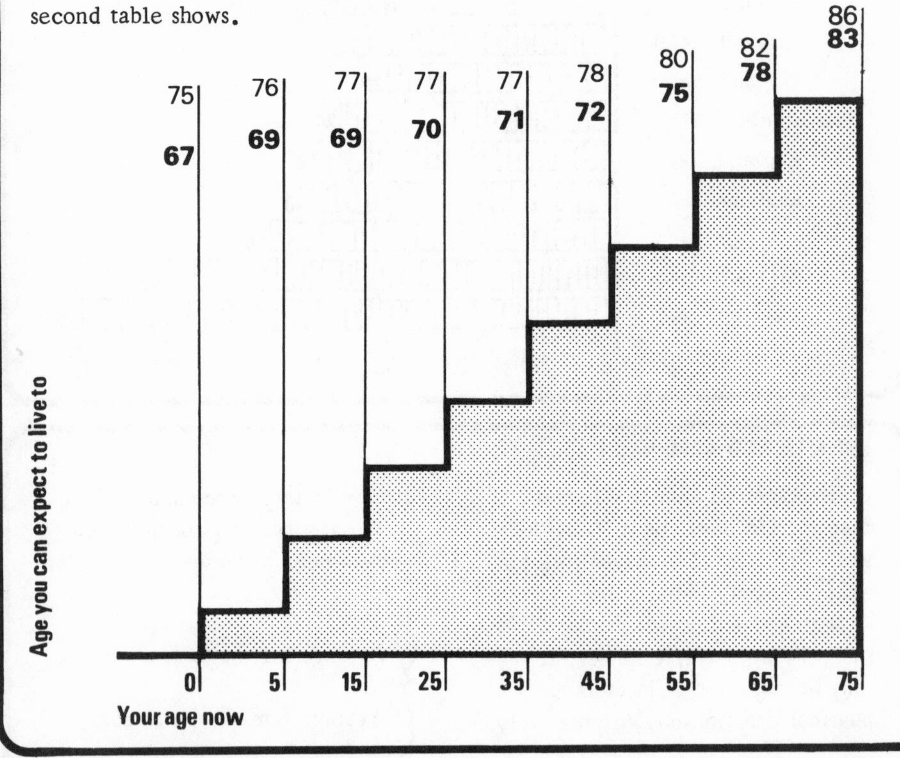

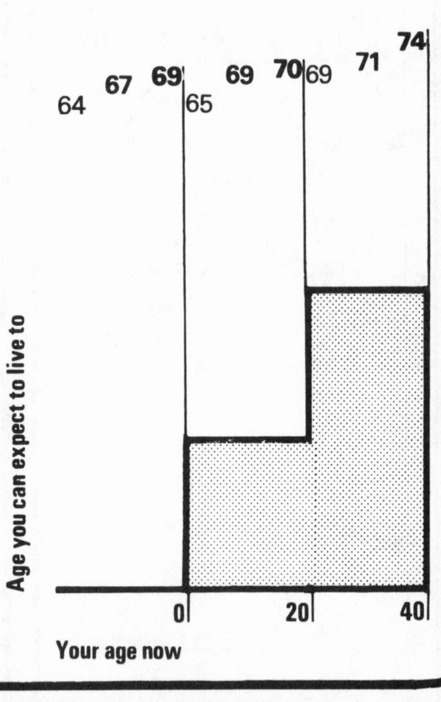

B07 PAST PATTERNS OF DYING
in a developed country.

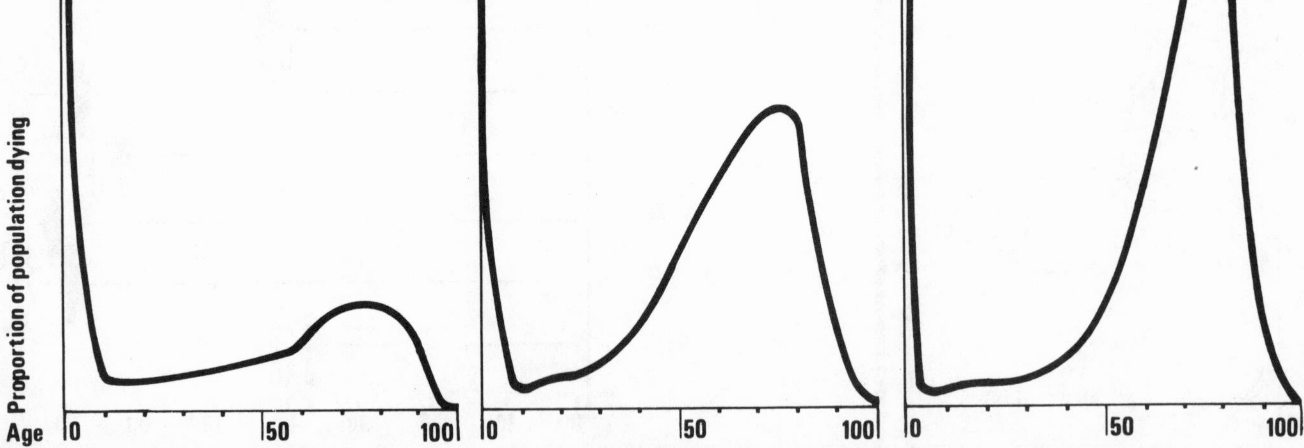

Life and death

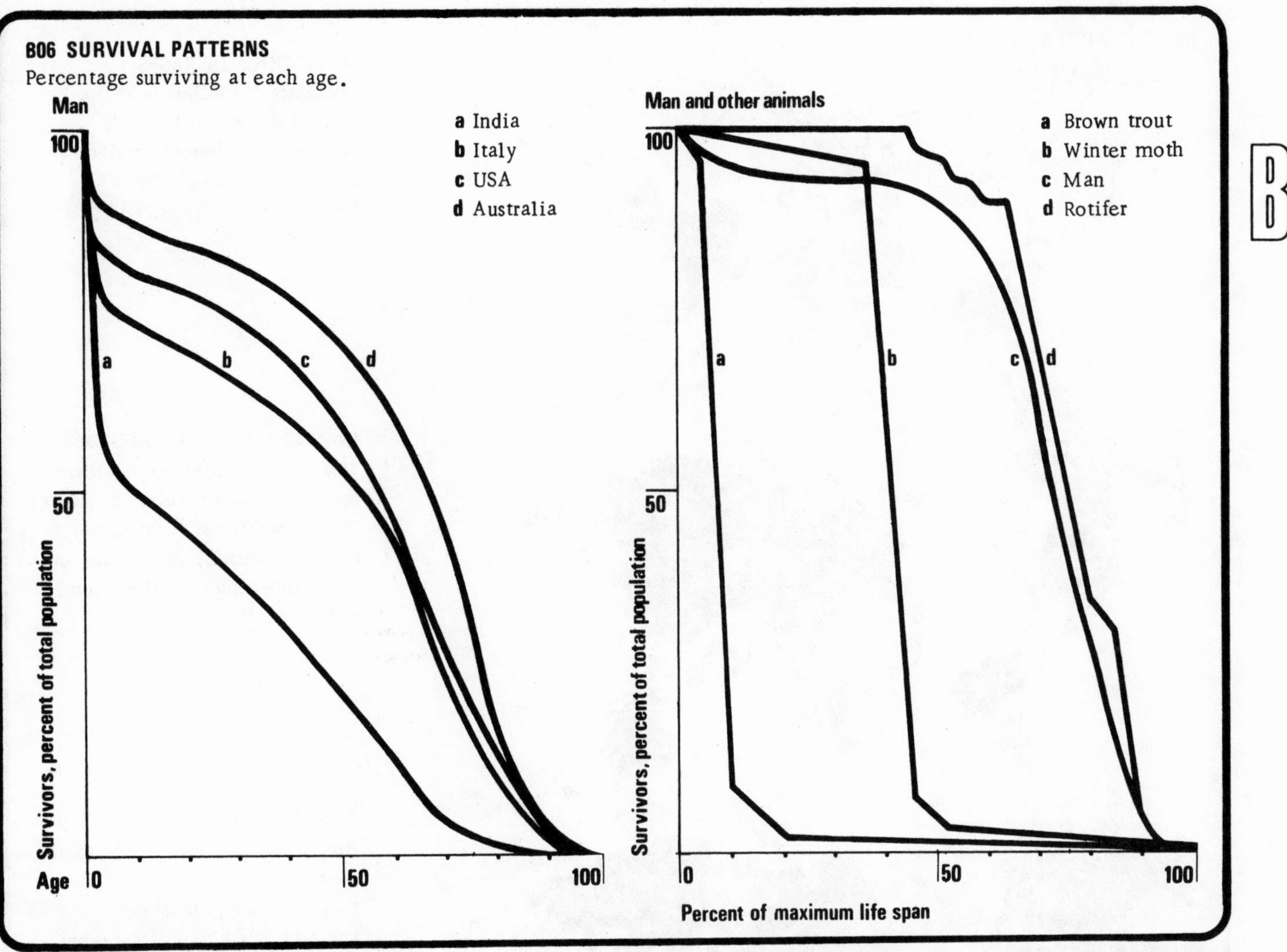
B06 SURVIVAL PATTERNS
Percentage surviving at each age.
Man
a India
b Italy
c USA
d Australia
100
50
Survivors, percent of total population
Age
0
50
100
Man and other animals
a Brown trout
b Winter moth
c Man
d Rotifer
Percent of maximum life span

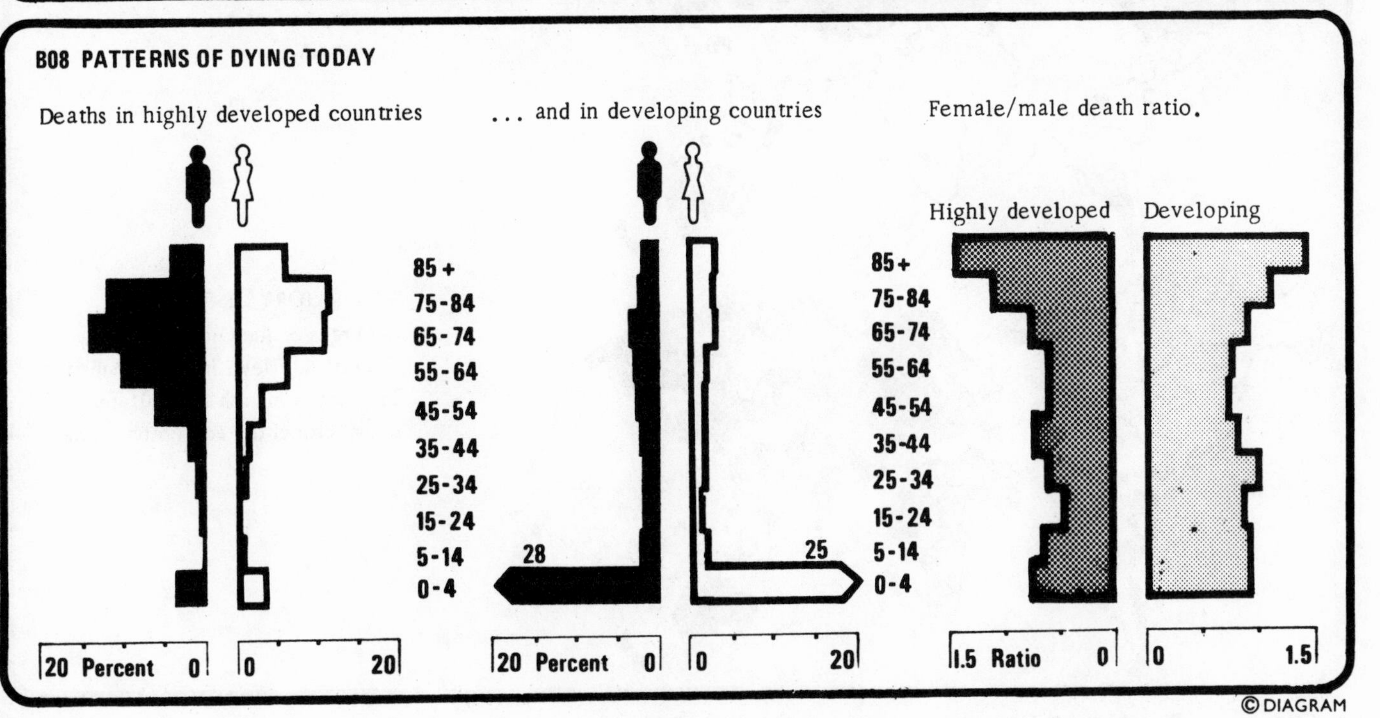
B08 PATTERNS OF DYING TODAY
Deaths in highly developed countries
... and in developing countries
Female/male death ratio.
Highly developed
Developing
85+
75-84
65-74
55-64
45-54
35-44
25-34
15-24
5-14
0-4
28
25
20 Percent 0
0 20
1.5 Ratio 0
0 1.5

CAUSES OF DEATH: World

B09 THE WORLD PATTERN

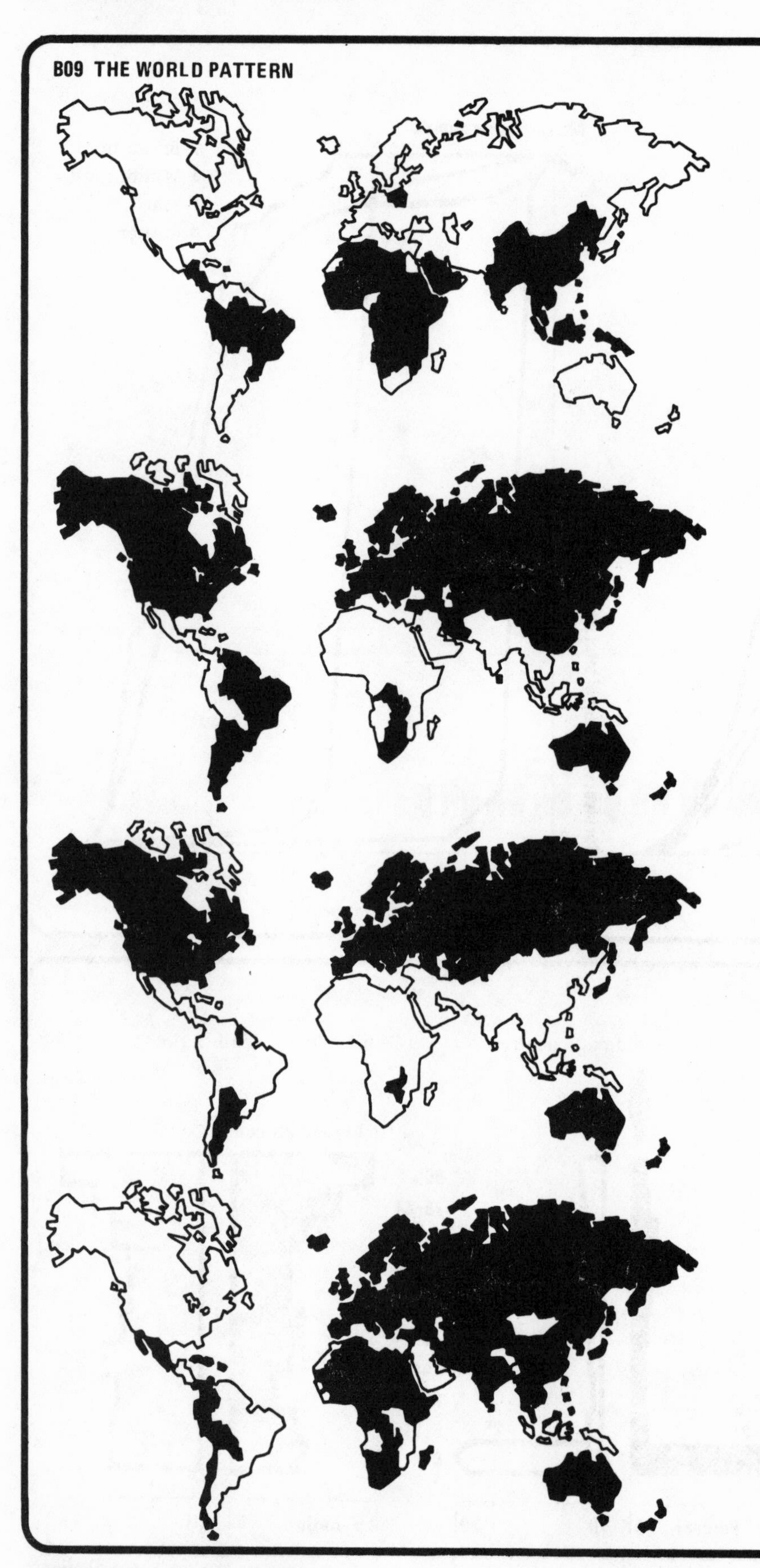

INFECTIOUS DISEASES
These are the killers in the poorer parts of the world: typhoid, paratyphoid, cholera, malaria, dysentery, tuberculosis, meningitis, smallpox, and yellow fever.

CARDIO-VASCULAR DISORDERS
The affluent world can deal with infection, but its life-style creates its own problems: degeneration of the blood vessels, thromboses and embolisms, high blood pressure, and heart failure.

CANCER
Another of the main problems of western society: cancers of the lung, stomach, intestines, pharynx and larynx; cancers of the breast, cervix, and uterus in women; and leukemia.

RESPIRATORY DISORDERS
Scourges of the Old World rather than of the New: in poor countries, influenza; in rich but polluted ones, bronchitis and emphysema.

B10 RICH DEATH AND POOR DEATH

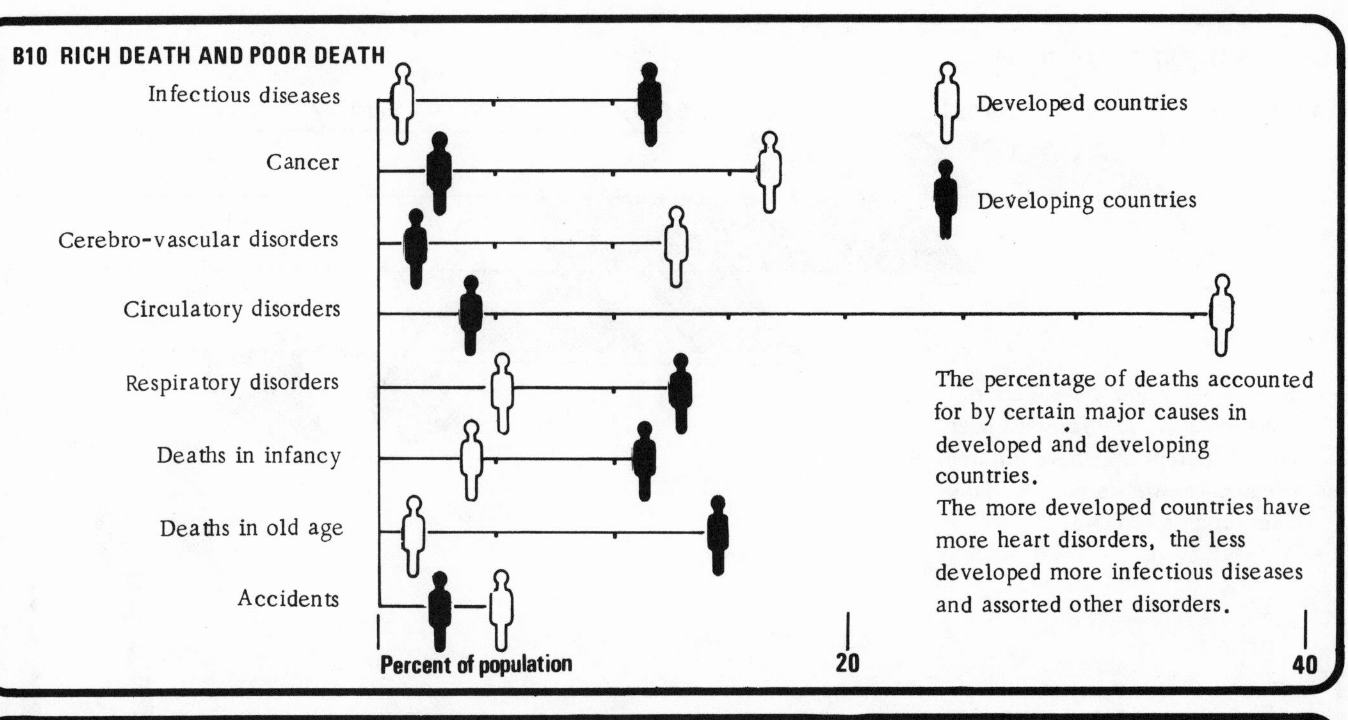

The percentage of deaths accounted for by certain major causes in developed and developing countries.
The more developed countries have more heart disorders, the less developed more infectious diseases and assorted other disorders.

B11 EVERY TEN DEATHS

What every ten dead men, and ten dead women, are likely to have died from, in selected countries

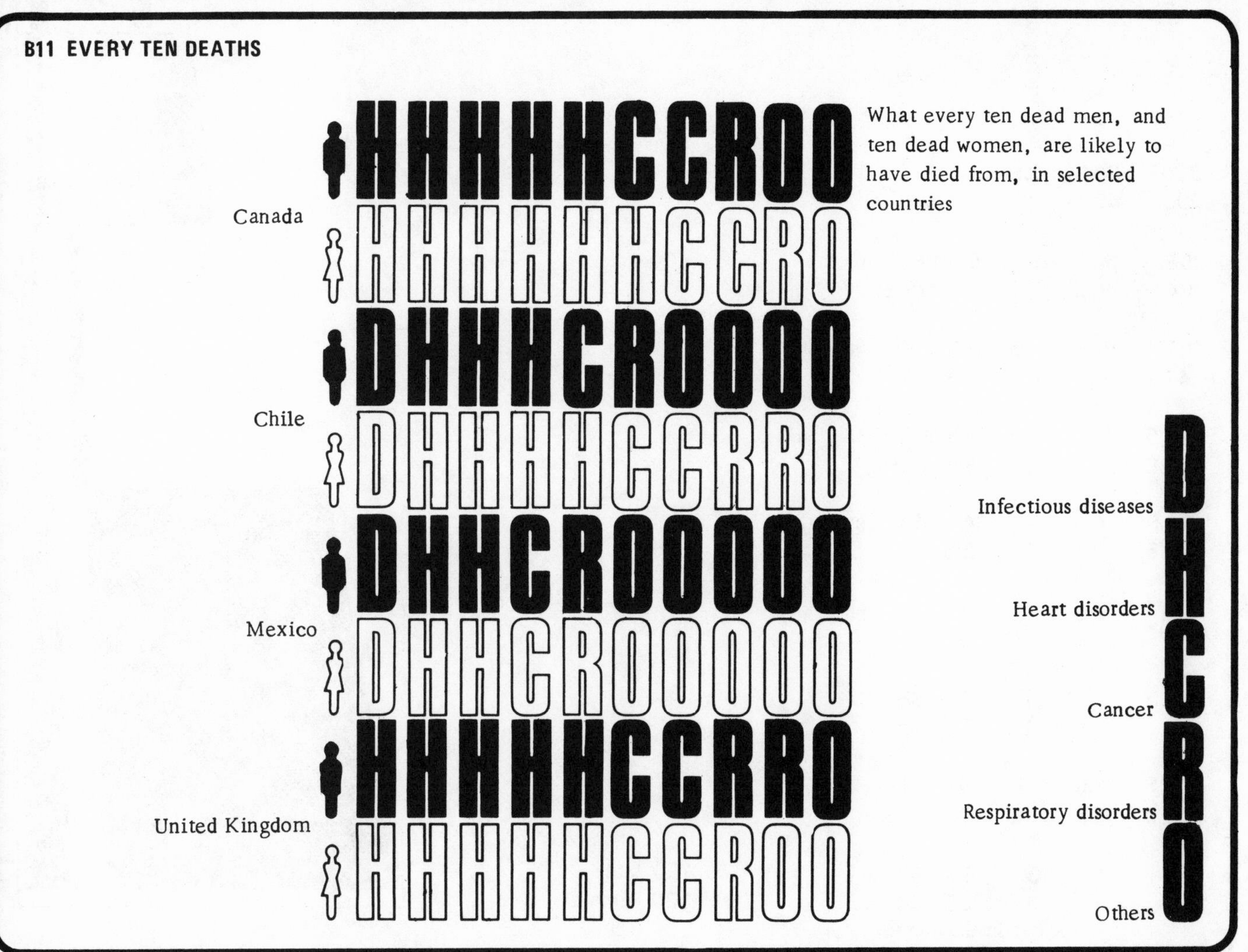

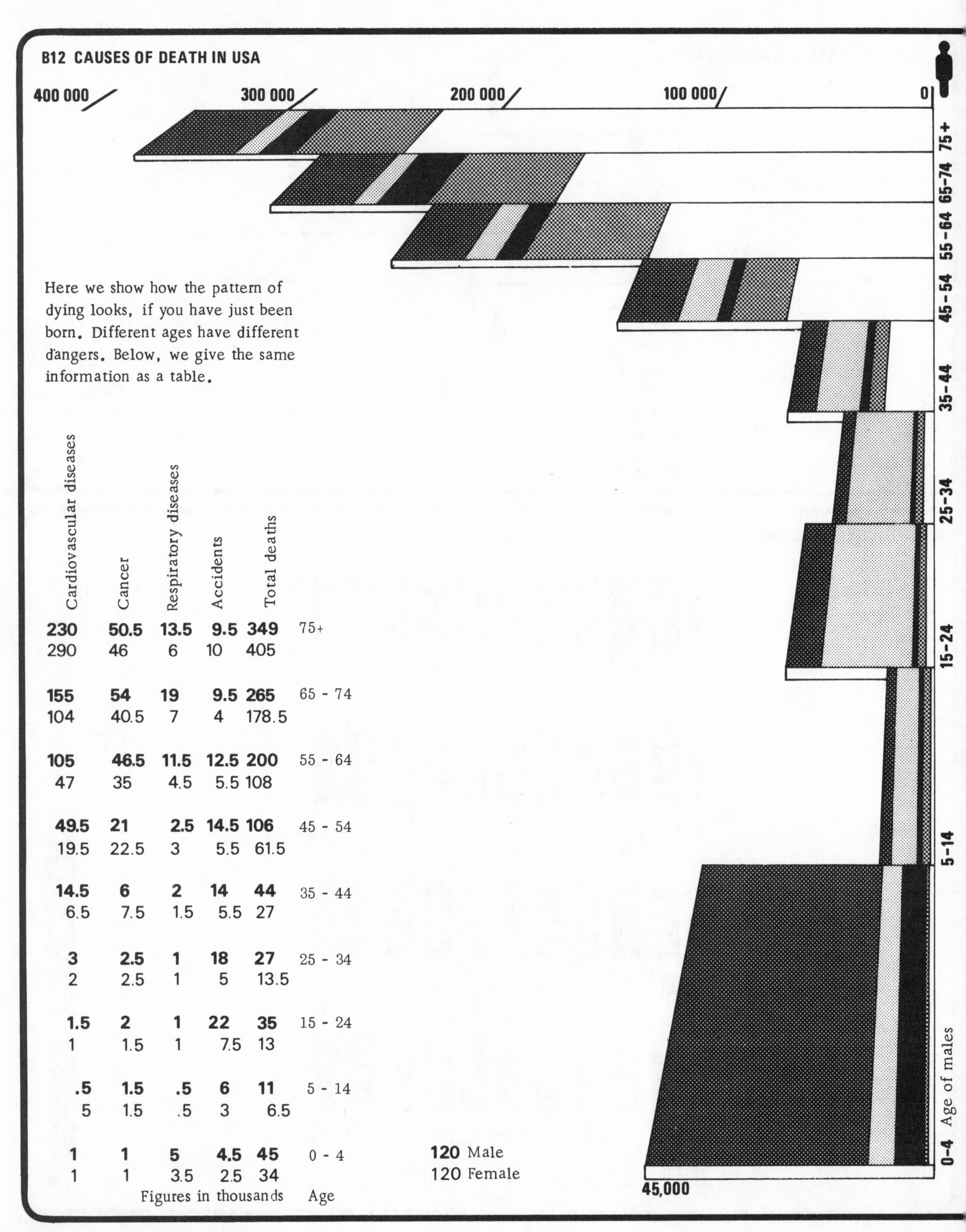

Here we show how the pattern of dying looks, if you have just been born. Different ages have different dangers. Below, we give the same information as a table.

Cardiovascular diseases	Cancer	Respiratory diseases	Accidents	Total deaths	Age
230	**50.5**	**13.5**	**9.5**	**349**	75+
290	46	6	10	405	
155	**54**	**19**	**9.5**	**265**	65 - 74
104	40.5	7	4	178.5	
105	**46.5**	**11.5**	**12.5**	**200**	55 - 64
47	35	4.5	5.5	108	
49.5	**21**	**2.5**	**14.5**	**106**	45 - 54
19.5	22.5	3	5.5	61.5	
14.5	**6**	**2**	**14**	**44**	35 - 44
6.5	7.5	1.5	5.5	27	
3	**2.5**	**1**	**18**	**27**	25 - 34
2	2.5	1	5	13.5	
1.5	**2**	**1**	**22**	**35**	15 - 24
1	1.5	1	7.5	13	
.5	**1.5**	**.5**	**6**	**11**	5 - 14
5	1.5	.5	3	6.5	
1	**1**	**5**	**4.5**	**45**	0 - 4
1	1	3.5	2.5	34	

Figures in thousands — Age

120 Male
120 Female

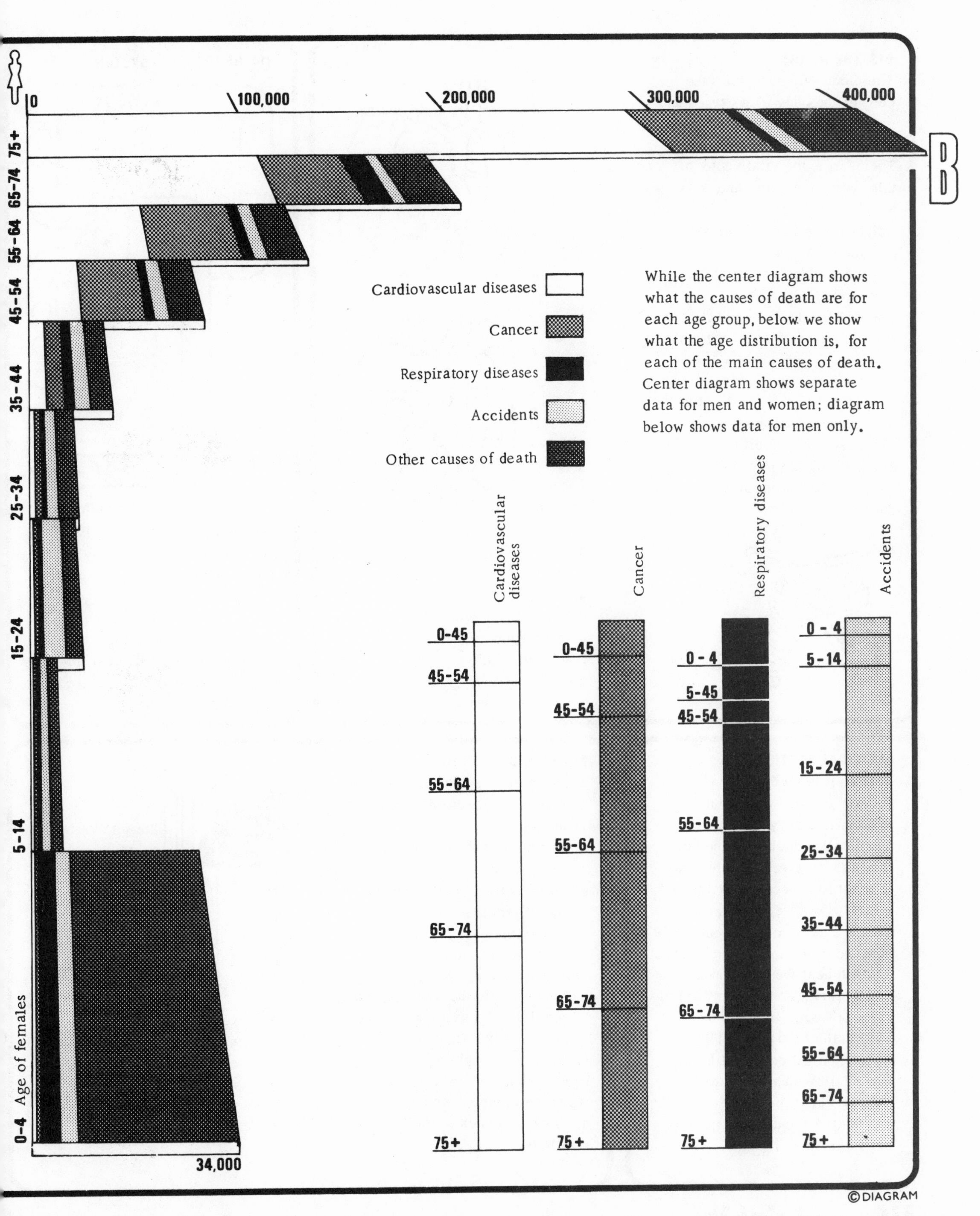
0
100,000
200,000
300,000
400,000
75+
65-74
55-64
45-54
35-44
25-34
15-24
5-14
0-4 Age of females
34,000
B
Cardiovascular diseases
Cancer
Respiratory diseases
Accidents
Other causes of death
While the center diagram shows what the causes of death are for each age group, below we show what the age distribution is, for each of the main causes of death. Center diagram shows separate data for men and women; diagram below shows data for men only.
Cardiovascular diseases
0-45
45-54
55-64
65-74
75+
Cancer
0-45
45-54
55-64
65-74
75+
Respiratory diseases
0 - 4
5-45
45-54
55-64
65-74
75+
Accidents
0 - 4
5-14
15-24
25-34
35-44
45-54
55-64
65-74
75+

B13 THE HEART

The blood system supplies the cells of the body with oxygen and nutrients, and carries away waste materials.
The heart is the vital center of this, being the pump that drives blood through the body. It weighs under a pound, measures on average about 5 inches long by 3½ inches wide, and comprises four muscular chambers.
The heart is positioned under the rib cage and in front of the lungs. It lies on the center line of the body, but not symmetrically: one end slants out to a point just to the left of the breastbone (sternum). The heartbeat is most noticeable here, giving the impression that the heart lies on the left side of the body.

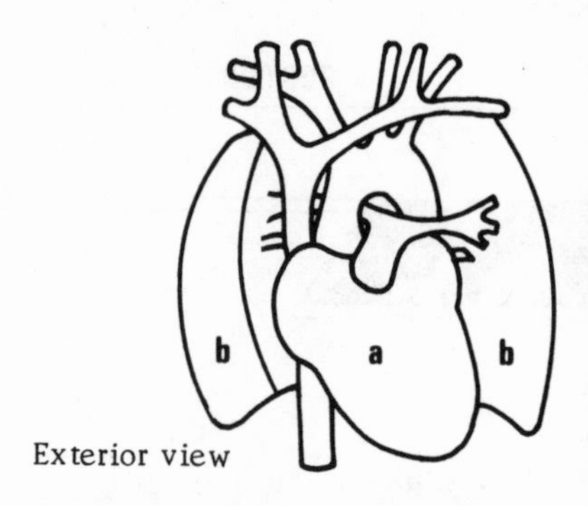

Exterior view

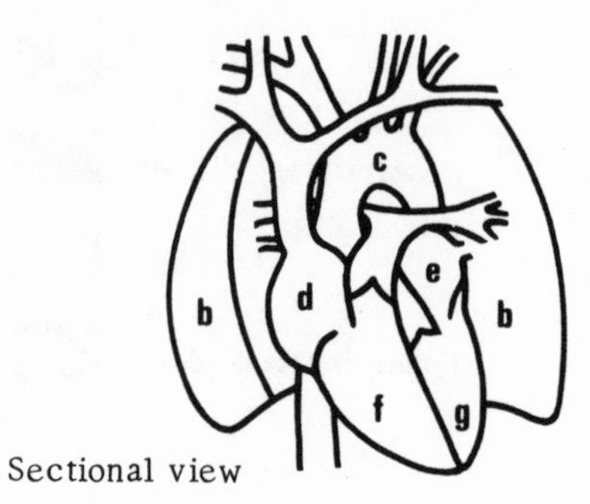

Sectional view

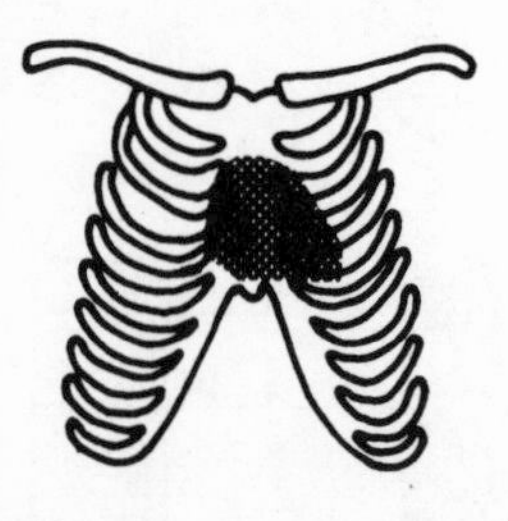

a Heart
b Lungs
c Aorta
d Right atrium
e Left atrium
f Right ventricle
g Left ventricle

B14 HEART-LUNG SYSTEM

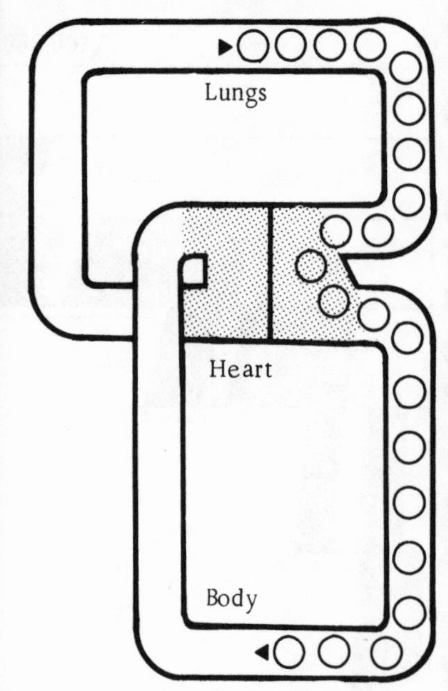

The heart is really two pumps. One pump receives blood from the body and sends it out to the lungs, where the waste product, carbon dioxide, is exchanged for fresh oxygen. The other pump receives back the oxygenated blood from the lungs, and speeds it on its way to the rest of the body.

B15 VITAL STATISTICS

The adult heart beats 60 to 80 times a minute, and about 40 million times a year.
The smaller the heart, the faster it beats. An average male heart is about 10 ounces in weight, and a female heart 8 ounces. So a woman's heart makes about 6 to 8 more beats a minute than a man's.
At each beat the heart takes in and discharges over ¼pint (US) of blood (130cc). It pumps over 2000 gallons a day, and 50 million gallons in a lifetime.
In a healthy man during exercise, the heart beat may increase to 180 beats a minute, pumping 40 pints a minute.

B16 BLOOD PRESSURE

Blood pressure is expressed in two figures that indicate the pressures in the aorta:
a) on contraction, called the systolic pressure;
b) on relaxation, called the diastolic pressure.
For a healthy young man at rest the systolic pressure is usually between 100 and 120mm Hg, and the diastolic between 70 and 80 mm Hg. These are expressed as 100/70 or 120/80.
Pressure in the right ventricle only rises to about 20 mm Hg. This is enough to send blood through the lungs and back to the left ventricle.

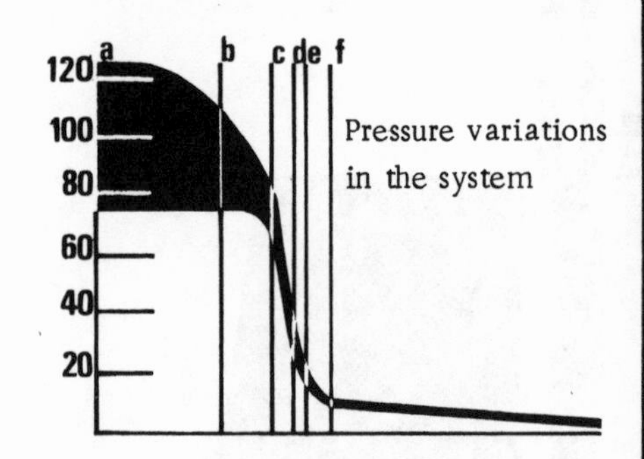

a Large arteries
b Small arteries
c Arterioles
d Capillaries
e Venules
f Veins

B

B17 HOW THE HEART WORKS

The heart beat is in two stages: contraction and relaxation.
As the heart begins to contract, both atria and both ventricles are already full of blood.
The left atrium and ventricle contain oxygenated blood, the right contain deoxygenated blood.
a) The atria contract slightly before the ventricles. This builds up the pressure in the ventricles.
b) Eventually back pressure closes the valves between the atria and ventricles.
c) The ventricles contract, and pressure forces open the valves between the ventricles and the arteries that lead from them. From the right ventricle, deoxygenated blood is sent into the lungs. From the left, oxygenated blood from the lungs is sent out to the body.
d) When most of the blood has passed, the valves close, because there is no longer enough pressure to keep them open. The heart relaxes, and atria and ventricles begin to fill with blood.
After about 0.4 seconds, a nerve impulse triggers off the next contraction.

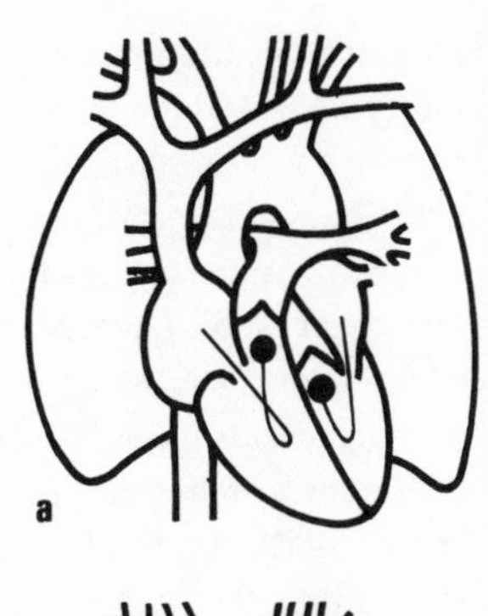

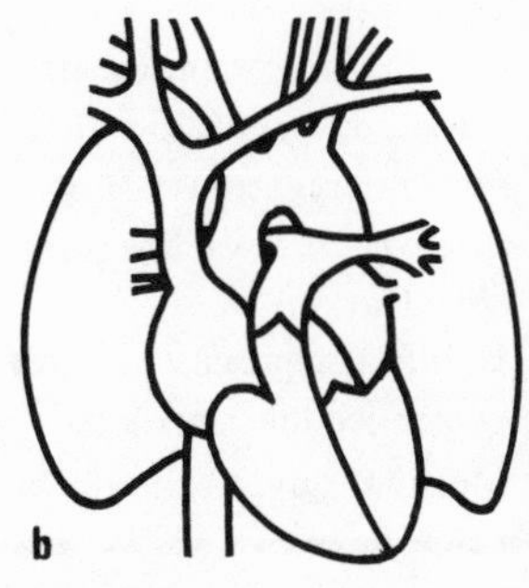

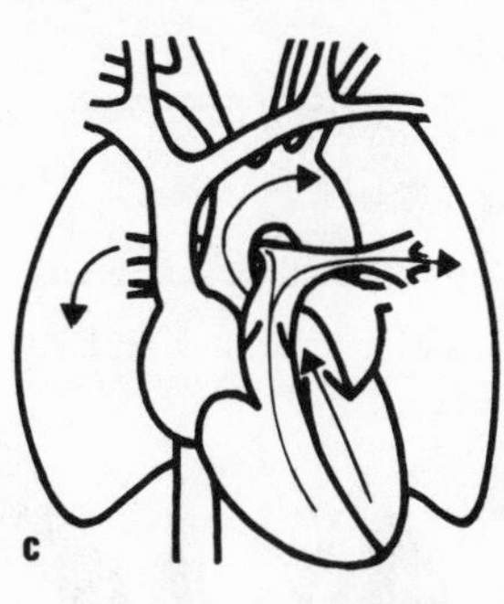

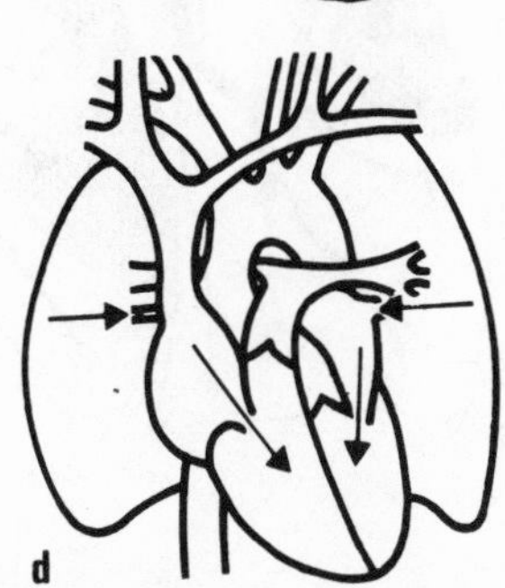

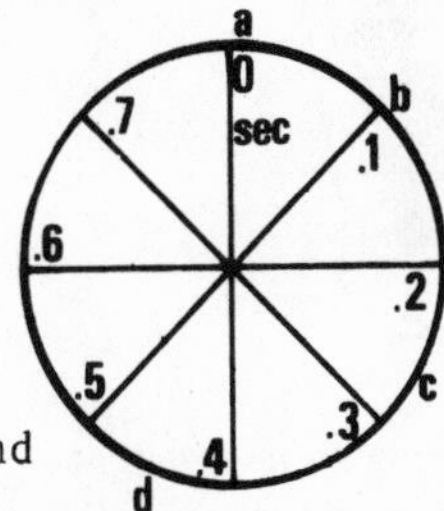

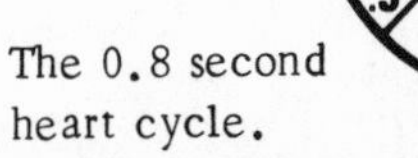
The 0.8 second heart cycle.

B18 BLOOD VESSELS

Blood vessels are of three types: arteries, veins, and capillaries. Arteries carry oxygenated blood from the heart to all parts of the body. They have strong elastic walls that squeeze the blood along with waves of contraction.
After profuse branching the blood passes through the tissues of the body in tiny capillaries, where nutritive substances and oxygen are exchanged for waste products. The blood is then conveyed back to the heart along veins. These have thinner walls than the arteries, and contain valves to prevent a back flow of blood.

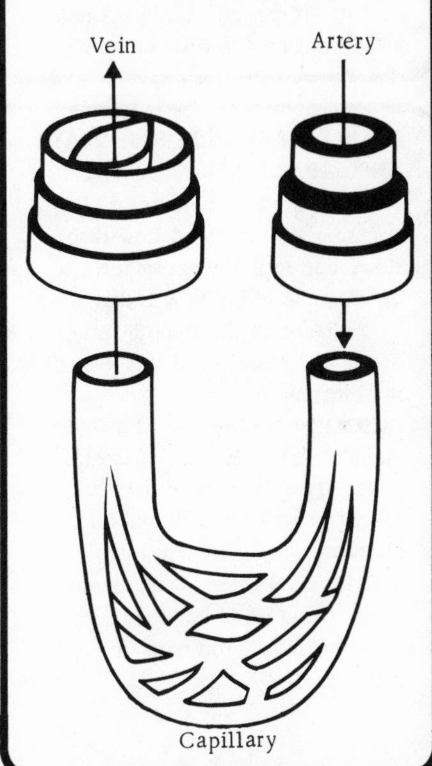

B19 WHERE THE BLOOD GOES

This shows the relative distribution of blood to the various organs of the body, when at rest. During exertion, the distribution changes. At rest, the heart-lung-heart route takes 6 seconds, the heart-brain-heart route, 8 seconds, and the heart-toe-heart route, 16 seconds.

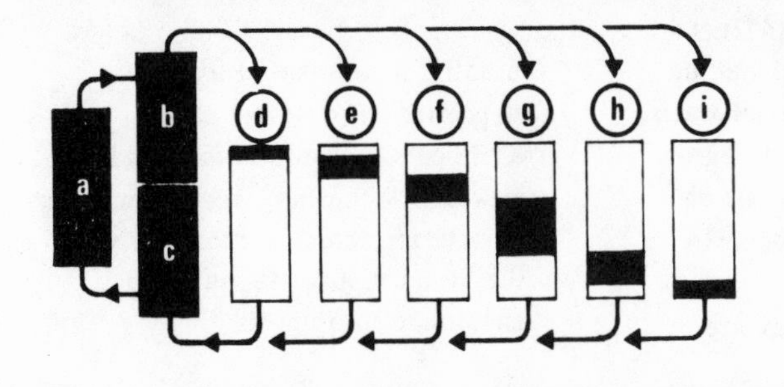

- **a** Lungs
- **b** Heart (right)
- **c** Heart (left)
- **d** Heart blood vessels 5%
- **e** Brain 15%
- **f** Muscles 15%
- **g** Intestines 35%
- **h** Kidneys 20%
- **i** Skin, skeleton etc 10%

CARDIO-VASCULAR DISORDERS 1

B20 HEART DISORDERS

ANGINA PECTORIS

Angina is any pain caused by muscular spasm. Angina pectoris is a pain in the chest caused by an increased demand for blood that the heart muscle is unable to meet. It can be caused by any activity that requires an increased heart rate. For example, those prone to it may suffer an attack after eating a heavy meal. It is not an illness in itself, but the possible symptom of other cardio-vascular malfunctions.

HEART FAILURE

This occurs when the heart cannot keep pace with the demands made upon it. It can be caused by: heart attacks; intense fevers; chronic lung disease; high blood pressure; faulty heart valves; or strain on the heart muscle in extreme physical exertion.

The symptoms are breathlessness and chest pain. Usually one side of the heart fails first, and then pressure builds up as the other side continues to function. Legs and ankles swell and the lungs flood with fluid.

The rhythm of the heartbeat is affected, becoming abnormally fast (tachycardia), slow (bradycardia) or irregular (fibrillation).

Unless the process is arrested and controlled, death results.

Medical advice should be obtained as quickly as possible. If the heart has stopped completely, external cardiac massage should be applied within three minutes - but only if it is certain that the heart has stopped.

Rest is an important factor in recuperation. A physician prescribes drugs for sedation, and to clear the lungs and tissues of excess fluids by increasing urinary output. When there is complete disruption of the rhythm between the atria and ventricles, a surgeon will implant an electronic pacemaker in the patient which will act as a generator for cardiac impulses (heart beats).

B21 BLOCKAGE AND TISSUE DEATH

THROMBOSIS is blockage of a blood vessel by a blood clot. It occurs when the blood flow is too slow, due to prolonged inactivity; or when the blood flow is disturbed by a change in the smooth lining of a blood vessel, and this sets off the clotting process.

EMBOLISM is blockage of a small blood vessel by a mass of foreign material, eg a mass of bacteria, or fragments from a thrombosis elsewhere.

INFARCTION refers to the death of living tissue when its blood supply is cut off by a thrombosis or embolism.

Thrombosis

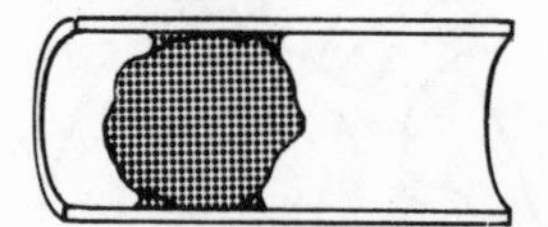

Embolism

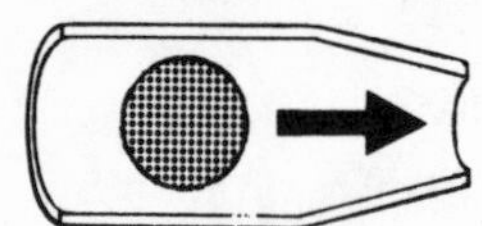

Three pulmonary embolisms: their areas of effect

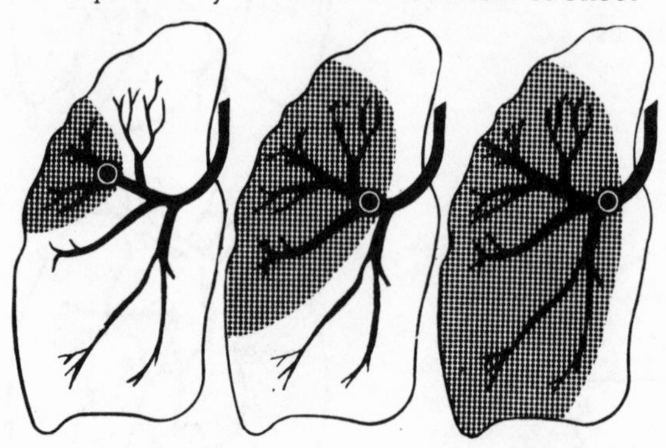

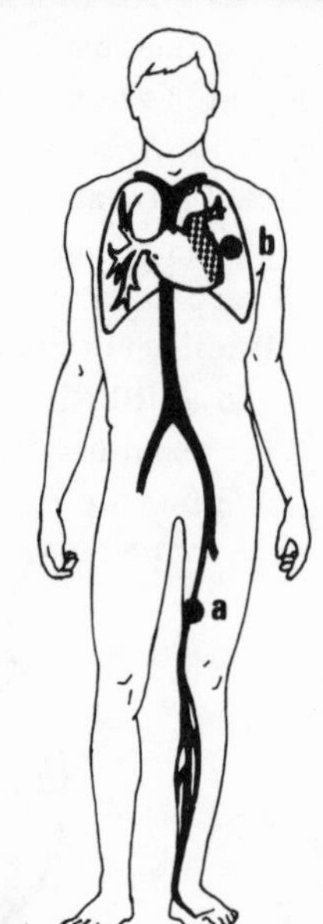

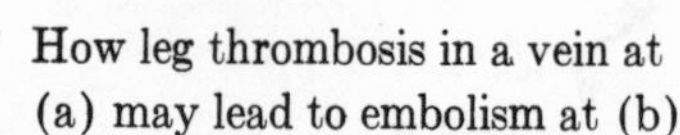

How leg thrombosis in a vein at (a) may lead to embolism at (b)

B23 ARTERIAL DEGENERATION

ARTERIOSCLEROSIS is thickening and hardening of the arterial walls. It particularly occurs in old age.

ATHEROMA is a fatty deposit on the arterial walls. Such deposits contain large amounts of cholesterol. With age they are usually accompanied by the deposition of calcium salts.

ATHEROSCLEROSIS is the condition in which atheroma, accompanied by arteriosclerosis, interferes with the blood supply. It may also encourage thrombosis.

ANEURYSM is a bulge in the wall of an artery at a weak point. Under the pressure of blood, the aneurism may balloon out, and finally break, spilling out blood.

HEART ATTACK
A "coronary thrombosis" is a thrombosis in the arteries that supply the heart muscle itself. It may result in a cardiac or "myocardial" (muscle of the heart) infarction. When these two disorders have occurred, the person has suffered a heart attack, which may result in a cardiac arrest (stoppage of the heart).
The severity of the attack depends on:
a) whether or not the blood can find an alternative route;
b) the size and position of the area affected; and
c) whether or not the nerves that regulate the heartbeat are affected.

The dead tissue of the infarction is gradually replaced by scar tissue. This cannot contract, and weakens the heart.
The chance of serious infarctions increases with age. They happen suddenly and are accompanied by severe pain, cold sweating, breathlessness and faintness. As with all heart disorders, rest, to allow repair, is necessary.

RHEUMATIC HEART DISEASE
As the result of the wide use of antibiotics, the incidence of acute rheumatic heart disease has sharply declined throughout the world, and is now relatively rare.
Rheumatic heart disease may cause inflammation of joints and/or the lining of heart chambers and valves. Resulting deformities of the valves may later cause heart failure. Surgical techniques are now available that correct valve deformities and protect the heart against failure.

B22 HIGH BLOOD PRESSURE

High blood pressure (hypertension) is associated with arteriosclerosis, kidney diseases, glandular disorders, obesity and anxiety. It can also occur without such factors. The cause is obscure at present, but is linked with contraction of the small arteries
Hypertension often starts in the early 30s, but no age is exempt, and it is not caused by ageing. Heredity seems to be one factor. Hypertension is usually controlled effectively by drugs.
For the role of high blood pressure in heart disorders, see B28 and B30.

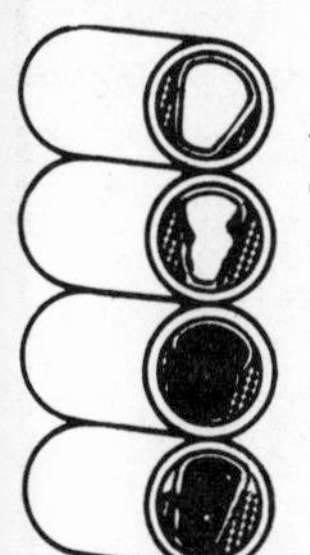

Atheroma is deposited. Clots of blood adhere to it. Finally a large thrombus blocks the artery. But blood may find ways through, or take alternative routes.

B24 HEART SURGERY

The main reason for heart surgery is the heart's importance to the body - and that is also the main difficulty. Till a few years ago, surgeons could only carry out operations that did not interfere with the heart's pumping action. For if the flow of oxygenated blood to the body stops, brain damage and death follow within 4 minutes due to lack of oxygen.
But the development of the heart-lung machine has changed the situation. For a short time, this machine can take over the functions of the heart and respiratory system, while the heart is being operated on.
Usually, the two large veins that lead into the right atrium are connected to the machine instead. Deoxygenated blood flows into the machine, where it is mixed with oxygen, in a way similar to the lungs' processes, and the blood flows back into the body through a connection to one of the branches of the aorta.
This allows sufficient time for certain procedures, especially:
a) closure of atrial or ventricular septal defects (see B26); or
b) replacement of diseased valves, such as the aortic or mitral. (The mitral valve is that between the left atrium and left ventricle, and is often damaged in cases of rheumatic fever.)
Difficulties that can arise afterwards, especially when the machine is used for longer than normal, include:
a) kidney damage; and
b) psychological psychosis (from which recovery usually occurs).
Both are possibly due to the pressure output of the machine being too low for pumped blood to reach some tissues.
Other surgical techniques include:
a) replacement of segments of coronary artery or aorta;
b) artificial pumping aids for the left ventricle; and
c) use of artificial "pacemakers", to stimulate the heartbeat.

B25 BRAIN DISORDERS

ARTERIOSCLEROSIS PSYCHOSIS

This results from a generally impaired blood supply to the brain. It is usually associated with old age, but may occur earlier. The person feels restless and emotional, is inclined to wander at night, and complains of headaches, giddiness, and momentary blackouts. Memory may fail and strong personality traits become exaggerated. These symptoms fluctuate.

As the physical change is permanent, treatment concentrates mainly on creating a relaxing environment. Sedative drugs may be used if the person is overactive or worried, anti-depressants if he is depressed. Drugs are also used to try to increase cerebral circulation (but this usually has little effect).

"STROKE"

Technically known as a cerebrovascular accident, a stroke results from failure of the blood supply to a part of the brain. This may be due to a thrombosis or embolism, or to a hemorrhage in the brain from a ruptured blood vessel. Infarction (death) of part of the brain may occur.

A stroke is more common in men than women. It can vary in severity from a minor disturbance, forgotten in a few minutes, to a major attack causing unconsciousness and death. The severity depends on the position and extent of the damage. In a severe attack, the patient loses consciousness almost immediately. Death may then follow in a matter of hours; alternatively, consciousness is regained, but there is usually lasting damage. An attack may also show itself in sudden paralysis of one side or part of the body, without loss of consciousness. Or, again, it may develop over several hours, with persistent throbbing headache, vomiting, dizziness, and numbness of the limbs.

Recovery depends on age, general health, and the site and size of damage. Even if recovery is possible, it may take years; but in other cases, control of the body has suffered permanent damage, with muscles paralyzed or very weak. The effects occur in the opposite side to the side of the brain affected (because one side of the body is controlled by the opposite side of the brain). A stroke in the side of the brain that is "dominant" may also affect speech. Mentally, concentration may be impaired, but judgement and basic personality need not be.

Treatment consists mainly of rest and prolonged convalescence, with careful nursing, physiotherapy and (if needed) speech therapy. Drugs are sometimes used to lower the blood pressure, if it is high, and so help prevent further damage.

B26 CONGENITAL HEART DEFECTS

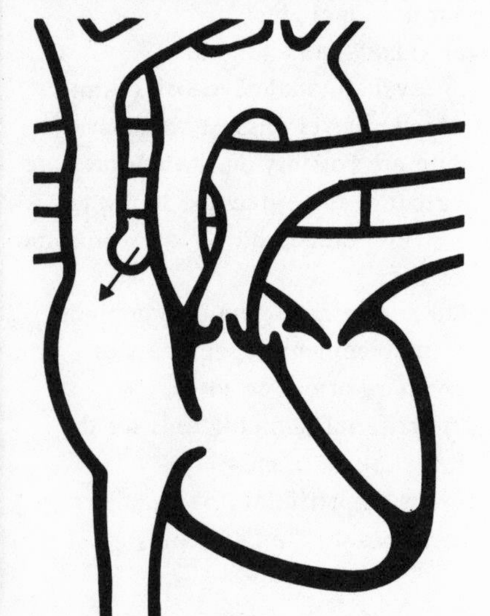

Atrial septal defect

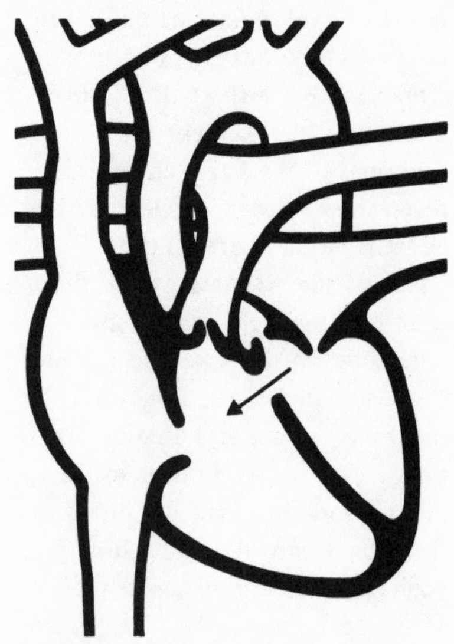

Ventricular defect

Two common types of congenital heart defect are shown here:

a) atrial septal defect, which is the presence at birth of a large hole between right and left atria; and

b) ventricular septal defect, which similarly is the presence of a hole between right and left ventricles.

In each case, because pressure in the left side of the heart is higher, the result is that oxygenated blood from the left passes through and mixes with deoxygenated in the right.

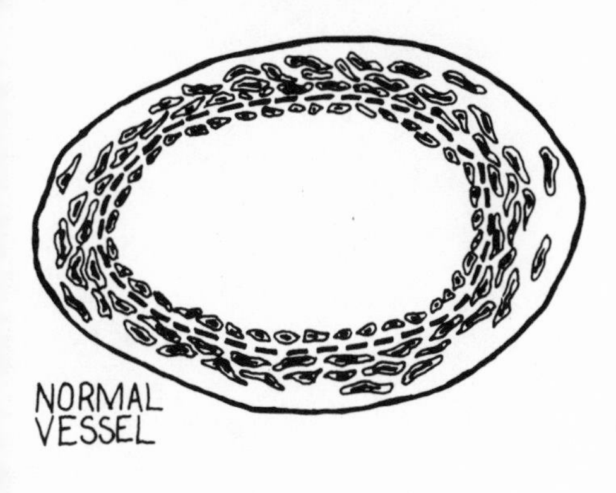

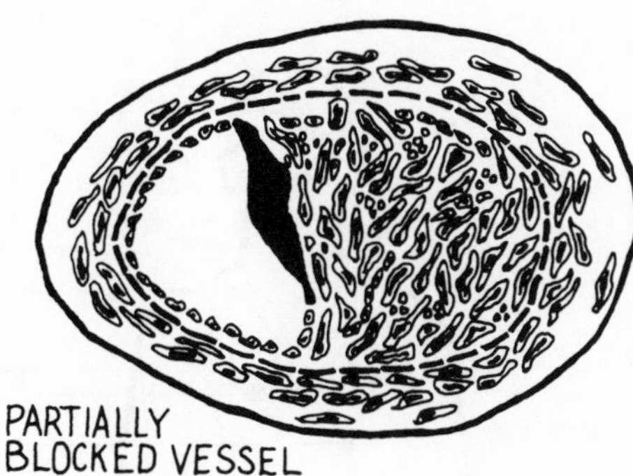

ATHEROSCLEROSIS
Atherosclerosis is the condition in which atheroma, accompanied by arteriosclerosis, interferes with the blood supply. When a vessel becomes blocked (see diagrams left), the results can be a change in heart rhythm, a heart attack, and even death.

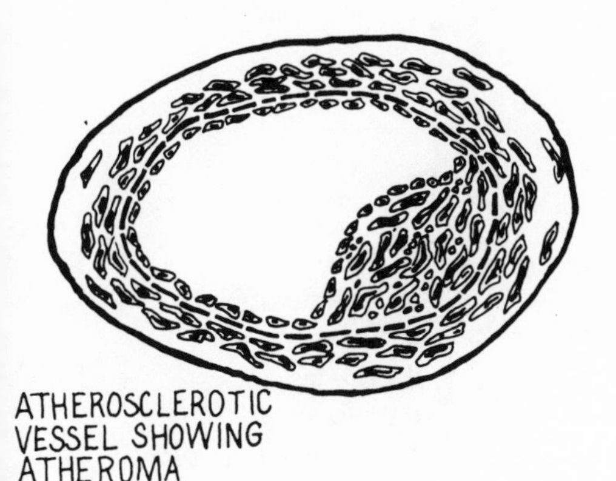

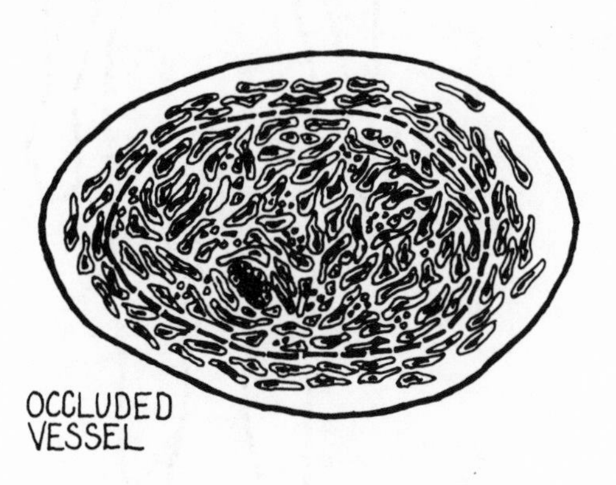

EVOLUTION OF OCCLUSION

B27 OTHER DISORDERS

THROMBOSIS can occur in arteries in the pelvis or legs, causing gangrene.
THROMBOPHLEBITIS is inflammation of a vein due to damage or infection resulting in a clot.
PULMONARY EMBOLISM is blockage of one of the arteries of the lungs, caused by fragments of a thrombosis elsewhere. It is a serious condition frequently causing death.
DEEP VEIN THROMBOSIS is a thrombosis of the veins deep in the legs. The superficial veins take over, as the main route for blood returning to the body; but the condition is dangerous because of the chance of a pulmonary embolism.
Because of inactivity and tissue damage, both deep vein thrombosis and pulmonary embolism are more likely after an operation. (Any pain deep in the calf muscle should be reported at once.)
VARICOSE VEINS
Varicose veins are dilated veins in the legs, that stand out above the surface and can be acutely painful. Their exposed position also makes them vulnerable to bleeding and ulceration.
Varicose veins develop if the valves in the leg veins fail to prevent the back flow of blood. They are more likely in occupations involving long periods of standing - and also where there is a swelling of the abdomen, as in obesity, chronic constipation, and pregnancy. This last is why 1 in 2 women over 40 suffer from varicose veins, but only 1 in 4 men of the same age. Treatment ranges from wearing pressure bandages and resting with the legs in an elevated position as often as possible, to surgical tying or removal of the vein, making the blood find alternative routes.

B28 RISK FACTORS

Risk factors in cardio-vascular disorders include high blood pressure, elevated blood cholesterol levels, obesity, smoking, lack of exercise, stress and anxiety. Genetic factors play a debatable role. High blood pressure is a major risk factor in cases of strokes. Successful treatment of high blood pressure with diuretics and, if necessary, other anti-hypertensive drugs has definitely reduced the incidence of strokes, but the effect of the treatment of hypertension on heart attacks is still uncertain.

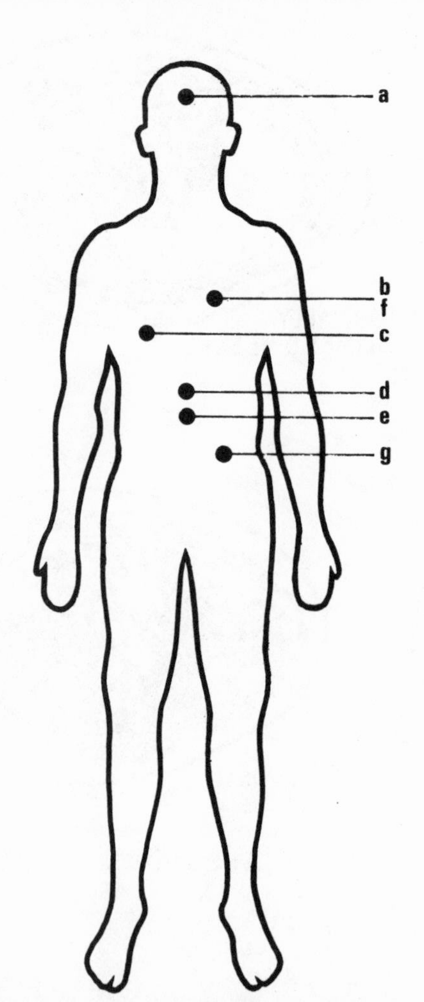

a Stress
b Cholesterol
c Smoking
d Drinking
e Overeating
f High blood pressure
g Obesity

B31 CHECKS FOR HEART DISEASE

BLOOD PRESSURE
A doctor will use an instrument called a sphygmomanometer (see right) to measure the pressure of the blood in the arteries. When the heart muscle is contracted, it is called systolic blood pressure. When the heart muscle is relaxed between beats, it is known as diastolic blood pressure. When blood pressure measurements are given (eg 120/80), the first number indicates systolic pressure; the second number represents diastolic pressure. 120/80 represents a normal blood pressure for a man or woman.

AUSCULTATION
A doctor will listen with a stethoscope to the sounds within the body, especially of the heart and lungs. This is known as auscultation. Heart murmurs are so discovered, as are the signs of pneumonia, pleurisy and paralysis of the intestinal tract.

ELECTROCARDIOGRAM
A doctor will use a cardiograph to make a visual picture of the electrical activity of the heart. The tracing produced on graph paper with this machine is known as an electrocardiogram. It provides information on the extent and location of injury sustained by the heart because of a heart attack, and is of great value in analyzing disturbances in cardiac rhythm. The electrocardiogram is used in

DIABETES
According to the National Institutes of Health of the U. S. Department of Health and Human Services, a diabetic's risk of developing cardio-vascular disease is higher than that of the nondiabetic. In addition, about 75% of deaths among diabetics are due to cardio-vascular disease. To make himself healthier, the diabetic should stop smoking (or never start); control high blood pressure if it develops; limit the amount of cholesterol and saturated fats in his diet; and exercise regularly.

B29 CHOLESTEROL
Cholesterol is a waxy substance produced in the liver, and also acquired from outside in certain foods, especially animal fats, milk products, and eggs. It is found throughout the body, but especially in the brain, nervous tissue, and adrenal glands. It is important in the repair of ruptured membranes, and in the production of sex hormones and bile acids.
Blood cholesterol level varies with age, sex, race, hormone production, climate, and occupation, and is thought to depend mainly on the amount manufactured in the body. Surplus adrenalin, due to stress situations, may be one cause of excess cholesterol.
However, nutrition does affect the level to some extent - though in this the cholesterol content of the diet seems less significant than the fat content. A diet rich in "polyunsaturated fatty acids" (i.e. those of most vegetable oils) can lower the blood cholesterol level. if saturated fat consumption is reduced.

B30 HIGH BLOOD PRESSURE
Blood pressure depends on the resistance of the arteries to the heart's pumping efforts. It falls if the heart pumps less and/or if the arteries are dilated. It rises if the heart pumps more and/or if the arteries are constricted.
Heart output can be raised temporarily by exercise*, but this is only dangerous in some cases of existing heart disorder - it does not cause disorder. Other temporary high blood pressure is caused by excitement, stress, or apprehension, and whether these are dangerous probably depends on their duration and frequency and how high they go.
Consistent high blood pressure is certainly dangerous. Its causes are discussed in B22. In the absence of a specific causative disorder, blood pressure can be kept low by exercise, elimination of body fat, and limiting salt intake.

B

exercise tolerance tests, which evaluate the ability of the heart to function normally under the stresses imposed by certain levels of exercise. Abnormalities in the electrocardiogram under such testing are an index to the degree of damage to the heart muscle and its ability to function.

Based on information from the U.S. Department of Health and Human Services, National Institutes of Health

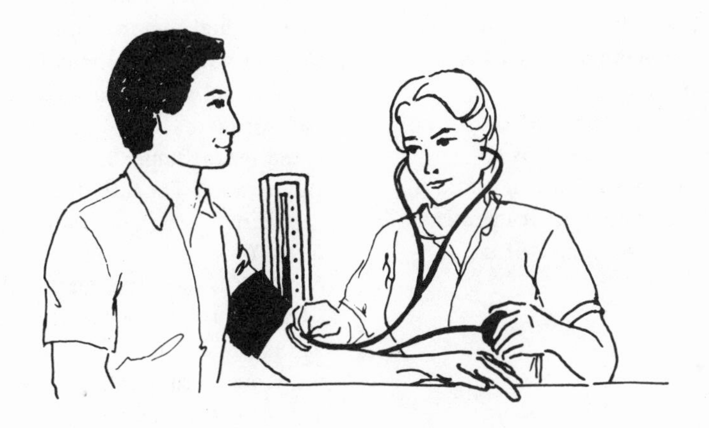

B32 WHAT IS CANCER?

Cancer is one of several disorders which can result when the process of cell division in a person's body gets out of control. Such disorders produce tissue growths called "tumors". A cancer is a malignant kind of tumor.

Cancer attacks one in every four people.

NORMAL CELL DIVISION

The body is constantly producing new cells for the purposes of growth and repair - about 500,000 million daily. It does this by cell division - one parent cell divides to form two new cells. When this process is going correctly, the new cells show the same characteristics as the tissue in which they originate. They are capable of carrying out the functions that the body requires that tissue to perform. They do not migrate to parts of the body where they do not belong; and if they were placed in such a part artificially they might not survive.

TUMORS

In a tumor, the process of cell division has gone wrong. Cells multiply in an unco-ordinated way, independent of the normal control mechanisms. They produce a new growth in the body, that does not fulfill a useful function. This is a tumor, or "neoplasm". A tumor is often felt as a hard lump, because its cells are more closely packed than normal.

Tumors may be "benign" or "malignant". A cancer is a malignant tumor. That is, it may continue growing until it threatens the continued existence of the body.

BENIGN TUMORS

In a benign tumor:

the cells reproduce in a way that is still fairly orderly;

they are only slightly different from the cells of the surrounding tissue;

their growth is slow and may stop spontaneously;

the tumor is surrounded by a capsule of fibrous tissue, and does not invade the normal tissue;

and its cells do not spread through the body.

A wart is a benign tumor. Benign tumors are not fatal unless the space they take up exerts pressure on nearby organs which proves fatal. This usually only happens with some benign tumors in the skull.

MALIGNANT TUMORS

In malignant tumors, the cells reproduce in a completely disorderly fashion.

The cells differ considerably from those of the surrounding tissue. (Generally, they show less specialization.)

The tumor's growth is rapid, compared with the surrounding tissue.

The tumor has no surrounding capsule, and can therefore invade and destroy adjacent tissue.

The original tumor is able to spread to other parts of the body by metastasis,* and produce secondary growths there.

A malignant tumor is usually fatal if untreated, because of its destructive action on normal tissue.

BIOPSY

A biopsy is the most certain way of distinguishing between benign and malignant tumors. A piece of the tumor is surgically removed. and then studied under a microscope.

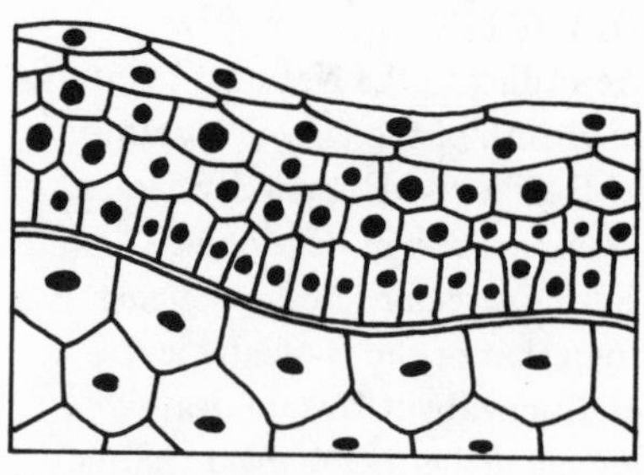

Normal body tissue

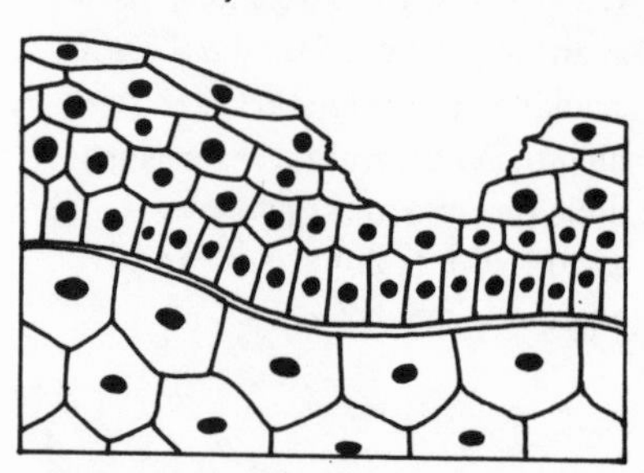

Damaged body tissue

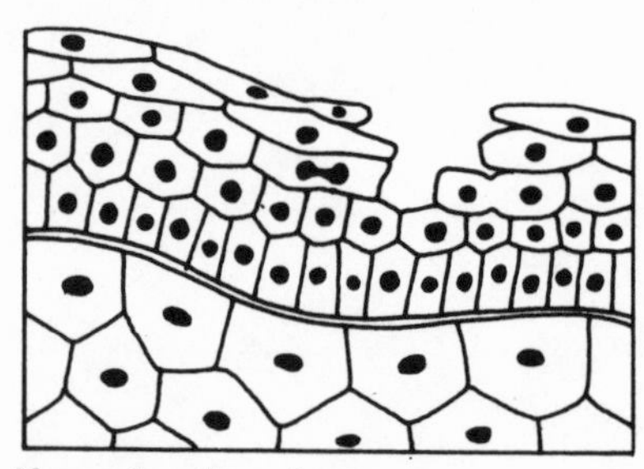

Normal cell replacement

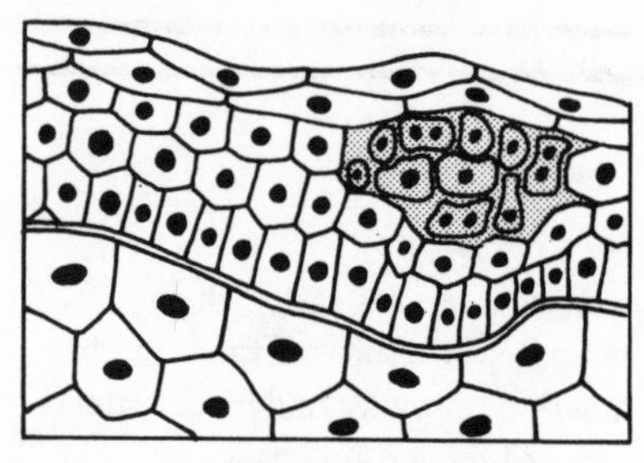

Abnormal malignant growth

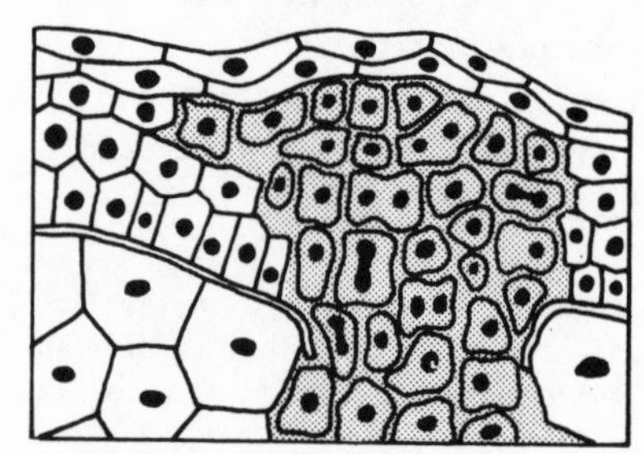

Loss of basement membrane integrity

B33 HIGH RISK FACTORS

The following table, based on epidemiological studies, lists major risk factors for some common cancers:

COLON—RECTUM:
- History of rectal polyps.
- Rectal polyps run in family.
- History of ulcerative colitis.
- Blood in stool.
- Over age 40.

LUNG:
- Heavy cigarette smoker over age 50.
- Started cigarette smoking age 15 or earlier.
- Smoker working with or near asbestos.

SKIN:
- Excessive exposure to sun.
- Fair complexion.
- Work with coal tar, pitch or creosote.

ORAL:
- Heavy smoker and drinker.
- Poor oral hygiene.

PROSTATE:
- Aged 60+.
- Difficulty in urinating.

STOMACH:
- History of stomach cancer among close relatives.
- Diet heavy in smoked, pickled or salted foods.

B34 CANCER BY COUNTRY

In all the sample, with the exception of Iceland, more men than women die of cancer.

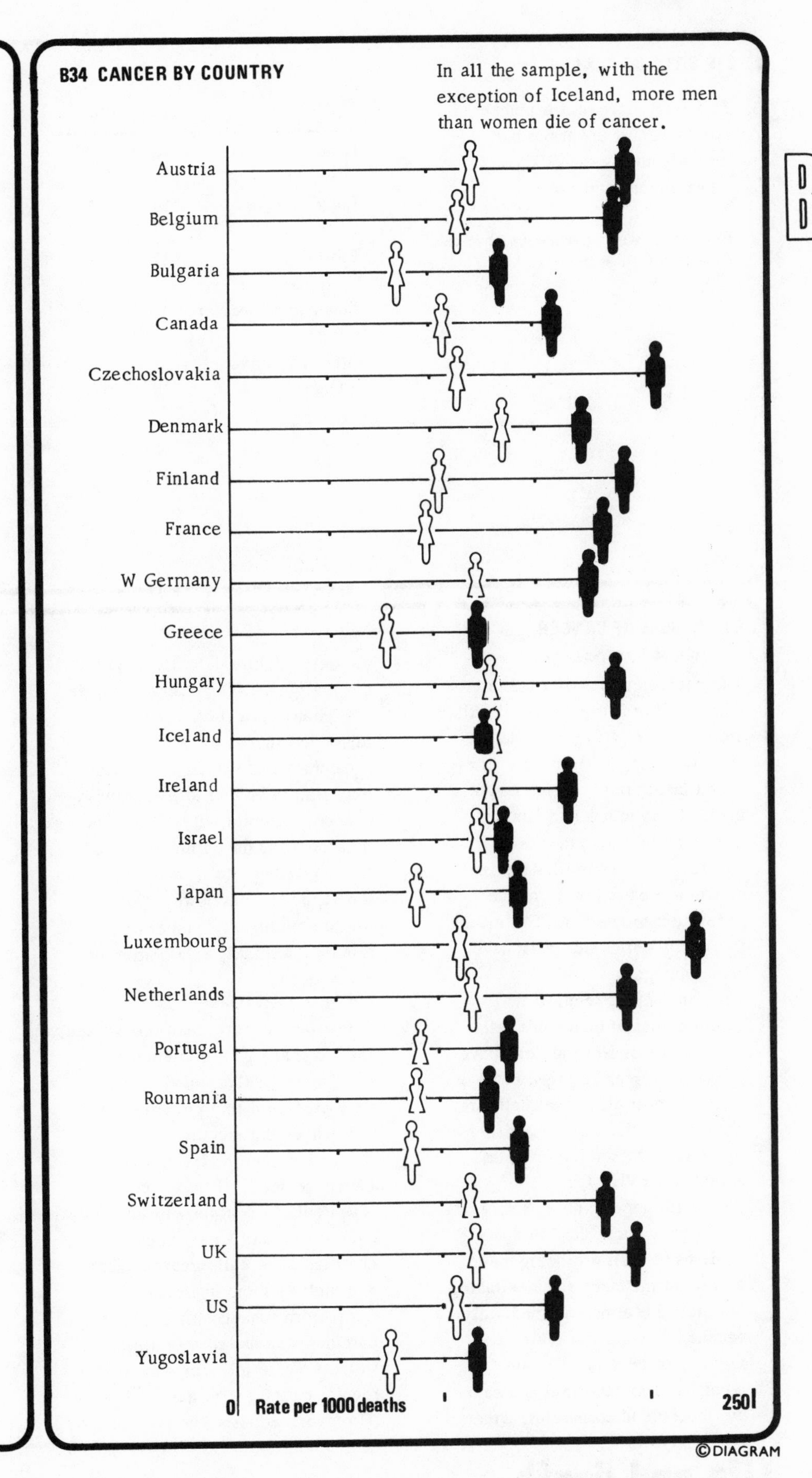

B35 SITES OF CANCER

This chart indicates the number of cases of cancer in various parts of the body among each 100 cases of cancer in men and women.

Reprinted with permission by the American Cancer Society.

Site	*Men*	*Women*
Breast	—	27
Lung	21	7
Prostate	17	—
Colon and Rectum	15	15
Other Digestive Organs	10	8
Uterus	—	14
Urinary Tract	9	4
Leukemia and Lymphoma	8	7
Oral	5	2
All other	15	16

B37 CAUSES OF CANCER

CHROMOSOME DAMAGE

The characteristics of a cell are inherited from its parent cell. They are passed on in the DNA* in the chromosomes. This forms a set of coded instructions, which controls the cell's structure and function.

In cancerous cells, the characteristics of malignant growth are passed on from one generation to another. This means that the genetic code must have been damaged.

This, in fact, is seen, if the chromosomes of cancerous cells are examined. Normal cells have 46 chromosomes arranged in 23 pairs. Almost all cancer cells are abnormal in the number and/or structure of these chromosomes.

NORMAL DEVIANCY

Cells with genetic defects appear in the body every day: so many millions of cells are being made, that some mistakes are inevitable. But most die almost immediately, because they are too faulty to survive, or because they are recognized as abnormal and eaten by white blood corpuscles. Others are only slightly defective, and not malignant. Only very rarely do malignant cells survive and reproduce successfully.

Appearance of cancer in a person may simply be due to this unlucky chance. Alternatively, it may be that the body has "immunity" to such malignant cells, and that this sometimes breaks down. This would explain why cancer can remain "dormant" in a person for many years.

SPECIAL FACTORS

A few factors have been recognized, that do make genetic damage in cells more likely. But they can only explain a tiny proportion of the cancer that occurs.

a) Certain chemicals can cause cancer to form, if they are repeatedly in contact with the body over a period of time. Such chemicals are called carcinogens, and include some hydrocarbons. Apart from tobacco smoke, these carcinogens usually only affect workers whose job brings them into regular contact with them. (However, atmospheric pollution may also be slightly carcinogenic.)

b) Certain viruses can pass malignant tumors from one animal to another, and the same may occur in man. But so far only one rare form of cancer is thought to be caused this way.

Apart from this, human cancer seems not to be virus induced - and therefore not infectious.

c) Ionising radiation. Without correct protection, X rays can cause skin cancer, and radiation can cause leukemia. Also ultraviolet rays (as in sunlight) may cause skin cancer in some circumstances.

d) Continued physical irritation. There is disagreement over this, but some experts believe that continued physical disturbance of the skin or mucous membrane can cause cancer. If so, the sharp edges of a broken tooth, for example, could eventually cause a cancer in the mouth.

Others argue that such irritation can only accelerate an existing cancerous growth.

Cancers can grow almost anywhere in the body, but the most common sites are shown here.
Cancers are classified by the kind of tissue in which the primary growth occured. Tumors originating in the "epithelial" cells (eg skin, mucous membrane, and glands) are called carcinomas; those in connective tissue (eg muscle and bone), sarcomas. Secondary sites are classified by the kind of primary tumor that they came from. This is possible because metastasized growths still show some of the characteristics of the tissue from which they originally came.

B36 CANCER SITES BY COUNTRY

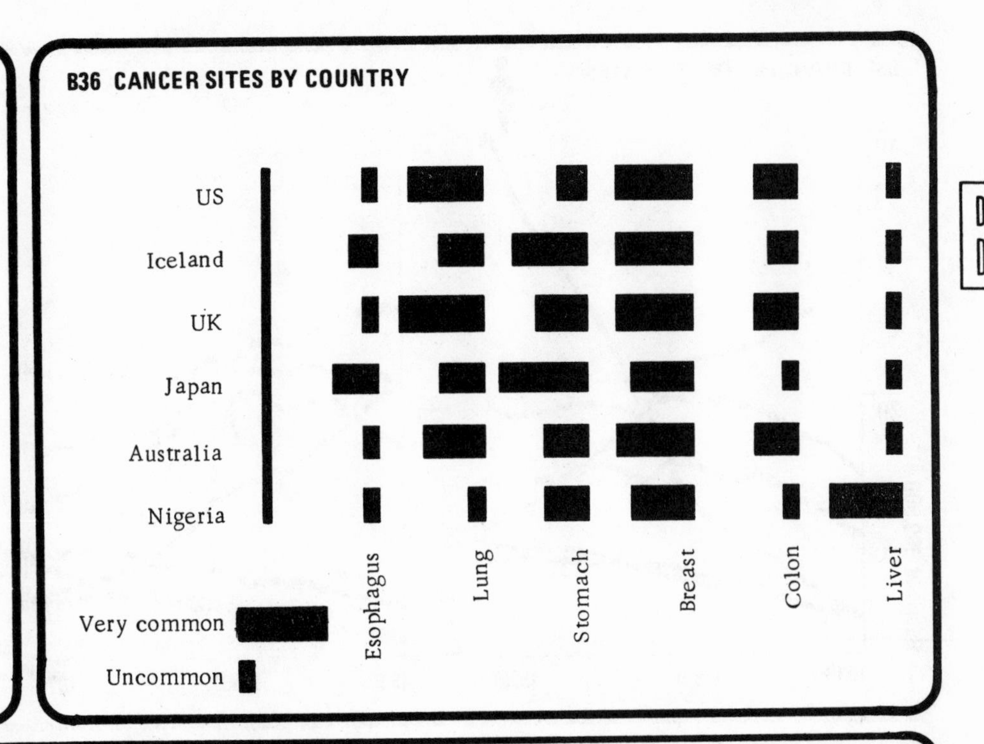

CORRELATIVE FACTORS
Some individuals are more likely to develop cancer than others.
a) Heredity. Actual cancerous growths are not inherited. But a predisposition for cancer can be passed on. It may be that some inherited characteristics make a person's cells more likely to become malignant.
b) Age. Most cancers occur in the 50 to 60 age group. However, children and adolescents are susceptible to leukemia, brain tumors, and sarcomas of the bone.
c) Sex. In almost all countries, cancer occurs more frequently in men than in women.
d) Geographical location. Eg, for some unknown reason, gastric cancer is most frequent in coastal countries with cold climates.
e) Cultural habits. Eg, cancer of the penis is less common in societies where circumcision is usual.

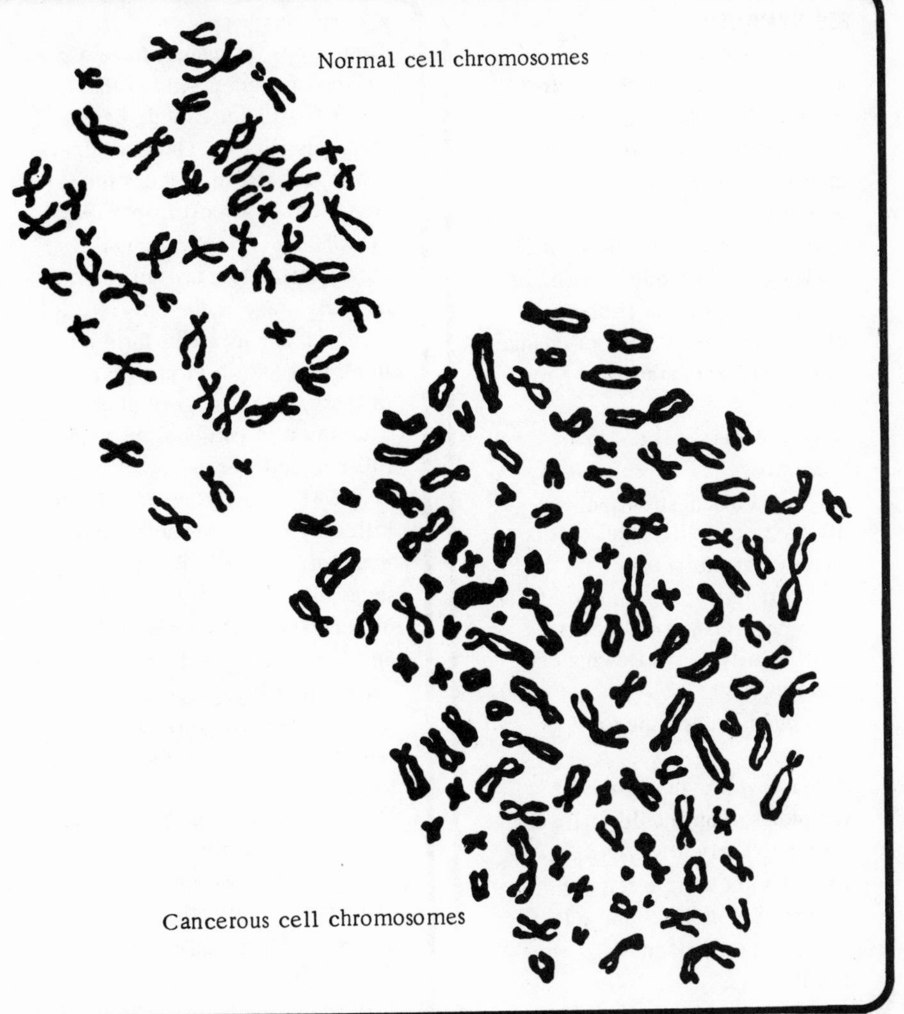

B38 CHANGING DEATH RATES

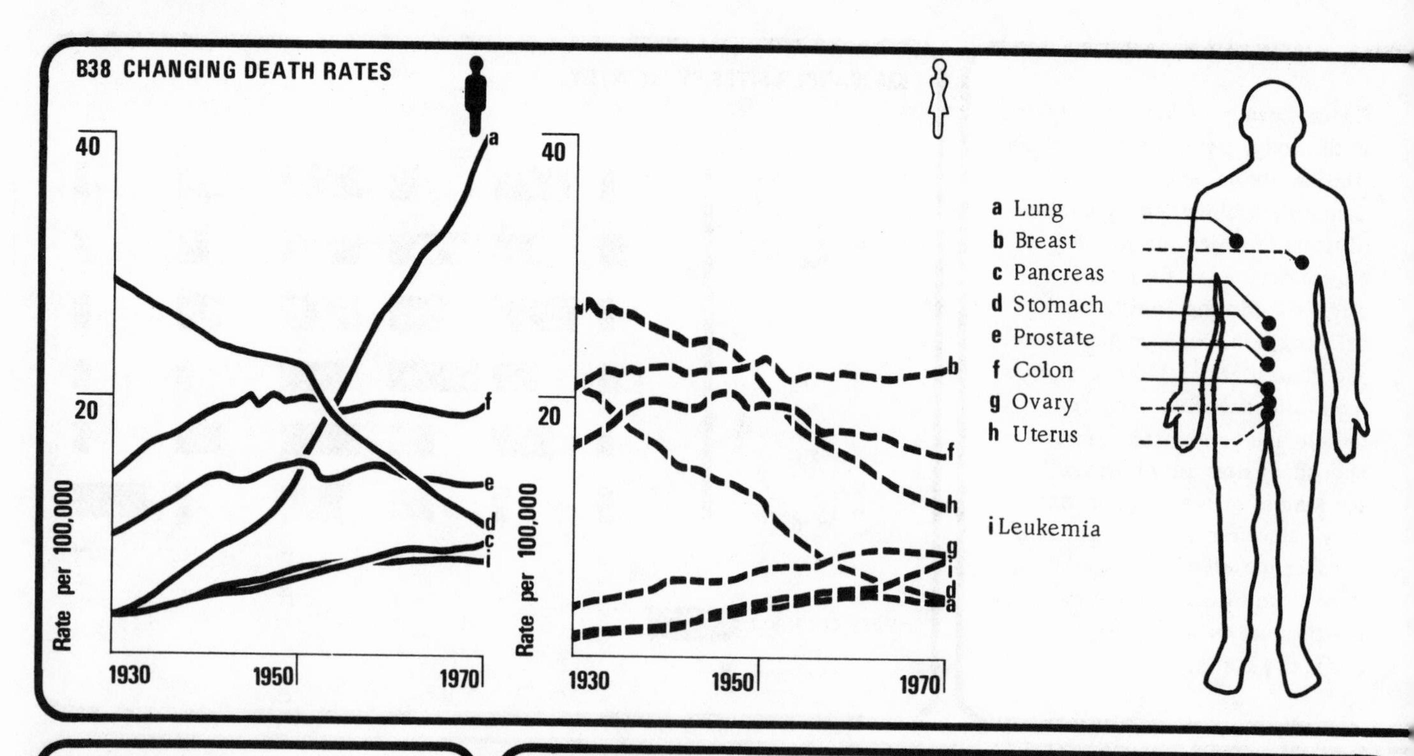

B39 SYMPTOMS

a) Any unusual bleeding or discharge from mouth, genitals, or anus (including, in women, bleeding from the breast and menstrual bleeding between periods).

b) Any lump or thickening or swelling on the body surface, or any swelling of one limb.

c) Any increase in size or change in color or appearance in a mole or wart.

d) A sore that will not heal normally.

e) Persistent constipation, diarrhoea or indigestion that is unusual for the person.

f) Hoarseness or dry cough that lasts more than three weeks.

g) Difficulty in swallowing or urinating.

h) Sudden unexplained loss in weight.

If you develop any of these symptoms, you should visit your doctor. Nearly always, the cause will be something else, not cancer. But do not delay. If it is cancer, quick diagnosis is essential.

B40 TREATMENT

Treatments for cancer have a good chance of success only if the tumor is still localized. Early diagnosis is vital. Once a tumor has metastasized, successful treatment is almost impossible.

SURGERY Surgical removal of localized malignant tumors at an early stage is the only completely successful form of treatment known at present.

In later stages, surgery may be attempted in conjunction with other techniques.

RADIOTHERAPY Cancer cells are killed by radiation more easily than normal cells. Radiotherapy seeks to destroy cancerous tissue by focussing a stream of radiation on it. This can be done only if the cancer is still localized, and can be destroyed without causing radiation damage to the rest of the body.

The rays used are either X-rays or those of radioactive materials such as radium or cobalt.

CHEMOTHERAPY This is treatment by the administration of chemicals. Again, the major difficulty is finding drugs that will destroy cancer cells without harming normal cells. Three main types of chemical are used:

those that interfere with the cancer cells' reproductive processes;

those that interfere with the cells' metabolic processes;

those that increase the natural resistance of the body to the tumor cells.

These chemicals can affect the whole of the body, specific regions, or the tumors themselves, depending on how they are applied.

HORMONE THERAPY is used mainly for tumors of the endocrine glands and related organs. It is also useful in the treatment of metastases originating from these areas (eg in women, against disseminated breast cancer). Success depends on whether the cancerous cells still have the specialized relationship with the hormone that the original tissue had.

Cancer is not a modern disease - it has been found in dinosaur fossils, and in the remains of Java man who lived about 500,000 years ago. But in the present century it has become vastly more prevalent. In 1900 it was the seventh main cause of death in the USA. Today it is the second. Some experts, though, believe this is simply because people are living longer - for likelihood of cancerous growth increases with age.
However, some types of cancer have shown a dramatic fall in recent years, eg stomach cancer. (This particular example may be linked with changes in techniques of food preservation.)

B41 LUNG CANCER

This is one of the most deadly forms of cancer, for it is not usually diagnosed until too late. The tumor begins in the walls of the bronchial passages or sometimes in the body of of the lung, and usually produces no symptoms until it has become firmly entrenched in the lung tissue and even metastasized. Only one in twenty cases live for more than two years after lung cancer has been diagnosed.
Lung cancer is very much associated with cigarette smoking. Most lung cancer patients are smokers.

Lung cancer metastasis

Primary site:
a Lung

Secondary sites:
b Liver
c Spine
d Lymph nodes

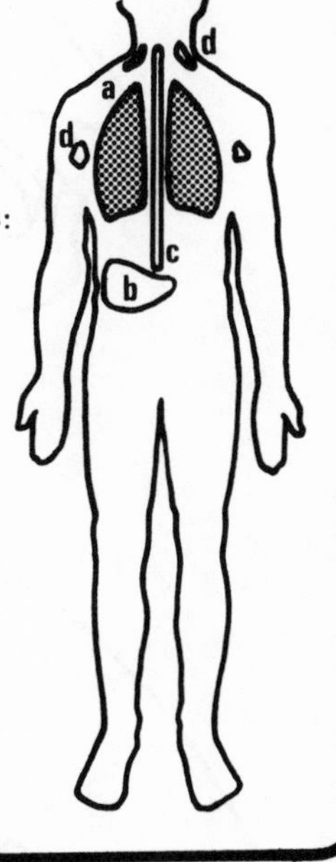

B

B42 LEUKEMIA

Leukemia is a cancerous disease of bone marrow and of tissues that produce blood corpuscles. It results in an abnormally large number of white corpuscles at the production site, or in the bloodstream, or both. There may be up to 60 times the normal number, and also many immature forms that never appear in healthy blood.

TYPES OF LEUKEMIA

There are two main types: acute, in which the onset is sudden, the duration usually only a few weeks, and the termination fatal; and chronic, in which the onset is gradual, and the duration up to 20 years before death ensues.
Each type subdivides according to the type of corpuscle that multiplies.
a) Acute lymphoblastic leukemia is the most common form. It is most frequent under the age of five, and rare after 25, but appears again in the old.
b) Acute myeloblastic leukemia can occur at any age, but it is most common in the middle aged.
c) Chronic lymphatic leukemia occurs most often after the age of 50. It is almost three times more common in men than in women.
d) Chronic myeloid leukemia is most frequent between 20 and 40, and more common in men.

CHARACTERISTICS

Shortage of red blood corpuscles make the patient pale, tired, and anemic. Shortage of normal white corpuscles* means that their protective work is undone, and the body is open to infection. Shortage of blood platelets reduces blood clotting ability. Swellings of feet and legs are common, and there may also be diarrhoea.
In chronic forms there are enlarged spleen, liver, and lymph nodes, and often a high temperature.

TREATMENT

Drugs and radiotherapy are used to try to hold it in check. Modern chemotherapy has succeeded in curing a substantial percentage of cases of acute lymphoblastic leukemia in young children.

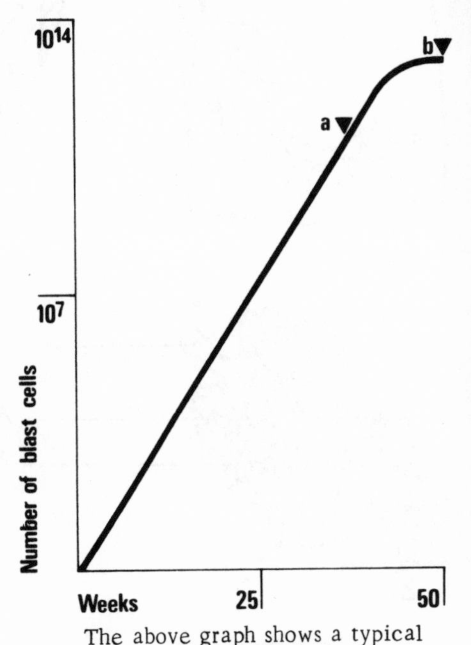

The above graph shows a typical growth rate for leukemia cells in the bone marrow.
The leukemia cell population doubles 40 times before the disorder can be properly diagnosed.
Diagnosis (a) occurs after 37 weeks, death (b) after about 50.

RESPIRATORY DISORDERS 1

B43 THE RESPIRATORY SYSTEM

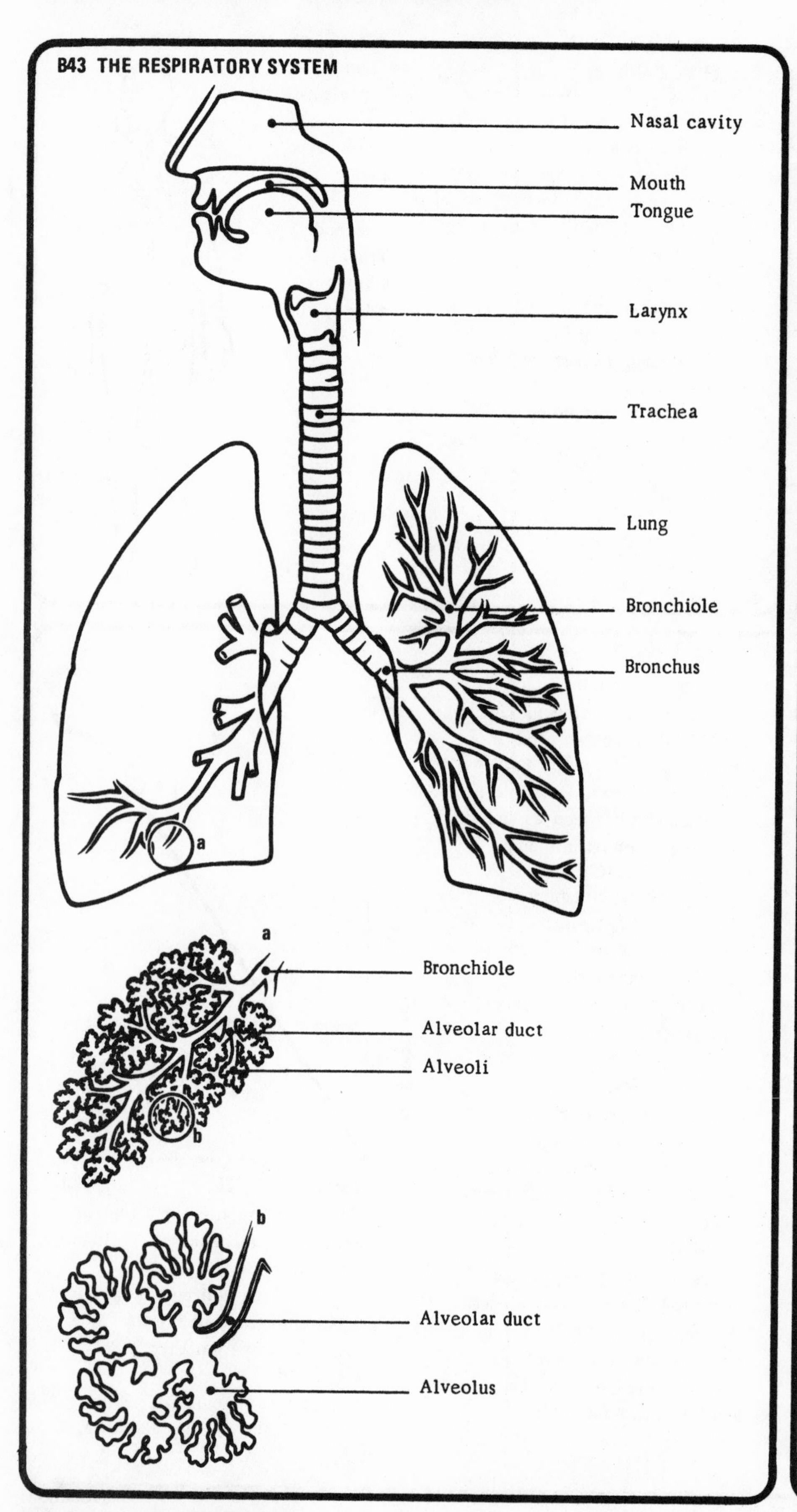

B44 LUNGS AND BREATHING

The two lungs lie in the chest (pleural) cavity, bounded by the ribs and the chest muscles and back muscles, and beneath by a muscular wall called the diaphragm.

Breathing occurs because muscular effort enlarges the chest cavity: the diaphragm moves down, and the cavity skeleton forward and outward. This threatens to create a vacuum in the cavity, so air rushes into the lungs under atmospheric pressure, and the lungs enlarge and fill out the cavity. Breathing out also occurs through muscular effort: the chest cavity contracts, forcing air out of the lungs.

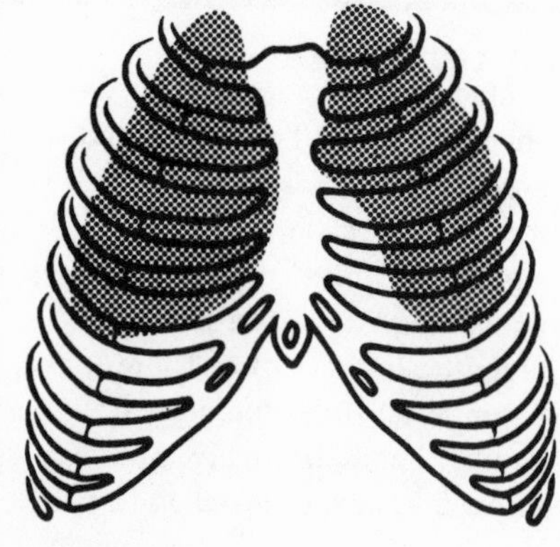

Inhaling

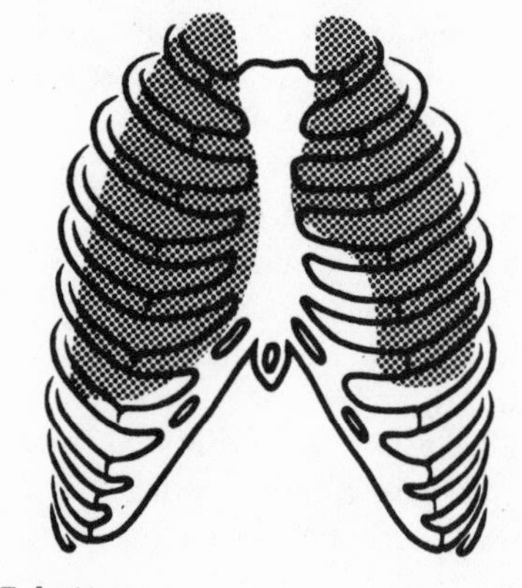

Exhaling

B

B45 BRONCHITIS

Bronchitis is an inflammation of the bronchi - though the bronchioles and smaller passages are often involved too. Its severity varies. Mild cases may seem like a severe chest cold. Severe cases lead to pneumonia and death. Bronchitis is most prevalent in the UK, where it kills over 30,000 people a year. There are two forms, acute and chronic.

ACUTE BRONCHITIS

This results from:
viral and bacterial infection following colds and flu;
exposure to damp cold air;
inhaling irritating dust or vapors;
or from combinations of these.

The attack begins with a short, dry, painful cough, and a general feeling of acute illness. There may also be slight fever. After two or three days the cough begins to bring up sputum (mucus from the lungs) in increasing quantities. The symptoms then begin to subside. The cough may last for three or four weeks, but the more distressing symptoms pass off in about ten days.

The condition is most dangerous in the old, especially if emphysema is also present.

Treatment consists of antibiotics, bedrest, warmth, hot drinks, inhalation of steam preparations, and abstention from smoking.

CHRONIC BRONCHITIS

Chronic bronchitis mainly affects the middle aged and the old. It can lead to emphysema and heart failure. It usually develops after repeated respiratory infections.

There are several major contributing factors:
excessive cigarette smoking;
exposure to a cold, damp climate;
damp living conditions;
exposure to irritating environmental dust and fumes, eg from industrial pollution;
obesity;
and, probably, constitutional predisposition.

The disease produces a constant cough which is worse during the night and in the mornings. The mucous membranes of the bronchial tubes become thickened, and the nutritional blood supply to the lungs may be impaired.

Emphysema and other complications may lead to constant breathlessness.

Treatment depends on the patient's age, the severity of the illness, and whether there are complications. It may include:
expectorants to loosen the mucus in the air passages;
steam inhalations;
and antibiotics if there is any bacterial infection.

To prevent recurrence, a sufferer should avoid cold, dusty, or polluted air, and should not smoke. Care must be taken to prevent colds from developing into bronchitis.

B46 PREVENTING CHRONIC LUNG DISEASE

From the Division of Lung Diseases, National Heart, Lung, and Blood Institute, U. S. Department of Health and Human Services come the following suggestions:

See your doctor if you have any of the symptoms listed below.

- A persistent or recurring cough, one that hangs on or goes away only to return
- A feeling of tightness or pain in the chest
- Shortness of breath, sometimes accompanied by dizziness
- General weakness or a tendency to tire easily

B47 EMPHYSEMA

Emphysema is linked with bronchitis, and with cigarette smoking. It is mainly seen in older people. Due to infection, inflammation, and obstruction of the air passages, the lungs lose their elasticity. The small alveolar air spaces become enlarged: the dividing walls are stretched thin and break down, and large air sacs are formed.

This greatly reduces the surface area available for gas exchange, so the blood and body get less and less oxygen for each breath. Breathing becomes increasingly labored, as more breaths are needed to take in the necessary oxygen.

The lung's deterioration often also hinders the passage of blood through the arterioles. This puts a strain on the right side of the heart. It becomes weakened and dilated, and death from heart failure can result.

RESPIRATORY DISORDERS 2

B48 PNEUMONIA

Pneumonia is a disease in which parts of the lungs become inflamed and filled with exudate.

TYPES OF PNEUMONIA

Bacterial pneumonia results from infection by bacteria. When one or more lobes of one lung are infected, it is called lobar pneumonia.

Broncho-pneumonia occurs in patches of the lung tissue, not in whole lobes. It often comes about as a complication of bronchitis and other illnesses.

Hypostatic pneumonia occurs in bed-ridden people, especially the elderly. Fluid collects in the lungs because of lack of movement.

Primary atypical pneumonia is caused by viral infection.

Predisposing factors for pneumonia include the common cold, chronic alcoholism, malnutrition, and bodily weakness.

SYMPTOMS

In lobar pneumonia the illness begins with chest pains and shivering, closely followed by a rapid rise in temperature to 104°F. Breathing is difficult. A harsh dry cough brings up rust colored sputum which may contain blood in untreated cases. The temperature stays high for about a week. It then falls within 24 hours to normal, and pulse and breathing become regular. The patient recovers quickly (but may be fatigued for many weeks).

Broncho-pneumonia and other forms have similar symptoms, but do not end suddenly. The temperature tends to fall and rise, gradually returning to normal over a number of weeks.

TREATMENT

Treatment includes antibiotics and measures similar to those for severe bronchitis. Oxygen is used in extreme cases. Convalescence should last for a month or two.

Pneumonia can be fatal in weak or aged people; in cases where the extent of inflammation prevents respiration; and in those whose resistance is low for other reasons (eg because of other illness, or alcoholism). Because of this it is often quoted as a cause of death for old people who could not withstand the illness or the accompanying fever and fatigue. But apart from these and other extreme cases, it is not normally fatal.

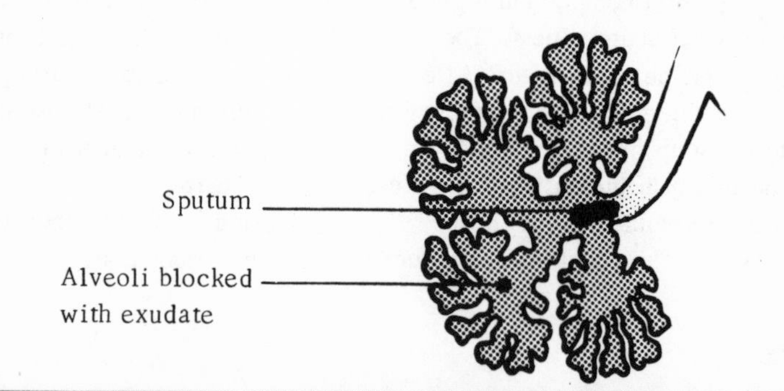

B49 PLEURISY AND EMPYEMA

Pleurisy is inflammation of the pleura - the membrane which lines the chest cavity and covers the lungs. It nearly always accompanies pneumonia and other lung inflammation. In dry pleurisy the inflamed membranes rub against each other as the patient breathes, causing acute pain. In wet pleurisy the pleural cavity fills with fluid - there is no pain, but breathing is impaired.

Pleurisy is seldom fatal in itself, but may increase the risk of fatality in the diseases it accompanies.

Empyema is any condition in which there is pus in the pleural cavity.

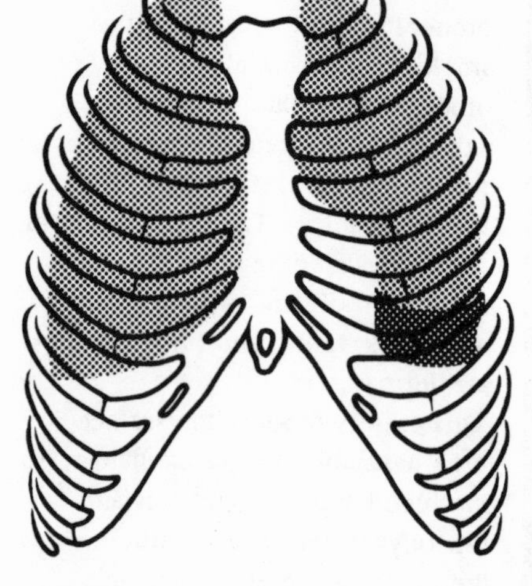

Pleurisy

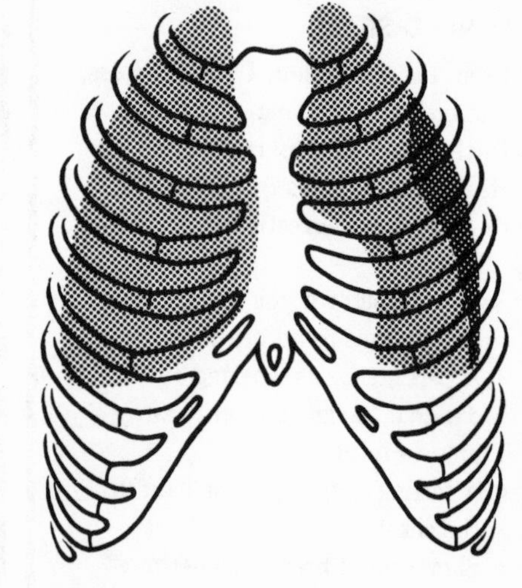

Empyema

B

B50 TUBERCULOSIS

Tuberculosis (TB) is not just a respiratory disorder. It is a general term for diseases caused by the bacterium "myobacterium tuberculosis". These are contagious: the bacteria are carried in the sputum of the patient, and are spread when he sneezes or coughs. They enter other bodies by being breathed in or swallowed. Since the bacteria are also very hardy, and can survive for a long time in dried sputum and dust, everything within the vicinity of a patient soon becomes infected.

The most common form of tuberculosis is pulmonary tuberculosis, because the lungs, in adults, are the most common point of entry into the body. But tuberculosis can also affect bones, joints, skin, lymph nodes, larynx, intestines, kidneys, testes, prostate gland, and nervous system.

PROCESS OF THE DISEASE

The bacteria enter the body through the lungs or through the intestines (most common in children). They are carried around in the lymph or blood vessels, settle in an organ, multiply, and produce small greyish nodules (or "tubercles") around themselves - big enough to be almost visible to the naked eye. When adjacent tubercles touch they fuse, forming a larger, yellow tubercle. This has a soft, yellow, cheesy substance inside.

As fusion spreads, the healthy tissue is broken down, to be replaced by the diseased substance of the yellow tubercles. In pulmonary tuberculosis this infected substance will eventually burst into a bronchial tube and be coughed up, leaving a hole in its place.

Often areas of fibrous scar tissue are built up as the body tries to surround and contain the infection.

SYMPTOMS

These depend on the organ attacked. In all cases the bacteria disrupt and then destroy the organ and its functions.

In pulmonary tuberculosis the first infection is often unrecognized, and thought of as a bad cold or flu. There is a cough, fever, and possibly chest pain. This often clears up, leaving a hardened, scarred area called the primary complex. Many people have signs of this primary complex with no further trouble.

Secondary infection occurs when the bacteria spread to the rest of the body. The patient spits blood and has a chronic cough.

He loses appetite and weight, is constantly tired, and sweats profusely, especially at night.

TREATMENT

Since the discovery and use of streptomycin and other drugs, the dangers of tuberculosis have been greatly reduced. Surgical treatment is now seldom needed, though a healthy diet and plenty of rest are still essential to full recovery. Early diagnosis is important.

B51 PNEUMOTHORAX

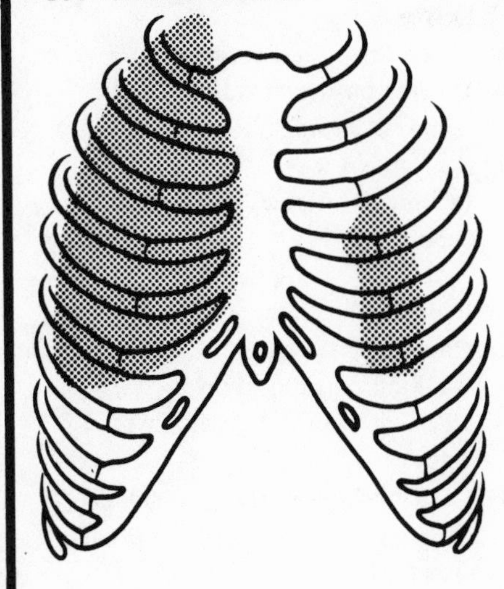

This is air in the chest cavity. It may have come from outside through a wound, or from inside through a hole in the lung. The lung on that side collapses as a result, causing sudden severe pain and breathing difficulties. It often reexpands again in a short time, because air in the chest cavity is quickly absorbed. When more severe, a doctor may tap the air by inserting a needle.

Pneumothorax may be induced surgically, in cases of tuberculosis for example, to allow the collapsed lung to rest and heal.

B52 SOUNDS OF DISORDER

As air passes in and out of the lungs, it makes sounds that can be heard through a stethoscope. In a healthy person these have a sighing or rustling character. But in an unhealthy person, unusual sounds and their location can tell of lung disorders. Tubes that are constricted but dry cause whistling and "snoring"; those narrowed by mucus, sibilant sounds; those filled with fluid, bubbling noises. In each case the coarseness and loudness of the sound suggests the size of the tube involved.

B53 ACCIDENTS

Accidents are a leading cause of death in all modern societies. In the USA they claim over 100,000 fatalities every year, ranking only beneath heart disease, cancer, and strokes in the number of their victims. And in the age groups up to 24 years accidents are by far the most important cause of death, outnumbering all the other top ten causes put together.

Men are far more likely to suffer accidental death than women (69% of all accidental deaths are male) - and this is true for all causes and all ages. In the 15 to 24 age group, in fact, there are four such male deaths to every one female. Only in the over 75 age group are there rather more female accidental deaths in absolute numbers - and this is only because women so much outnumber men in this category. So, even at this age, an individual man remains far more susceptible to accidental death than an individual woman.

The overall distribution of fatal accidents by age is fairly even, rising only in the 75 and over and 15 to 24 age groups. (The great predominance of death from accident for all ages under 25 is, of course, because there are not many other things that young people often die from.)

CAUSES

By far the most important causes of accidental death are motor vehicle accidents. They account for almost half of all such deaths, and are the leading cause in all age categories except 75 and over. Motor vehicle accidents, in fact, account for over ⅔ of accidental deaths in the 15 to 24 age group. The next main cause is accidental fall (16% of deaths) - and this by itself accounts for the significance of accidental death in those 75 and over. Fifty-five per cent of all fatal falls are in this age group, and they account for 63% of the group's accidental deaths.

The other leading causes of accidental death are: fires and burns (6% of deaths), drowning (6%), choking on food and objects, (2½%), firearm accidents (2%), poisoning by solids and liquids (2½%), and gas poisoning (1%). Fires and burns are notable for fatalities in the old and the under fives; choking in the under fives; and drowning in the 5 to 24 age group. Other causes are spread out fairly evenly over the age categories.

The male predominance reaches its highest in firearm deaths (86% male). It is lowest in falls (50% male), due to the large number of women over 75 dying this way.

Comparing today with fifteen years ago, death rates from motor vehicle accidents have risen, and those from falls and fires have gone down.

B54 MOTOR ACCIDENTS

The main types of fatal motor vehicle accident are, beginning with the most important: collisions with other motor vehicles (42%); overturning or going off the road (28%); hitting a pedestrian (17%); collisions with fixed objects (7%); collisions with trains (2½%); and collisions with bicycles (1½%).

Most causes distribute over the age groups to coincide with the general age pattern of motor vehicle fatalities i.e. they are much more common in those of working age (15 to 65).

However, pedestrian deaths are spread much more evenly over all age groups - with the result that almost half of those killed under 14 are pedestrians. Also over a third of those 75 and over are pedestrian deaths - but even more, in this age group, are deaths in motor vehicle collisions.

Driver

- **a** Exceeding speed limit
- **b** Driving on wrong side of road
- **c** Reckless driving
- **d** No right of way
- **e** Driving off highway
- **f** Others

Pedestrian

- **a** Crossing intersection with signal
- **b** Walking on rural highway
- **c** Crossing intersection against signal
- **d** Crossing intersection, no signal
- **e** Crossing from behind parked car
- **f** Others
- **g** Crossing between intersections
- **h** Not on roadway
- **i** Children playing in street

INJURY
Accidents also cause, every year, in every 100 people, about 31 injuries that limit activity for a time and/or need medical attention. The rate for men (37 per 100) is half again as high as that for women. Among these accidental injuries, those at work are least common (about 4 per 100), those at home next (about 12 per 100), and others, including motor vehicle accidents, highest (about 19 per 100). Comparing men and women, men are equally likely to be injured at home, more likely to be injured in a motor accident, and (because of job differences) over 6 times more likely to be injured at work.

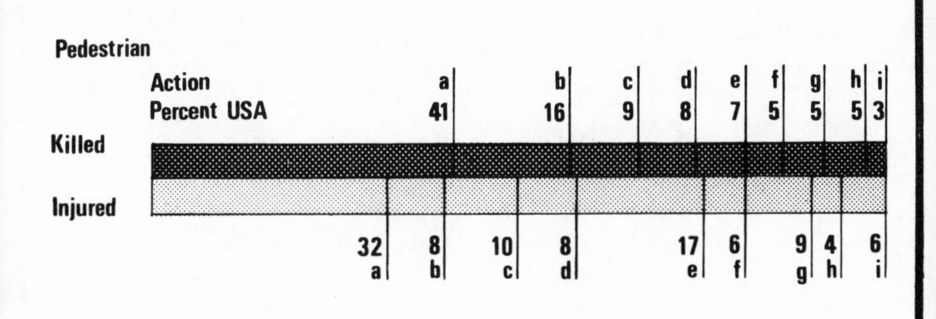

B55 HOME ACCIDENTS

Home accidents claim over 25,000 victims every year in the USA. About a third of these are 75 or over, and almost a quarter of the remainder are in the 0 to 4 age group.

The main types of accident in the home are, beginning with the most important: falls (36%); deaths associated with fire (21%); poisoning by solids and liquids ($9\frac{1}{2}$%); choking ($8\frac{1}{2}$%); firearms and poisoning by gas (each $4\frac{1}{2}$%); and "mechanical" suffocation (4%). Falls are most prevalent in the old; suffocation in the under fives; and poisoning with solids and liquids in the 25 to 44 age group, as well as in the under fives. Also, among other, unspecified causes of fatal home accidents, one third of the victims are children under five. Other causes distribute comparatively evenly over the age groups.

B56 SIGNAL DEVICES AND CARDS FOR IDENTIFYING HIDDEN MEDICAL PROBLEMS

Many people - one out of every five Americans - have medical problems that are not visible (allergies, epilepsy, diabetes), but which can seriously endanger their lives. Such persons can identify themselves in case of a serious accident or illness by wearing a signal device and/or carrying a wallet card with their medical problem(s) engraved or imprinted on it. The following two organizations can provide such devices and cards.

MEDIC ALERT FOUNDATION, INTERNATIONAL is a non-profit, charitable, tax-exempt organization which provides a complete system for individuals with serious medical problems. For a once-in-a-lifetime $10 fee, participants receive a metal signal device which can be worn as a necklace or as a bracelet. Engraved on the device is the member's medical problem, the member's Medic Alert number, and Medic Alert's emergency telephone number which can be called collect, 24 hours a day, any day of the week. In addition, the member will also receive a wallet card with more medical information printed on it. Members can update their records for $3. For more information, contact Medic Alert, Department ZE, P.O. Box 1009, Turlock, California 95380.

THE AMERICAN MEDICAL ASSOCIATION provides an emergency wallet card and signal device with important medical information. Write to the American Medical Association, Order Department OP-2, 535 North Dearborn Street, Chicago, Illinois 60610.

B57 THE TENTH CAUSE OF DEATH

Suicide is killing yourself. There are 365,000 suicides in the world each year - and about 3 to 4 million attempts. In the United States there is one suicide every twenty minutes, and about 25 to 30,000 a year i.e. about 13 to 14 per 100,000 people of all ages. It is the tenth leading cause of death.

B58 SOCIETY AND SUICIDE

Suicide occurs in almost all societies - but in some far more than others, and in some eras more than others. Two things seem to explain the differences.

One is prosperity. Suicide is a phenomenon of prosperous countries, prosperous regions, even, within cities, prosperous neighborhoods - while in many poor lands suicide is so rare that the word, and the concept, are barely understood. Suicide does not occur when the outside world makes it a struggle for us to keep alive. It appears when the world leaves us alone with our consciousnesses.

The other factor is society's attitude to suicide - including the effect of religion and moral belief. Our decline in religious fear of suicide is hard to separate from the impact of prosperity: the most traditionally Christian countries are also among the most rural and most poor. In any case, when a suicide rate seems to rise, as attitudes change, it may only mean that suicide is more openly admitted. But the importance of society's attitude is more clearly seen when the story goes the other way. In imperial Rome, and modern Japan, suicide declined as prosperity rose, because an ancient code that valued suicide was broken.

B59 THE INDIVIDUAL AND SUICIDE

Suicide is a product of social isolation - of loneliness and the sense of uselessness. Single people are more likely to kill themselves than married; widowed than single; and divorced than widowed. The products of broken homes are more likely to kill themselves than the products of happy homes; and those with no religious convictions than those who have.

Hence suicide accompanies modern prosperity. The familiar features of industrial society - the geographical and social mobility, the separation of young and ageing adults from the family, the pressure to achieve, the lack of a role for those who can no longer work (where school is compulsory, grandparents are no longer needed to look after the children) - all these, and the other features that they create, such as the failure rate of modern marriages, leave individuals and even family units struggling to persuade themselves that they have a place that they belong to, and a value to others.

So suicide rates reach their highest in the managerial and professional classes, in cities, and in "bedsitter land". And - despite the general link with prosperity, from one month and year to another the suicide rate keeps in step with the level of unemployment. Suicide is a hopeless admission of defeat: it happens when a isolated person cracks under the strain of his isolation, and it happens mostly to those who have already shown signs of their defeat, in psychic depression and perhaps in alcoholism. It is only rarely a dramatic gesture, and very rarely a rational preference to a painful death from incurable disease.

SEX AND SUICIDE

Successful suicide is a male achievement. Today, and historically, men are twice as likely to kill themselves as women are.

AGE AND SUICIDE

In some societies - such as imperial China - suicide among the old was rare, because the old were revered. But in most cultures the likelihood of suicide grows with age. It is rare in children. Then, in the 15 to 24 age group, it suddenly leaps to prominence, as the fourth main cause of death. But this is because there is not much else - except road accidents - that they often die from. (The exception is among students, where the suicide rate is genuinely high.) Thereafter, the rate rises steadily, reaching a peak in men in the 75 to 84 years age group. (In women, the peak is earlier, in middle age.) Men over 65 have three times the suicide rate of male teenagers.

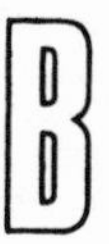

B60 ATTEMPTED SUICIDE

There are ten times more attempted suicides than suicides; and most are not trying to kill themselves. Suicide is typical of men and of the old. Attempted suicide is typical of women and of the young - and especially of young women. Of every four men who try suicide, three kill themselves; of every four women, only one.

Of course, some genuinely wish to commit suicide, and fail - just as others wish only to attempt suicide, and unhappily succeed. But, in general, those who attempt suicide, and live, have different motives from those who kill themselves. Suicide happens among those who are socially isolated; attempted suicide among those who are socially - in fact, emotionally - involved. Suicide is a way of ending your pain for yourself. Many who genuinely think of suicide are deterred by the thought of the pain and grief they would leave behind. Attempted suicide is a way of trying to call on those emotional ties: it is an appeal for help, or a blackmail note for it.

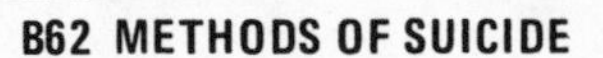

But never ignore someone who talks of suicide. Talking of it does not mean he only wants to attempt it: talking of it need not be a plea for sympathy. Two-thirds of those who kill themselves have told someone beforehand what they intended to do; and those, who have tried once, are not safe from trying again and succeeding.

B61 SUICIDE RATES

... for selected countries.

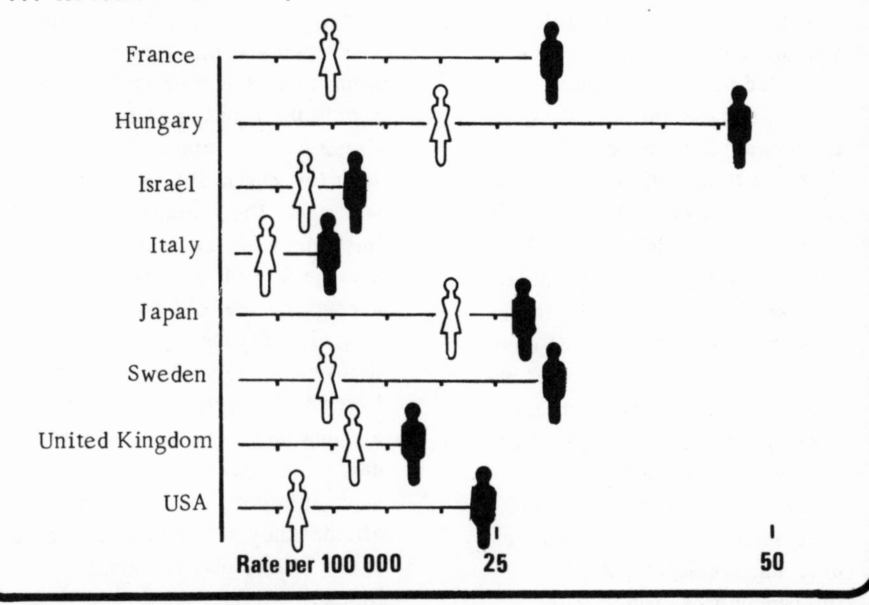

B62 METHODS OF SUICIDE

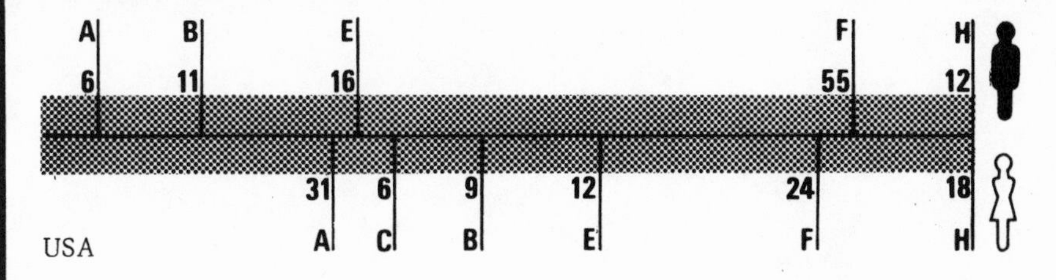

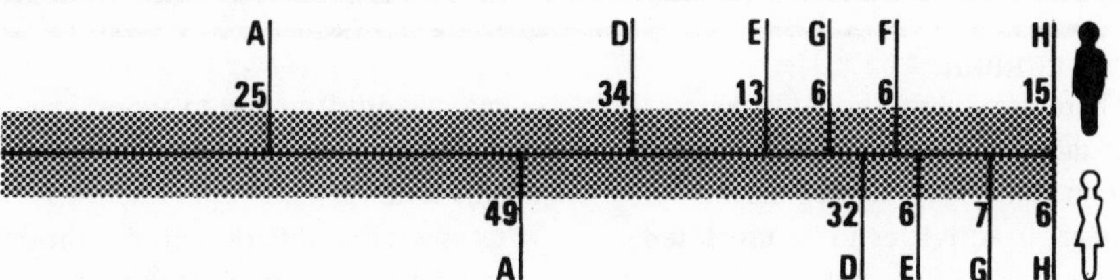

Methods vary between countries, depending on habit and availability. In the UK, self-asphyxiation with domestic gas has begun to give way to "the overdose", as coal gas is replaced by non-poisonous natural gas, and as a pill-taking and pill-prescribing culture grows. In the USA, pills are also important, especially among women, but male suicide still reflects the American familiarity with firearms.

- **A** Analgesics and Narcotics
- **B** Non-Domestic Gas
- **C** Other Poisons
- **D** Domestic Gas
- **E** Hanging and Strangulation
- **F** Firearms and Explosives
- **G** Drowning
- **H** Others

C01 ILLNESS

Every year, the population of the USA loses about 3,500 million days with normal activities restricted because of illness. Over a third of these are actually spent ill in bed. The number of entire days lost from work due to illness (i.e. days on which the person did no work at all), is almost 500 million. Almost 250 million entire days are lost from school. The average person has about 6½ days in bed ill every year, and has over 5 entire days off sick from either work or school. There is a slight difference between men and women. The average male (all ages) spends 5½ days a year ill in bed, the average female 7½.

In all countries, illness is by far the main cause of loss of working activity. In the UK, for example, about twice as many days are lost from injuries as from strikes, and about nine times as many from illness as from injury.

Days lost due to illness rise steadily with age. The average 40 year old loses almost twice as many as the average 20 year old, and the average 60 year old over 7 times as many. Yet the number of illnesses per person is higher in the lower age groups. In other words, a young man has several separate days off ill, scattered over the year; an old man has more days off, but they are more likely to be in one block, due to a single illness.

C02 ACUTE

Frequency of different sicknesses changes with medical advances and social habits. This table shows some sicknesses for which frequencies have changed most in the last 25 years. Measles, whooping cough, poliomyelitis, and tuberculosis have been greatly reduced by immunization. Better drugs and careful control have kept syphilis in check. But hepatitis has risen with drug abuse, salmonella food poisoning with the rise of carry-out cooked food, and gonorrhea with changing sexual behavior.

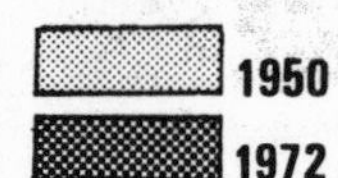

C03 SICKNESS AND AGE

Showing the percentage with incidents of illness in a year in different age groups.

a Infective illnesses
b Upper respiratory illnesses
c Other respiratory illnesses
d Illnesses of the digestive tract
e Injuries

C04 CHRONIC

There are over 25 million people in the USA who suffer badly enough, from some long-lasting disability, for their activities to be restricted. Of these people, 73% are restricted in their major activity (whether work, school attendance, or housework) - including 18% who cannot carry it out at all.

There are slightly more disabled men than women, but much more dramatic is the way in which disablement increases with age. About a third of all disabled are 65 or over. This age rise applies both to those restricted in their major activity, and to those suffering from less significant limitation.

Causes of disability include: the standard causes of death (heart conditions, cancer, respiratory disorders, etc); sensory disorders (eyesight and hearing); impairments of movement (paralysis, arthritis, back disorders, etc); mental and nervous conditions; isolated "trouble spots" (ulcers, hernias, varicose veins, hemorrhoids, etc); and disorders of certain body systems (ranging from diabetes to digestive trouble and asthma).

The main causes of disability are (listing the most important first): heart conditions; arthritis and rheumatism; visual impairments; high blood pressure without any heart condition; and mental and nervous conditions. These are fairly equally distributed between the sexes, except that women are twice as likely to suffer from arthritis and rheumatism and (though it is far less important in both sexes) from high blood pressure without heart condition. (Men are rather more likely to suffer from visual impairment.)

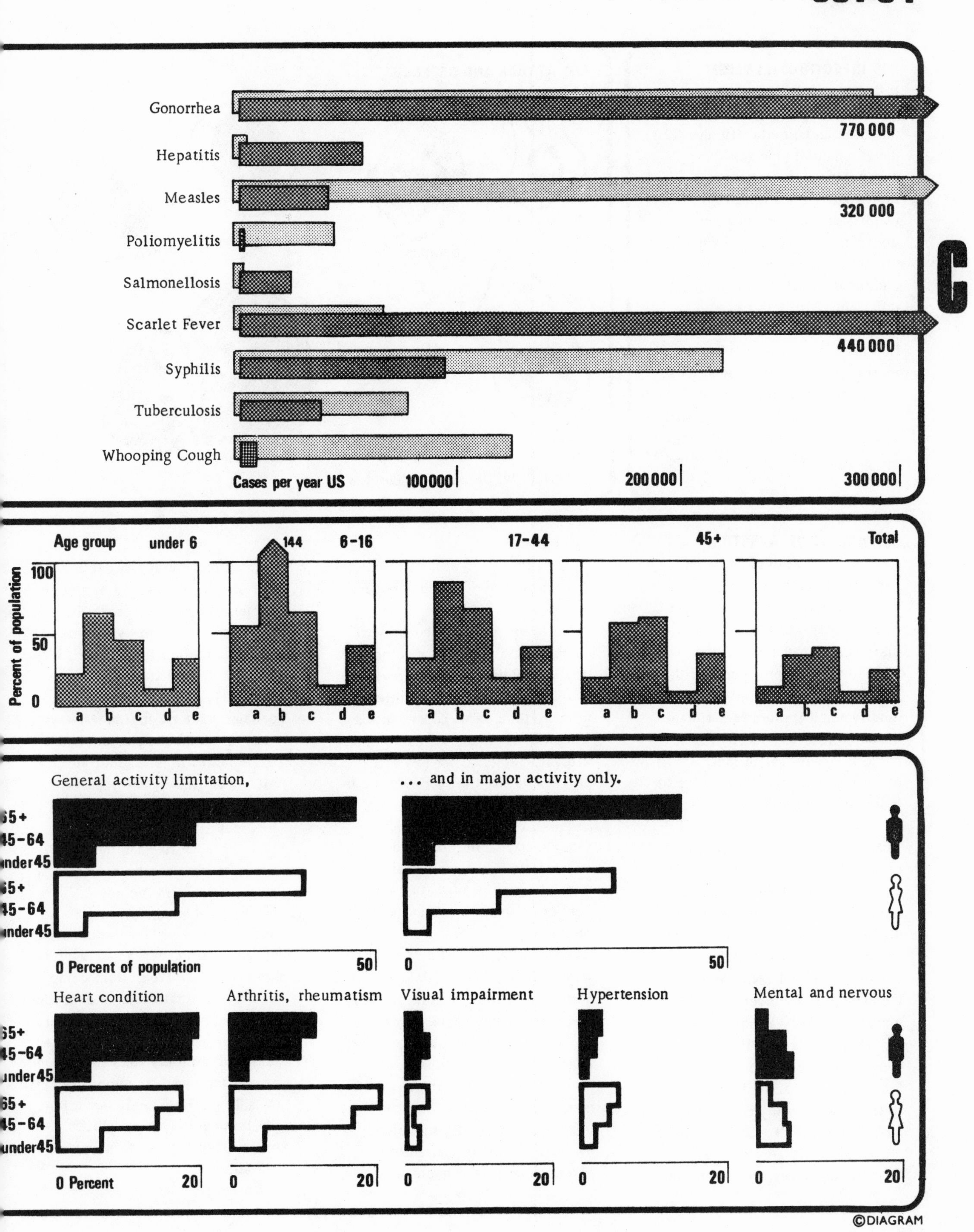

Gonorrhea
770 000
Hepatitis
Measles
320 000
Poliomyelitis
Salmonellosis
Scarlet Fever
440 000
Syphilis
Tuberculosis
Whooping Cough
Cases per year US
100 000
200 000
300 000
Age group
under 6
144
6-16
17-44
45+
Total
Percent of population
100
50
0
a b c d e
General activity limitation,
... and in major activity only.
65+
45-64
under45
0 Percent of population
50
0
50
Heart condition
Arthritis, rheumatism
Visual impairment
Hypertension
Mental and nervous
0 Percent
20

C

C05 INFECTIOUS ILLNESSES

Infection is not the only cause of illness. Other causes include: inborn defects; metabolic disorders; developmental changes; degenerative processes and malignant growths; nervous conditions; poisons; nutritional disorders; and irritation by external sources, whether mechanical, chemical, thermal, or from radiation. All these can also interact to support each other. However, the illnesses that we most expect to have to deal with, in day to day living, are the infectious ones; and they are still among the major causes of death, in the less developed parts of the world.

C06 ATTACK AND DEFENSE

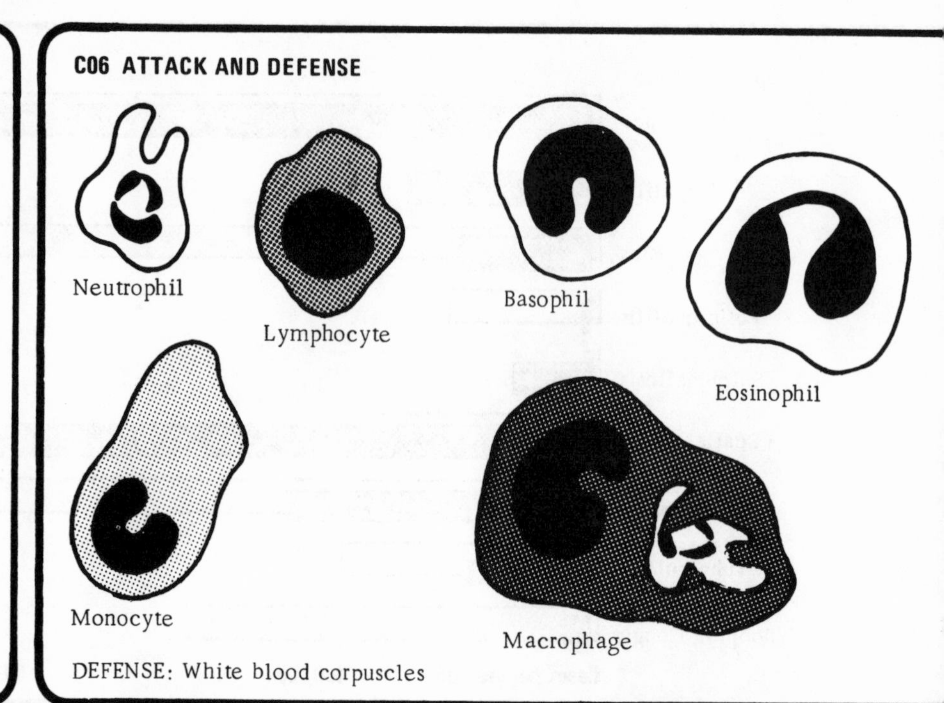

DEFENSE: White blood corpuscles

C07 AGENTS OF INFECTION

Infectious illnesses occur when certain microscopic living organisms gain access to the body. The symptoms of illness arise from their effect on the body, and from the body's attempts to cope with them. The creatures involved are usually single-celled rather than many-celled, and mostly either bacteria or viruses. In fact, bacterial infection is the source of most infectious illness.

BACTERIA

These are a form of tiny single-celled plant life, round or rod shaped, and each from one to 20 thousandth of a millimeter in diameter. They consist simply of an outer wall inside which there is protoplasm and DNA. Most are incapable of any independent movement. They almost always reproduce simply by dividing in two; and many can form themselves into spores - a seed-like inactive state, in which they can survive adverse conditions. The conditions they prefer vary greatly between the different types, but mostly they do not like too great heat or cold, and like moisture which is not too acidic.

Bacteria commonly occur in vast numbers in almost every corner of life - including on and in man's body. Most are utterly harmless to man, some he is dependent on, and some no life forms could exist without. Bacteria, for example, play a vital part in the body (eg in digestion, vitamin manufacture, and destruction of dangerous substances), while all life depends on bacteria in the air and soil, without which dead matter would not decay and return into the cycle of existence.

Illnesses from bacteria arise in two ways. Firstly, because bacteria that normally exist on, or in, the body - and may be very useful - get into the wrong part of the body. Examples of this include acne, pimples, and boils; some meningitis; and many urinary infections (especially in women). The first group are caused by normal skin surface bacteria gaining entry into a sweat duct or skin wound; the second by throat bacteria gaining access to the brain; and the third by bacteria from the rectum finding their way into the urinary tract.

Secondly, illnesses can occur because bacteria that are always harmful gain access to the body. Examples of illnesses that are always carried by one specific organism include scarlet fever, tuberculosis, whooping cough, typhoid, syphilis, and gonorrhea. Examples that can be caused by a range of bacteria include tonsilitis, dysentery, most pneumonia, and "food poisoning". In fact, certain types of bacteria have so far evolved, from being free living, that they are dependent on other living cells for their very existence. Some of these are useful or harmless - but others are among the most dangerous to man. Outside the living cell they either die immediately (eg syphilis bacteria) or have to form spores (eg tetanus).

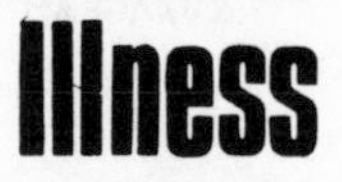

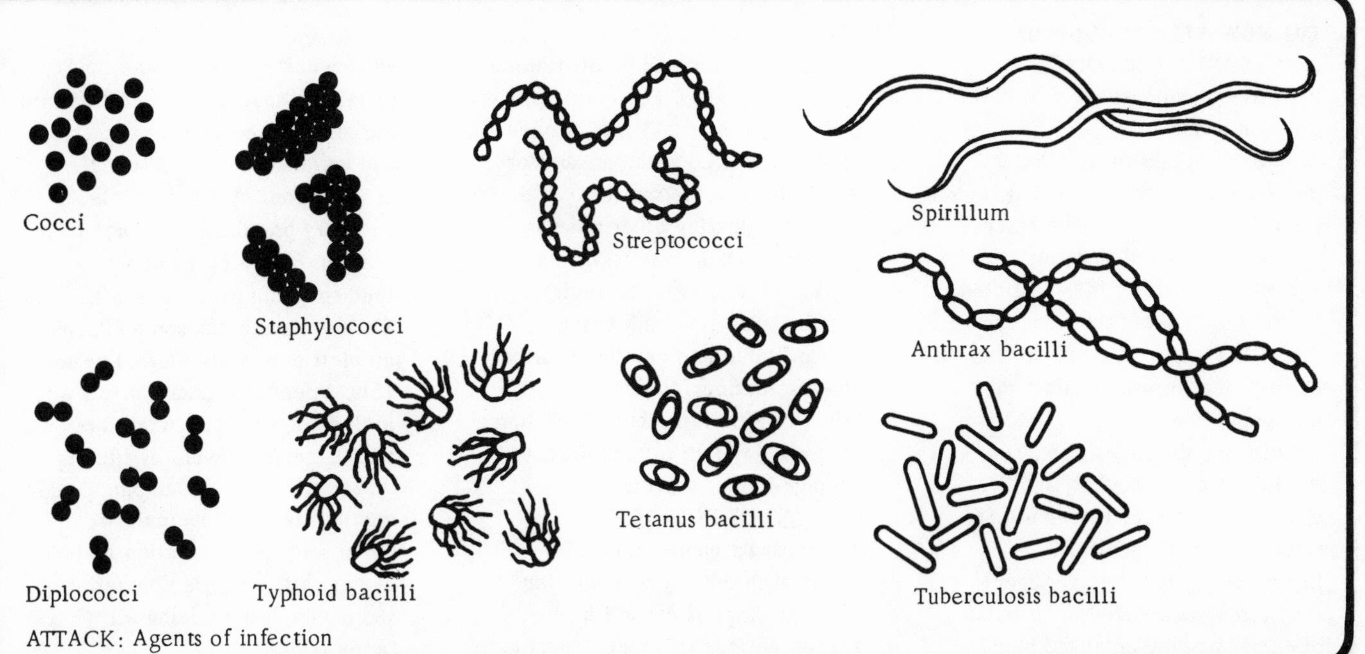

ATTACK: Agents of infection

VIRUSES
If bacteria seem small enough, they are giants compared with viruses. These are the most primitive form of life we know: each a minute quantity of nucleic acid, wrapped up in a protein sheath. They are also the ultimate parasites. They can survive well enough in many conditions, but can only become active and reproduce inside another living cell, where there are enzymes which they lack. Having gained entry to a cell (sometimes by a syringe-like injection process), a virus takes over the cell's chemical processes, and uses it to produce hundred of new viruses. Finally the cell breaks open and dies, spilling out the new viruses to enter into other cells. Sometimes the cells attacked are easily replaced - as in the nose lining, for example. But usually the viral attack at least interferes with the body processes, and may cause irreparable damage - for example, if nerve cells are destroyed.

Illnesses caused by viruses fall into two groups: those that attack particular organs (eg influenza and the respiratory system, mumps and the salivary gland, polio and the nervous system); and those that cause general symptoms, often with a skin rash (eg measles, rubella, chicken pox, smallpox, and yellow fever).

RICKETTSIAE
These are intermediate between viruses and bacteria. Most live in the intestines of insects, and can infect a human being if the insect is a parasitic blood-sucker. Typhus fever and Rocky Mountain spotted fever are both caused in this way.

TOXINS
Toxins are not organisms in themselves - they are immensely powerful chemical poisons, produced by certain bacteria when active in the human body. For example, it has been estimated that one 6,000th of an ounce of pure botulin (the cause of botulism food poisoning) would be enough to kill the entire population of the world. Other toxic infections include tetanus and diphtheria. In many toxic illnesses, the bacteria themselves are not harmful to the body - only the substance they produce, if it is not neutralized.

OTHER ORGANISMS
Other single-celled organisms, much larger than bacteria, can cause infection, but such illnesses are mostly found in tropical or subtropical climates, where they are often fatal.
Examples include amoebic dysentery, malaria, and sleeping sickness. Some of these are caused by parasites, which have developed a life cycle that depends on passing part of their existence in another creature, and part in man.
Multi-celled organisms may also infect man, eg pinworms, tapeworms, and flukes. More common are infections by fungi - a type of plant that has no chlorophyll, and so must obtain its food from organic material. One example is athlete's foot (ringworm).

BODY AND INFECTION 2

C08 HOW INFECTIONS OCCUR

ROUTES INTO THE BODY

Infective agencies have four main routes into the body:

a) through breaks in the skin, or in the mucous membrane that lines the mouth, nose, etc (the breaks may be wounds, that germs happen to enter, or bites inflicted by the insect that brings the infection);

b) down the respiratory tract into the lungs;

c) down the digestive tract, into the stomach and bowels; and

d) up the reproductive and urinary systems, via the genitals.

In all cases, the infective agent may remain localized at its point of entry, or may enter the blood or lymph system and be distributed through the body. For example, infection of a wound may result in an abscess filled with pus; and/or may spread to the surface, possibly infecting other flaws in the skin; and/or may travel up the lymph canals to the regional lymph nodes - perhaps being trapped there and causing a further abscess. Serious blood-borne infections are rare, but blood-borne bacteria do often attack already damaged heart valves.

SOURCES OF INFECTION

The most frequent source of common infections is inhalation of water droplets carried in the air. Breathing, speaking, coughing, and sneezing, all spread droplets of saliva, sputum, or secretion into the air. These can bear bacteria, and can be breathed in (or taken in with food) by other people. Ordinary breathing can spread droplets over a range of 4ft, and loud speaking over about 6ft, while a sneeze can spread 20,000 droplets over a distance of up to 15ft. Infections spread in this way include colds, influenza, sore throat, scarlet fever, diphtheria, measles, mumps, whooping cough, meningitis, and tuberculosis.

Other sources of infection include:

a) inhalation of dried bacterial spores, in dust-carrying air (anthrax);

C09 THE BODY'S DEFENSES

The body has three levels of natural defense to infection. It tries to prevent foreign organisms from entering the body's tissue. It tries to kill the ones that it cannot prevent. It tries to render harmless the ones it cannot immediately kill.

BARRIERS TO INFECTION

The main barrier to infection is the skin surface - a physical barrier that cell repair is constantly trying to maintain, and that few foreign organisms can penetrate when it is unbroken. The skin also secretes antiseptic substances in its sweat, so that not many infectious agents are able to survive on it for long. (Tear fluid does the same job for the crevices around the eyelid.) Where the orifices of the body form necessary openings, their lining of mucous membrane also presents a physical barrier and a trap, coated as it is with antiseptic substances in a layer of mucus. The digestive and respiratory tracts are also guarded by a ring of lymph tissue, around the pharynx, at the back of the mouth. Finally, if outside organisms do get beyond this, they are usually either caught in the layer of mucus that coats the respiratory tract, or destroyed by hydrochloric acid in the stomach juice.

PHAGOCYTIC CELLS

Certain cells in the body are "phagocytic" - they recognize and eat intruders. If infective agents do penetrate the body tissue, they may be of a kind that these cells can deal with. The white corpuscles in the blood are mobile phagocytes. Others are fixed at points throughout the body - especially in the spleen and liver, where they can filter infection out of the blood, and the lymph nodes, where they can filter the lymph circulation.

ANTIBODIES

Some foreign organisms the body cannot destroy immediately. But it may be able to neutralize them - the process is a chemical one. Bacteria and viruses have an outer sheath of protein. To neutralize them, the body manufactures another protein, called an

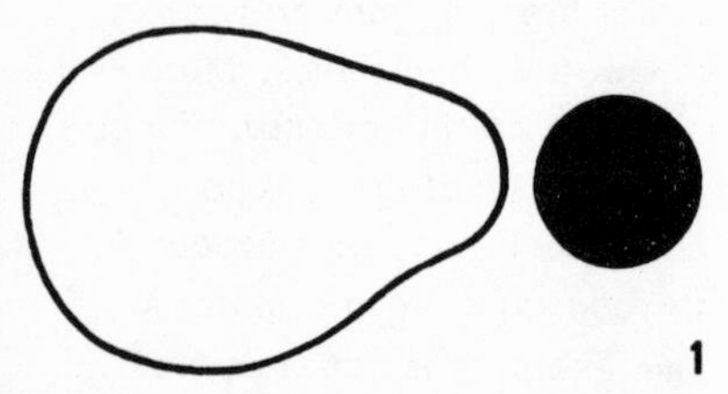

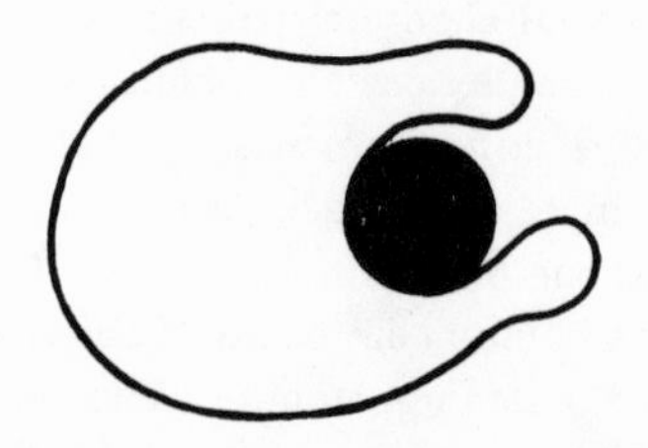

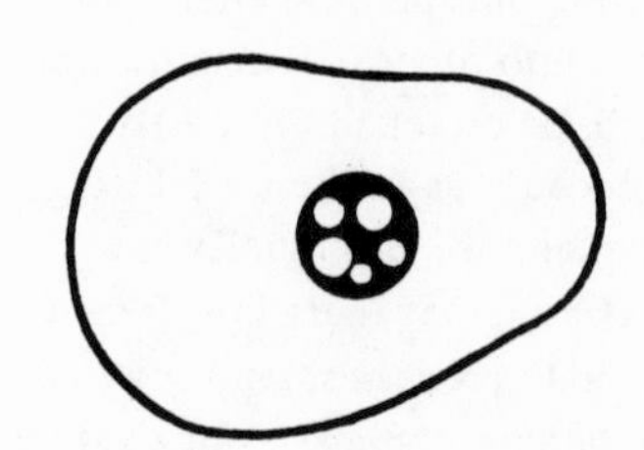

Stages in the phagocytic digestion of a bacterium

b) direct physical contact with an infected person (venereal disease, some skin conditions);
c) contact with "fomites", i.e. intermediate objects, such as clothing and eating utensils, that someone else has infected;
d) eating or drinking infected food and liquid (dysentery, typhus, cholera, brucellosis);
e) entry of soil or dust into a wound (tetanus, gas gangrene);
f) the bites of parasitic insects, such as the mosquito (malaria), tsetse fly (sleeping sickness), rat flea (bubonic plague), and louse (typhus fever);
g) the bites of infected animals (rabies), or contact with infected animals (brucellosis);
h) insufficiently sterile medical procedures, as in surgery and hypodermic injection (hepatitis);
i) infection carried by the mother in her blood stream and passed on to the fetus during pregnancy.

Infection from a human origin can come from someone who has no symptoms. With many infections, someone who has had, or is about to have, the infection, can infect others. With some, a person who never shows signs of the illness can infect others: the person is immune, but "carries" the infection (typhoid, diphtheria, cholera, dysentery).

The final cause of infection is self-infection: the transference of bacteria from a part of the body where they are harmless (such as skin surface or rectum) to a part where they can cause infection (such as a wound). This is mostly caused by lack of hygiene (especially of the hands), and is often compounded by scratching. Resulting illnesses are not usually passed on to others.

With all sources of infection, it is very important how long the organisms have to multiply, before they enter the body. The taking in of a few isolated bacteria is not normally going to cause illness.

antibody. Antibodies are formed in the lymphoid tissue, and released into circulation. The molecules of the antibody interlock with those of the protein sheath, as pieces of a jigsaw interlock. This is then coated with other proteins, called "complement", always present in the blood, and the whole mass can be eaten in the usual way by phagocytic cells. However, antibodies are "specific" - i.e. they can usually only cope with one particular organism.

For another organism is almost always sheathed in another protein; and another protein requires another antibody, for the correct chemical neutralizing reaction. Again, it is like a jigsaw - only certain pieces interlock; and complement, the general immunizer, cannot act until this interlocking has been done.

This means that the body has to learn anew how to neutralize each new threat; and if the threat comes in overwhelming numbers, the body has no time to learn.

Sometimes the response of producing the correct antibody has been acquired from the mother. But otherwise the body needs mild contact with the threat first, so it has time to set up the right process. Then, in the face of a serious threat, it can immediately put the relevant antibody into mass production. For the body does not have to learn anew how to neutralize old threats as they recur. It recognizes them, and remembers what was done before; and sometimes the memory lasts for life.

Incidentally, allergies are over-violent antibody reactions to organisms that are not dangerous but that the body regards as foreign.

CELL DEFENSES

Antibodies are carried in the body fluids, not in the cells. But some cells can produce substances that will attack organisms that enter them. Chemicals for destroying the cold virus, for example, are produced in the mucous membrane of the nose.

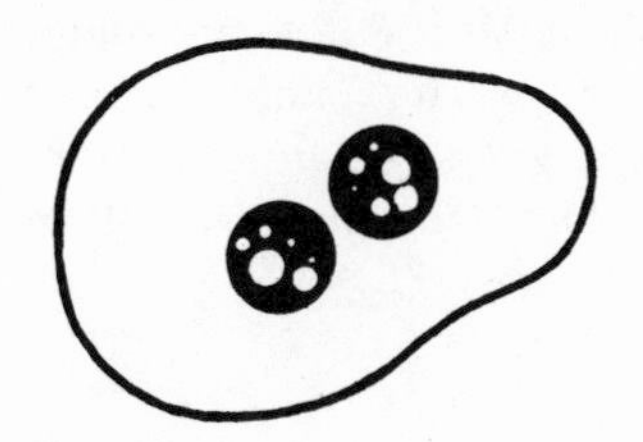

4

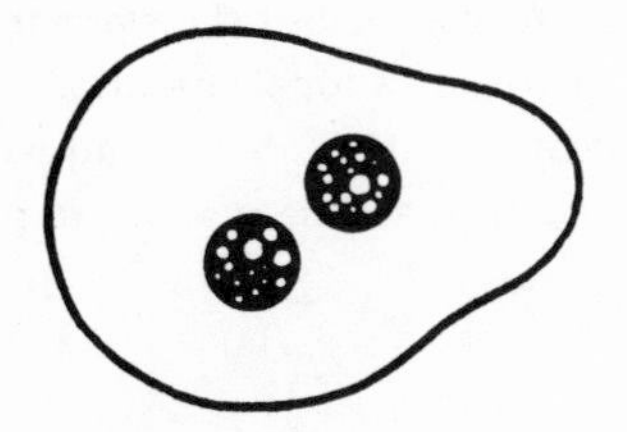

5

6

C10 HEPATITIS

Hepatitis means inflammation of the liver. In the United States, most hepatitis cases are caused by viruses; hepatitis virus type A, type B or type C. The virus causing hepatitis A, formerly known as infectious hepatitis, is passed predominantly from one person to another through close contact. Sometimes it is spread by contaminated water and food, including raw or inadequately cooked clams and oysters harvested from polluted waters. Hepatitis B, formerly known as serum hepatitis, can be acquired through the use of contaminated needles, including tattoo needles and other instruments used to puncture the skin, or through transfusions of blood or blood products containing the virus. Often, however, type B is contracted through personal contacts with contaminated body secretions. Type C hepatitis is usually transmitted through blood transfusions or contaminated needles. Type C is also known as the non-A, non-B type.

SIGNS/SYMPTOMS

Hepatitis A usually begins about four weeks after exposure, but it may occur as early as two weeks or as long as six weeks after exposure. The most common symptoms are mild fever, fatigue, sore muscles, headache, upset stomach (with or without vomiting), pain in the abdomen and dark urine. The most characteristic sign is a yellowing of the whites of the eyes. The skin also may develop jaundiced color. Some infected individuals, especially

C11 DEFENSE PROCESS

If the infective agent is not in the blood stream, the white corpuscles and antibodies must get to the point of infection and fight their battle there. The body brings this about by what is called the "inflammatory response". Any damage to body cells causes them to release "histamine" - a substance that automatically increases blood flow to the area, by widening the small arterial branches and the capillary openings. Also gaps appear, between the cells that form the capillary walls; and, through these gaps, blood plasma, containing white corpuscles and antibodies, escapes into the neighboring tissue, until the fluid pressure between tissues and capillaries is equalized.

The fluid dilutes the infectious organisms; the white corpuscles eat the organisms and damaged body cells; antibodies neutralize what organisms they can; and the mixture of cell debris and white blood cells forms the familiar fluid called pus. (If the amount of pus is large enough, and not drained away by the body, it forms a massive accumulation called an abscess.) Meanwhile the area is walled off by a blood clot, which gradually forms into connective tissue, completing the isolation of the area. Any organisms that escape into the blood or lymph vessels are killed off in the liver, spleen, and lymphatic nodes. Finally, after the infection is overcome, healing begins. The fibrous wall is digested away, and body tissue grows inwards to repair the damage.

It is the process of the inflammatory response that causes the standard symptoms of a local infection: redness, swelling, heat, and pain. The redness and heat arise from the increased blood supply, the swelling from the build-up of fluid, the pain from the swelling. Throbbing may also be felt, from the pulse of blood in the neighboring arteries.

All this is familiar for surface infections. But even in an infective invasion deep within the body, the same basic principles are involved.

More general effects may also be felt throughout the body, especially if the infection is serious. The numbers of a type of white blood corpuscle may increase rapidly from 3,000 or 4,000 up to 20,000 per cubic millimeter; the body temperature rises; and the pulse rate rises by about 10 beats a minute for every degree Fahrenheit rise in temperature. Together with flushing, as surface blood vessels enlarge, these give the familiar symptoms of illness.

children, do not show this sign. It is important that individuals with suggestive symptoms consult a physician.

Hepatitis B may begin within two to six months after exposure. The symptoms are similar to those of hepatitis A except that they develop more slowly and are more likely to include skin rash and joint pains. Recovery from hepatitis B usually takes longer than from hepatitis A because it is a more serious disease.

A vaccine against Hepatitis B is in the experimental stage.

Hepatitis C is increasing in frequency. In all respects, its clinical picture is similar to hepatitis B.

Information from the U.S. Department of Health and Human Services, Center for Disease Control.

C12 COURSE OF INFECTION

An infectious illness may be either acute or chronic. Acute illnesses are brief, with suddenly developing symptoms. They soon end with the illness defeated or the patient dead. Chronic illnesses are long drawn out. Most specific diseases always produce one type of illness rather than the other.

As all infections involve the same basic process - invasion by a foreign organism, and the body's response - so all tend to show a common pattern (though the stages are more obvious in an acute illness).

a) Incubation, beginning with the moment of infection. The organisms multiply inside the body.

b) Prodrome, a short interval of generalized symptoms (eg headache, fever, nasal discharge, irritability, and general feelings of illness). The infection at this stage is usually very communicable to others - but diagnosis is difficult.

c) Peak, when the illness is at its height. Each infection shows its own characteristic symptoms. Temperature is at its highest, and the rash appears where relevant.

d) Termination, the end of the illness. This is marked either by a "crisis" - a period of 12 to 48 hours in which the symptoms rapidly disappear - or by a "lysis", a more gradual termination.

e) Convalescence, after the illness. The patient regains health and strength.

Note that, from the micro-organism's point of view, a successful infection is one strong enough not to be killed by the body's defences, yet not strong enough to kill off its host. Chronic infections, such as syphilis and tuberculosis, show this pattern: the organism is just able to hold its own against the body's defences. Acute infections often spread rapidly through a population and then die out, because everyone is either dead or recovered.

C13 MEDICINE AND INFECTION

ARTIFICIAL IMMUNIZATION

The antibody process shows how our defences against an infection are strengthened if we have already met the infection in mild form. This principle underlies artificial immunization. A vaccine is given to the patient, usually by injection. It gives him only slight symptoms, if any, but makes him immune to a specific disease.

Vaccines may use:

a) a related, weak infection (eg using cowpox to immunize against smallpox);

b) the dead organism of the disease (eg whooping cough, influenza, and Salk polio vaccines);

c) a weakened organism of the disease (eg BCG tuberculosis, measles, plague, and Sabin polio vaccines); or

d) (where the threat is from toxin rather than infection) a "toxoid", i.e. a toxin that has been made non-poisonous, but can still stimulate anti-toxins in the body.

The protection of many vaccines lasts a lifetime. Immunization can also be achieved less efficiently and for a shorter period by injecting a ready-made antibody or anti-toxin (eg against diphtheria, or tetanus).

ANTIBIOTICS

Immunization protects against future infection; antibiotics fight an existing one. Micro-organisms have to compete with each other for scarce food supplies, so some have developed the ability to produce chemicals that kill off their rivals. These chemicals form the bases of antibiotics. However, resistant strains of bacteria often develop, helped by their rapid reproduction rate; and against viruses, less progress has been made, because their similarity to the human cell makes it hard to destroy one without the other.

C14 INFECTIONS

	Incubation	When contagious	Symptoms	Treatment	Quarantine?	Recurrence?
Chicken pox	4 to 7 days	From 5 days before rash till 6 days after it appears.	Chill, fever, headache, malaise. Red spots on face, chest, back; later contain clear fluid, burst, and develop brown crusts.	For symptoms only. Rest, and lotion for itching.	Yes, till crusts over lesions appear.	Uncertain
German measles	14 to 21 days	From 7 days before rash till 5 days after it appears.	Malaise, fever, headache, inflamed mucous membrane. Fine pink spots on face and neck, and spreading elsewhere.	Little or none. Lotion for itching.	Yes, till rash disappears.	No
Glandular fever	Not known	Not known	Headache, fever, sore throat, swollen lymph nodes. Loss of appetite.	For symptoms: rest, throat wash, aspirin. Also for complications if any.	Yes, till temperature has been normal for a week.	Uncertain
Measles	8 to 13 days	From start of rash till 4 days after main rash appears.	Fever, cough, conjunctivitis. Later, spots all over: white with red perimeter - background skin inflamed.	For symptoms: rest; protection from cold, damp, bright light; cough syrup; soft diet. Also for complications if any.	Isolation from infants.	Yes
Mumps	12 to 20 days	From 6 days before glands swell till 9 days after swelling.	Chill and fever, headache, temperature, swollen salivary glands (pain on chewing). Other glands may be swollen.	For symptoms: rest, soft diet, aspirin, perhaps sedatives. Also for complications if any.	No	Unlikely
Roseola	4 to 7 days	Not known. (Roseola usually only occurs in infants.)	High fever 3-4 days. Convulsions. Enlarged spleen. Later, purple-brown spots on chest, abdomen, face, and extremities.	For symptoms only: aspirin, water sponging to lower temperature.	No	No
Scarlet fever	1 to 3 days	During illness.	Chills, fever, vomiting. Rash 24 hours after fever: small red spots join to form redness on whole body. Strawberry tongue. Sore throat.	Penicillin, rest, soft diet, water sponging to lower temperature, lotions for itching.	Yes, for not less than 7 days from onset.	No
Whooping cough	7 to 14 days	7 to 21 days, beginning before symptoms	Sneezing, listlessness, and cough becoming convulsive with typical whooping breathing. Vomiting. May expel thick mucus.	Rest, fresh air, small meals, refeeding after vomiting. Mild sedatives and antibiotics. Hospital for serious cases.	Yes, till 8th week.	No

C15 IMMUNIZATION

	Injections	Spacing	Immunity	Boosters
German measles	1	-	Probably long	No
Measles	3	1 month	Probably life	No
Mumps	2	1 week	Life?	No
Polio (Sabin)	3 (oral)	1 month	Probably life	No
Smallpox	1	-	Several years	After 5 to 7 years and for foreign travel
Diphtheria	3	1 month	About 10 years	Diphtheria, tetanus, whooping cough, all similar (in fact, may be injected together in young children). 1st booster after 1 year, 2nd and 3rd after 2 year gaps, 4th and 5th after 3 year gaps and on exposure
Tetanus	3	1 month	Varies	
Whooping cough	3	1 month	About 10 years	
When traveling to infected areas...				
Cholera	2	7-10 days	Short	Every 6-12 months
Plague	2-3	1 week	Short	Every 6-12 months
Rocky mountain spotted fever	3	1 week	Short	Every 12 months
Typhoid	3	1-4 weeks	1-3 years	Every 1-3 months
Typhus	2-3	1 week	Short	Every 12 months
Yellow fever	1	-	Long	Every 6 years
When exposed to the infection ...				
Infectious hepatitis	1	-	4-6 weeks	If re-exposed after immunity ends
Influenza	2	1 week	1 year, for that variety of 'flu	If re-exposed after immunity ends
Rabies	14	Daily	3-6 months	If re-exposed after immunity ends
Scarlet fever	3	Daily	4-6 weeks	If re-exposed after immunity ends

C16 ROUTINE INJECTIONS

3 months
1st DPT*
1st oral polio

4 months
2nd DPT*
2nd oral polio

5 months
3rd DPT*
3rd oral polio

9 months
Smallpox

9 to 12 months
Measles
German measles

15 months
Booster DPT*
Booster oral polio

$3\frac{1}{2}$ years
Booster DPT*

6 years
Booster DPT*

9 years
Booster DT •

12 years
Booster tetanus
Mumps vaccine

* Diphtheria, whooping cough and tetanus combined
• Diphtheria and tetanus

C17 INHERITED DISORDERS

A few disorders exist that usually occur only in men but are always inherited through their mothers. These include hemophilia, red-green color deficiency, and two forms of muscular dystrophy.

Of course, many defects can be inherited. Each chromosome* inherited from a parent carries many thousands of "genes" or units of genetic information. If any one of these genes is faulty, it will not pass on the correct instructions, and a defect can occur.

However, these few disorders such as hemophilia are passed on in the odd way described because they are linked with the X chromosome*. This is one of the chromosomes that determine sex; but other genes on the same chromosome have other jobs - including helping to ensure normal color vision, blood clotting, and so on.

Both men and women have X chromosomes, and both men and women can have X chromosomes in which one of these genes is faulty. But whenever the defective chromosome is matched by another, normal X chromosome, the defect will not appear: the correct function (eg color vision) is guaranteed by the normal chromosome i.e. the normal gene is "dominant".

So in any woman the defective chromosome is normally masked by a healthy one, from the other parent. And a father with the defective gene cannot pass it on to his sons at all, because to them he contributes only his Y chromosome. But a mother can pass it on to her sons, because to them she contributes their X chromosome, which may be defective, and their other, Y, chromosome, will not "mask" it, because it does not have a gene responsible for the defective function.

The only way in which a woman can show the signs of one of these defects is if she has inherited defective X chromosomes from both sides of the family. This is very unlikely, but does happen rather more often in the case of color-vision deficiency.

A woman who does not herself show signs of the disorder, but can pass it on, is called a "carrier". Only chance decides whether or not any one of her children inherits the defective X chromosome: the child can equally inherit the healthy one. So if a carrier becomes pregnant, there is: a one in four chance of her having a normal son; the same chance of her having a normal daughter; the same of her having an affected son; and the same of her having a carrier daughter.

If a woman is found to be a carrier, there is risk not only to her own subsequent children, but also to those of her female relatives on the maternal side - because they may also have inherited the defective gene.

If no previous family history is discovered after careful check, it is likely to be an isolated mutation in either mother or child. If in the mother, she can still pass it on to subsequent children.

C18 HEMOPHILIA

Hemophilia is a term indicating two hereditary bleeding disorders, resulting from a lack of coagulation factors VIII (hemophilia A) and IX (hemophilia B). These disorders are sex-linked, occurring in males (in extremely rare cases in females). The mother is the carrier of the abnormal gene.

SYMPTOMS

In mild cases, the disorder may remain undiscovered until some trauma provokes bleeding. The hemophiliac must take special care in all he does, and in severe cases he must drastically curtail his activities.

The real danger is from internal bleeding. Bleeding in soft tissues, such as the kidney, is serious, and bleeding in large joints can eventually cripple them. Both occur spontaneously in severe cases. There is also a risk of hepatitis when the hemophiliac receives blood transfusions.

A young hemophiliac may miss school in severe cases; an adult hemophiliac may lose time on the job.

The hemophiliac should wear a medical identification tag or carry identification in his wallet (see page 57) in case he meets with a serious accident.

The symptoms may decline with age, and at any age there may be periods free from trouble.

TREATMENT

Proper management requires identification of the type and severity of the deficiency of the coagulation factor involved. The specific type is then treated with its specific factor by intravenous injection either as a prophylactic when blood levels are low or as a replacement to levels compatible with normal clotting when bleeding occurs unabatedly.

Factor VIII is now produced in a stable concentrate so it can be kept on a shelf at home until needed. Then the hemophiliac can give himself an injection (or if he prefers, a parent or friend can give the injection). This procedure makes life much more tolerable.

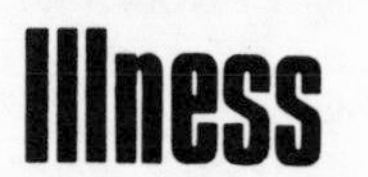

C19 CARRIERS AND SUFFERERS

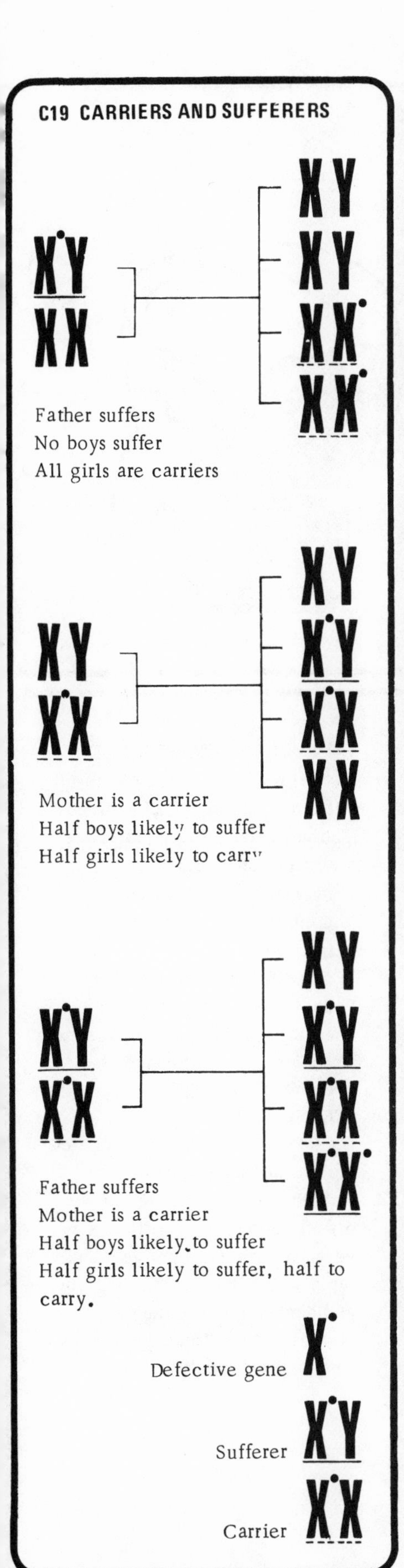

C20 MUSCULAR DYSTROPHY

This is a disease in which the muscles waste away. Muscle tissue does not replace itself, and slowly gives way to fibrous tissue and fat. It may be due to absence or excess of protein, or presence of abnormal protein. There are several forms of the disease. All are usually inherited, but two are sex linked - inherited almost only by men, and through female carriers. The carriers themselves may have slight muscle weakness, but are usually apparently normal.

DUCHENNE TYPE

This is the most common and most severe form. Half those with muscular dystrophy are boys with the Duchenne type. Most are dead by the time they are 25. It is invariably fatal.

The first symptoms develop between the age of 2 and 5. Walking is clumsy, running poor, falls frequent. Later, climbing stairs and getting up after falls become difficult. Weakness begins with certain muscles of the shoulders, upper arms, and thighs. Diagnosis is by measuring enzymes in the blood serum, and examining small muscle samples under a micro-scope. (If muscular dystrophy is suspected in a family, these tests can also diagnose it within a few days of a child's birth).

There is at present no cure or effective drug treatment.

Exercise and muscle stretching can slightly slow the progress of the disease, but eventually (usually between 8 and 11) the child has to take to a wheelchair. The spine curves, muscle weakness spreads, eventually affecting even eating and drinking, and muscle contraction distorts limb positions. Finally respiratory and heart muscles are involved, and death occurs, usually between 16 and 25.

There are tests that prove a woman is a carrier (though none can prove she is not).

BECKER TYPE

This is similar in the muscles affected and pattern of inheritance, but rarer, later, slower, and milder. Patients can usually still walk in their thirties and often into middle age.

C21 COLOR VISION DEFICIENCY

Color vision deficiency is much more common than is usually realized, and ten times more so in men than in women. Estimates range from 2 to 8% of all men, so millions suffer without realizing it. It usually results from a hereditary defect in the structure of the eye. There are various forms, but more than half of all cases have "red-green" color deficiency, and this is one of the types that are linked with sexual inheritance. In this condition, all three normal pigment responses occur in the eye, but there is difficulty in telling red, green, and yellow apart - all are likely to appear grayish. This can occur in varying degrees, ranging from slight graying from a distance to identical response to vivid colors close at hand.

An affected person will not normally realize for himself that he has this problem, but special tests can reveal the defect. Charts covered in colored dots are used. These show up a pattern or number to a person seeing them with normal vision, but no pattern (or a different one) to those with color defects.

The condition cannot be cured, but the newly developed X-Chrom contact lenses can give sufferers near-normal color perception.

C22 HERNIAS

A hernia has occurred if a body organ protrudes through the wall of the body cavity in which it is sited. This happens most often in the abdomen: part of the stomach or intestine is pushed through the abdominal wall.
Hernias occur where the cavity wall is weak; either because of a natural gap where a blood vessel or digestive tube passes, or because of scar tissue. They are often called "ruptures", but this really means any tearing or breaking of tissue, eg ruptured blood vessels.

C23 INGUINAL AND FEMORAL HERNIAS

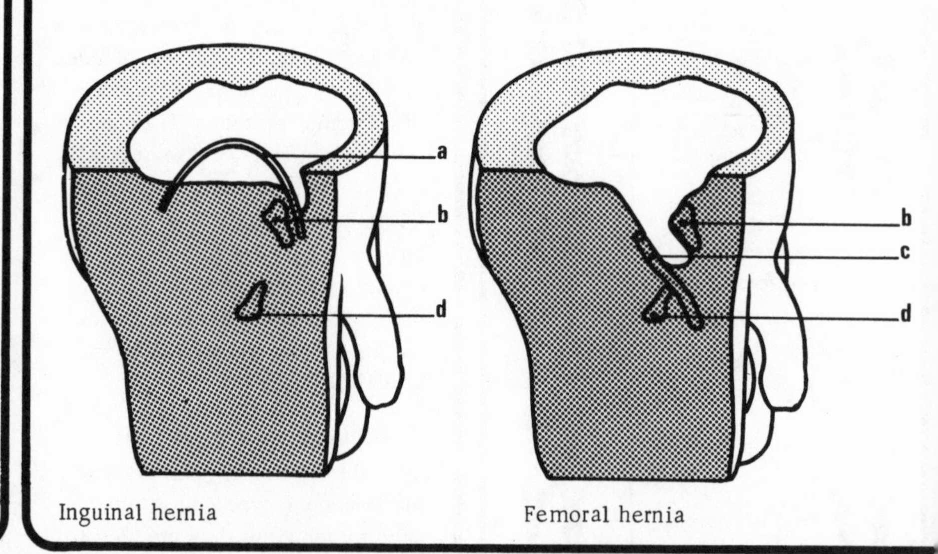

Inguinal hernia

Femoral hernia

C25 TYPES OF HERNIA

INGUINAL HERNIAS are by far the most common. In men, the inguinal canal is the pathway down which the testes descend just before birth. In later life it contains the spermatic cord and blood vessels. In an inguinal hernia, part of the intestine protrudes down this canal, into the scrotum. Since the inguinal canal is much smaller in women (containing only a fibrous cord), inguinal hernias are much more common in men.
FEMORAL HERNIAS are more often found in women. The femoral canal is the route through which the main blood vessels to the leg pass from the abdomen. In a femoral hernia, part of the intestine passes down the canal and protrudes at the top of the thigh.

UMBILICAL HERNIAS occur where the abdominal wall has been weakened at the navel by the umbilical cord. They are found mostly in young children.
VENTRAL HERNIAS occur where the abdominal wall has been weakened by the scar of a wound. (When the scar is due to an operation, it is called an incisional hernia.)
EPIGASTRIC HERNIAS are protrusions of fat and sometimes intestine through the abdominal wall between the navel and the breastbone.
OBTURATOR HERNIAS occur when part of the intestine passes through a gap between the bones of the front of the pelvis.
HIATUS HERNIA occurs when the upper part of the stomach protrudes upwards through the hole in the diaphragm occupied by the esophagus.
Hernias can also be classified in other ways.

CONGENITAL OR ACQUIRED
Congenital hernias exist at birth. All others are acquired hernias. The only congenital hernias are umbilical or inguinal, but congenital weakness in the abdominal wall may give rise to hernias later on.
REDUCIBLE OR IRREDUCIBLE
Reducible hernias can be pushed back into place in the abdomen. Irreducible hernias cannot - the opening is too small.
STRANGULATED OR UNSTRANGULATED Strangulated hernias are those in which the tightness of the opening has cut off the blood supply. This is a very serious condition, leading rapidly to tissue death, gangrene, and death. In unstrangulated hernias, the protruding tissue still has its blood supply.

a Spermatic cord
b Pubic bone
c Femoral canal
d Ischium

e Site of inguinal hernia
f Site of femoral hernia

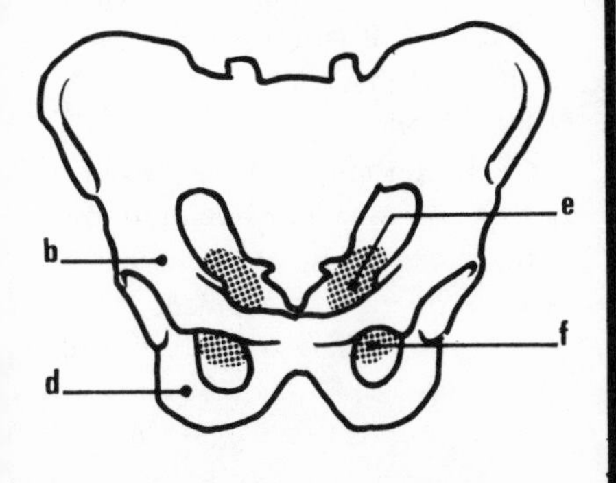

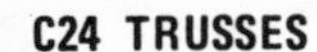

C24 TRUSSES

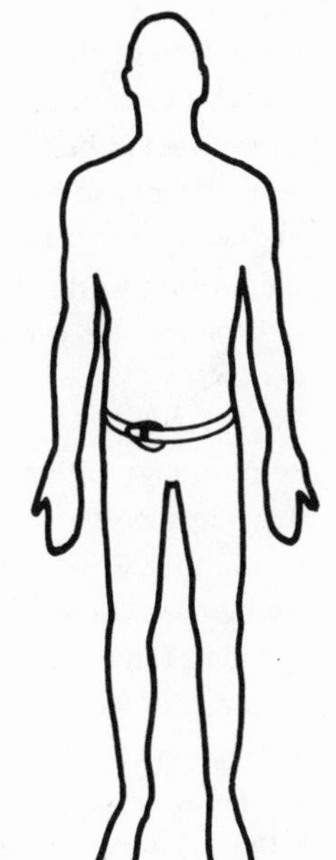

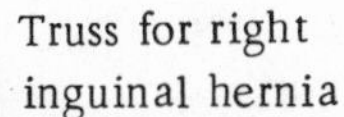

Truss for right inguinal hernia

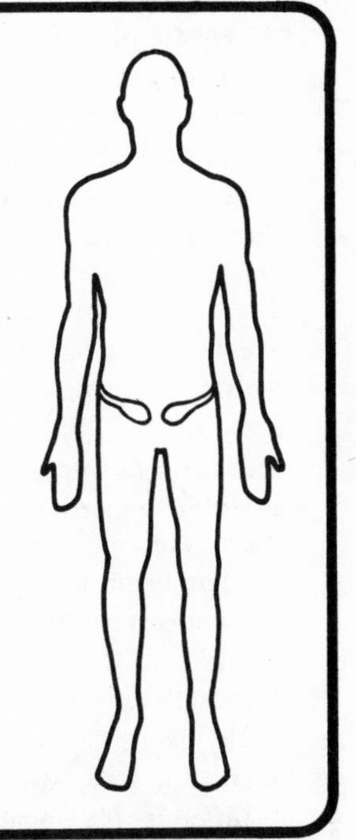

Double truss

C

C26 CAUSES, SYMPTOMS, AND TREATMENT

CAUSES

Congenital hernias are caused by the failure of some channels to close properly during fetal development. The intestine is either displaced at birth or easily becomes so.

Acquired hernias are caused by any form of straining or exertion that increases pressure in the abdomen, and forces it through a weak spot in the abdominal wall, eg physical work, straining at the bowels, violent coughing, etc. Strain and exertion equally act as predisposing factors, i.e. they weaken the abdominal wall, as also does any large, sudden gain or loss in weight (including pregnancy). Because of the use of men in heavy manual work, the male is much more likely to suffer from hernias.

SYMPTOMS

These depend on the type and condition of the hernia, the size and tightness of the opening, and the amount of the organ involved. Also the onset of the hernia may be gradual, with the symptoms increasing till they become noticeable; or sudden (perhaps whilst lifting a heavy weight), in which case the person is often aware of something having "given way", perhaps with varying degrees of pain.

In general there is a feeling of weakness and pressure in the area, occasional pain or a continual ache, and a gurgling feeling in the organ under strain. A swelling may be present all the time or may appear only under pressure. Swellings that are continually present may increase in size.

Digestion is disrupted, usually causing constipation.

Strangulated hernias produce special acute symptoms. When the blood supply is cut off the protruding tissue dies and swells, increasing the pressure in the opening. The hernia becomes inflamed and acutely painful and the skin over the area may redden. (With intestinal hernias, forward movement in the intestine ceases, and there may be vomiting.) The dead tissue in the hernia quickly becomes gangrenous, often within five or six hours, and this in turn causes peritonitis - inflammation of the abdominal lining and its contents. If untreated, death occurs within a few days.

TREATMENT

Reducible hernias are sometimes held in place by a truss - a belt with a pad which is fitted over the hernia. But as long as the hernia exists, the risk of future strangulation remains. Most hernias are therefore treated surgically. Any damaged tissue is removed, the protruding organ replaced in the abdomen, and the opening stitched up again.

Strangulated hernias require immediate operation.

C27 PEPTIC ULCER

An ulcer is a breach in the surface of the skin or in the membranes inside the body. The breach does not heal, and it spreads across, and through, the tissue.

PEPTIC ULCERS

These are ulcers of the stomach and duodenum (the first part of the small intestine). They occur if the lining of the stomach or duodenum fails to stand up to the digestive properties of the gastric juices, i.e. the stomach and intestine begin to digest themselves. Peptic ulcers rarely exceed ¾in across.

Duodenal ulcers form 80 to 90% of peptic ulcers, "gastric" (stomach) ulcers 10 to 20%. Men form 90% of all sufferers. (In women, gastric ulcers are slightly more common than duodenal ones.) Duodenal ulcers can occur at any time after the age of 20, gastric ulcers usually occur after 40.

CAUSES

The exact cause of peptic ulcers is not understood. It is thought that any small cut or tear in the lining is eroded and deepened by the action of the digestive juices. But why these ulcers do not occur more often (when such a cut or tear is likely to happen to all of us at one time or another), and why the erosion works through but not right across the surface, is just not known.

ASSOCIATED FACTORS

Some things are known to increase the likelihood of developing a peptic ulcer:

living under considerable stress;
drinking large amounts of alcohol;
eating rich food;
having excess acidity of the stomach;
suffering from frequent stomach or intestinal infection;
being of blood group "O";
having a family history of ulcers;
and being of "personality type A"*. The fact that women are much more likely to develop gastic ulcers after the menopause suggests that the female hormone, estrogen, may have some preventative value.

C28 SITES OF ULCERS

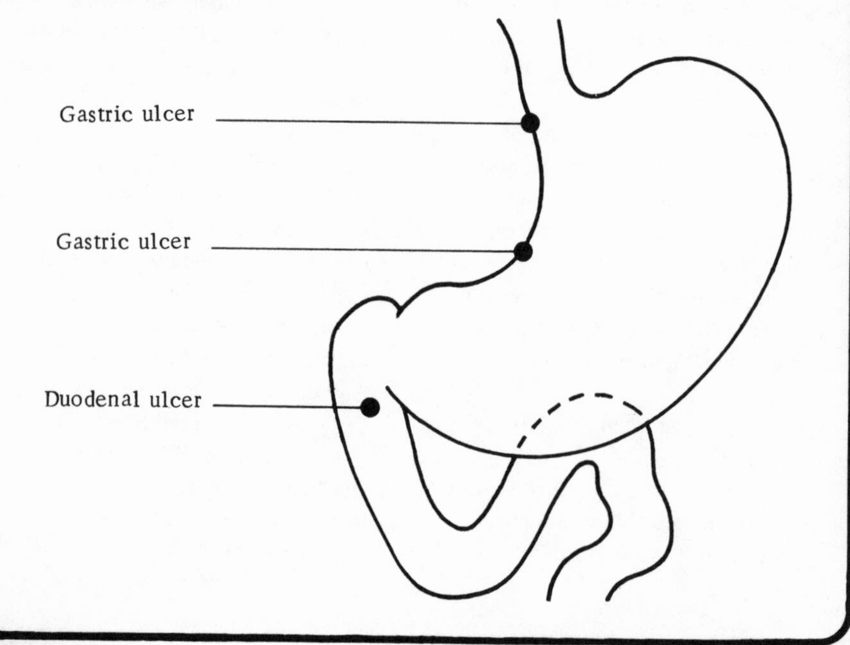

C29 SYMPTOMS AND TREATMENT

SYMPTOMS

There is pain in the upper abdomen, which gets worse when the stomach is empty and can often be relieved by taking more food. There is also tenderness in the area of pain. Indigestion, nausea, and vomiting may occur. If the cause is an ulcer, it can be seen on X rays.

TREATMENT

Antacids act to neutralize the stomach juices. Diet should be controlled: rich, strong foods, alcohol, tea, and coffee must be avoided. Frequent snacks of soft, bland food

When does pain occur?

Is it made better by food?

Vomiting?

Appetite?

C30 DANGERS

PERFORATION occurs when the ulcer eats right through the stomach or duodenal wall. This need not happen because there is a continual laying down of scar tissue during the process of erosion. But if it does happen it is extremely serious, because digestive juices are released into the abdominal cavity, threatening fatal peritonitis. Immediate surgery is needed: by 8 to 10 hours after perforation, the patient's situation is very grave.

Perforations are 8 to 10 times more likely with duodenal ulcers than with stomach ulcers.

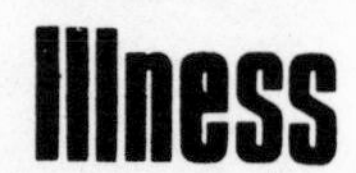

are taken, so the patient is eating about every two hours. This also helps to reduce stomach acidity. If the ulcer does not improve, surgery may be needed. With a stomach ulcer, the part of the stomach containing the ulcer is removed. With duodenal ulcers, the amount of gastric juice reaching the ulcer is reduced. This may be done by:
cutting some of the nerves that trigger gastric juice production;
or removing a part of the stomach where production occurs;
or diverting the outflow past the ulcer.

DUODENAL	GASTRIC
Before meals or 2 to 2½ hours after	½ to 2 hours after meals
Yes	Sometimes
Rare	Common
Good	Fair

OBSTRUCTION Peptic ulcers may block the passage of food through the stomach and/or duodenum, by causing swellings or muscular spasms. This is treated by administering special foods intravenously, in the hope that the obstruction dies down when irritation is removed. If this fails, surgery is needed.
HEMORRHAGE occurs when a blood vessel is ruptured by the ulcer. Blood is vomited, or passed in the feces. If the bleeding cannot be controlled within 24 hours, surgery may be needed.

C31 GOUT

Gout is a recurrent - and extremely painful - inflammation of certain joints. It is caused by overproduction of uric acid in the body. (Uric acid is produced during the breakdown of proteins, and is usually excreted from the body in the urine.) Excess uric acid is carried round in the bloodstream, and crystals of the acid and its salts (urates) are laid down in the cartilage of the joints - most often those of the feet (especially where the big toe joins the foot) and hands. The exact cause of the increase in uric acid is not known, but gout is associated with overconsumption of rich and high protein food, and of alcohol, and with sedentary living. It seldom occurs before the age of 45. In 80% of cases there seems to be a family history, so it may be partly hereditary. Men form 95% of all sufferers: women only develop gout after their menopause, so there is thought to be a connection with sex hormones.

ACUTE GOUT

Attacks of gout usually begin at night, with acute pain in the big toe or thumb. The joint becomes red, swollen, shiny and very tender, and the patient is feverish and irritable. He passes less urine than normal, but of a much thicker color. If untreated, the attacks can last from four to ten days. With drugs, the pain can be relieved within 24 hours. Large amounts of fluid - at least 5 pints a day - should be drunk, to flush the kidneys, with the aim of increasing the excretion of urates.

CHRONIC GOUT

The first attack of gout is very seldom the last. In the first subsequent attacks, the same site is usually affected, but later more joints become involved.
In chronic gout the acute attacks occur more often. They tend to be less painful, but the symptoms do not clear up completely in between. The joints affected become arthritic, as the deposits of crystal become permanent. The deposits gradually form stones ("tophi"), and the joints become swollen, disfigured, and fixed. Crystals are also deposited in the kidneys (which may lead to kidney failure), under the skin, in the eye, along the tendons, and in the cartilage of the ear.
In cases of long standing, gout is accompanied by degenerative changes in the heart, arteries, liver, and kidneys.
In treatment, drugs are used to combat the pain and to reduce the level of uric acid in the blood. Diet is also controlled: kidneys, liver, brains, fish roes, sardines, spinach, strawberries, and rhubarb should not be eaten. Also alcohol should not be drunk, and the weight is best kept below average.

C

BOWEL DISORDERS

C32 THE INTESTINES

The intestines are the long tube by which food leaves the stomach and is eventually excreted from the body. The tube is made up of sheaths of muscle, coated on the inside with mucous membrane.
The small intestine leads directly from the stomach. It is about 22 feet long, and up to $1\frac{1}{2}$ inches wide. It continues the process, begun in the stomach, of absorbing nutrients from the food.
The large intestine (the "colon") follows on from this. It is about 6 feet long and up to $2\frac{1}{2}$ inches wide. Its main function is the absorption of water from the waste products ("feces").

Many physiological disorders may affect the small intestine, eg bacterial infection, or fever. It can also be a site for ulcers* and cancer*.
However, the term "bowels" refers mainly to the large intestine - and often simply to the last 6 to 8 inches (the "rectum") and the surface opening (the "anus") through which the waste products are excreted, usually in a fairly solid form known as "stools." This is another potential cancer site. But it is also affected by certain well known disorders, linked with the physical process of waste evacuation, and dealt with on these pages.

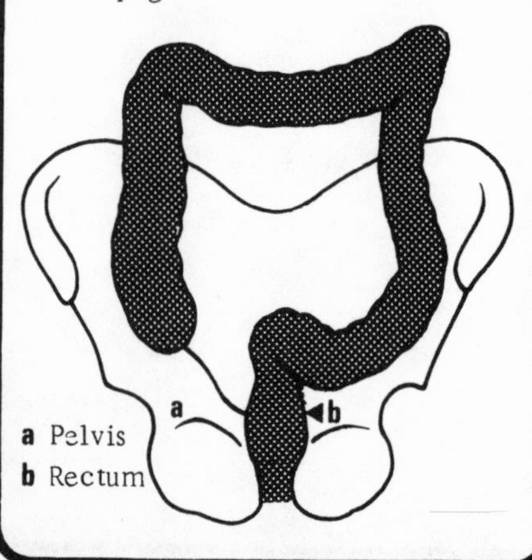

a Pelvis
b Rectum

C33 NORMAL BOWELS

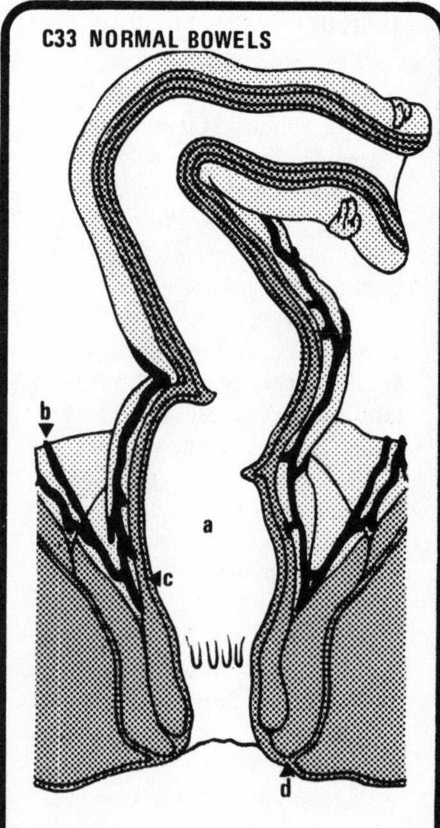

a Rectum
b Veins
c Mucous membrane
d Skin

C34 DISEASED BOWELS

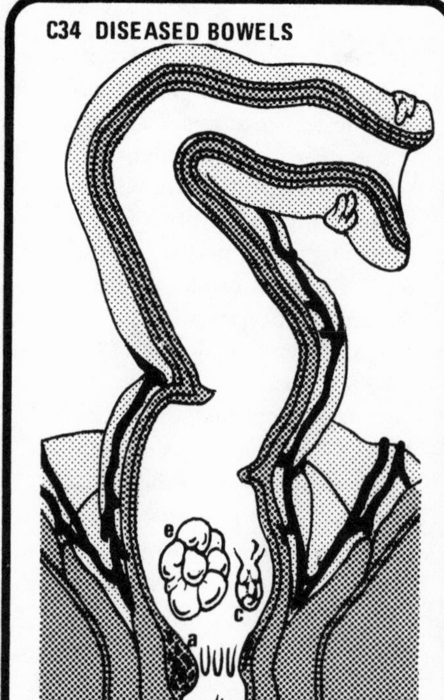

a Internal hemorrhoid
b External hemorrhoid
c Polyp
d Perianal abscess
e Rectal carcinoma

C35 DIARRHOEA AND CONSTIPATION

These common complaints are both usually caused by the failure of the colon to carry out its job of controlling the level of water in the feces.
This may be due to any one of many causes: a change of eating habits; gastritis (inflammation of the stomach); gastro-enteritis (inflammation of stomach and intestine); or bacterial or viral infection of the intestine.
DIARRHOEA
Diarrhoea is the excessive discharge of watery feces. The primary danger in serious cases is body dehydration, and this can be combated by an increased intake of fluid.
CONSTIPATION
Constipation is infrequent or absent defecation. It is usually caused by a poor diet, expecially one lacking in roughage*. But it may follow diarrhoea in the course of an infection- and is also sometimes caused by intestinal obstruction. However, much imagined constipation is only the consequence of judging bowel habits by an excessive norm of "regularity." In fact, "normal" bowel motions may occur as often as three times a day, or as infrequently as once every three or four days, depending on the individual.

C36 HEMORRHOIDS (PILES)

Hemorrhoids (piles) come about through the enlargement of veins in the wall of the rectum or in the anus.
This may be due to acute constipation, or overstraining during excretion. It can also result from tumors.
The swellings cause the mucous membrane to press against passing feces, causing discomfort, pain, and sometimes bleeding.
Internal hemorrhoids occur at or before the rectum's junction with the anus. If they protrude beyond the anal opening the pressure of the anal muscle (the "sphincter") often causes great and constant pain - this is known as "strangulation".
External hemorrhoids occur under the skin just outside the anus. In addition to the usual causes, they can also result from a ruptured vein, leading to a hemorrhage.
Internal hemorrhoids may eventually develop "polyps". This is a condition in which the hemorrhoidal protrusion becomes fibrous and elongated.

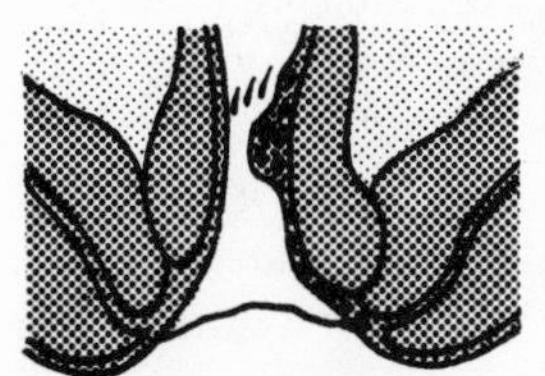
Internal hemorrhoid

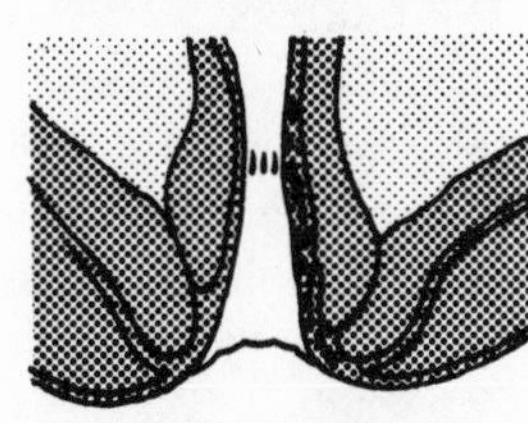
External hemorrhoid

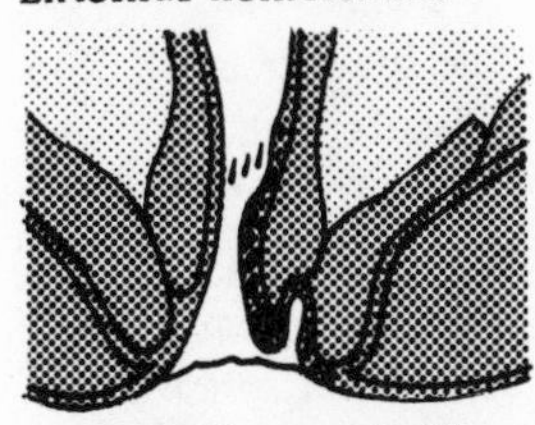
Enlarged hemorrhoid

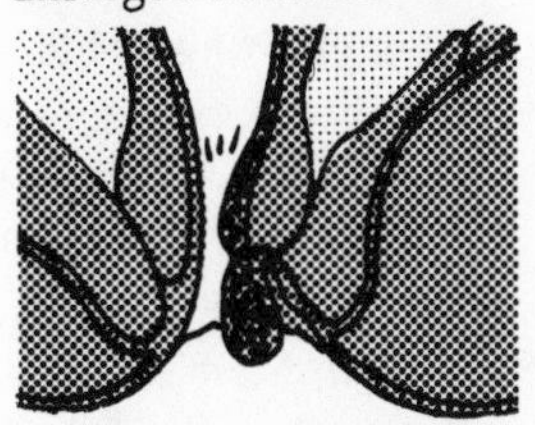
Strangulated hemorrhoid

C37 COLITIS

Colitis is inflammation of the colon - often with an associated ulcer*. The symptoms are abdominal discomfort, diarrhoea, blood in the feces, and fever. Anemia and even emaciation result. The first (acute) phase can be fatal if untreated. More usually, a prolonged (chronic) phase develops.
The causes are unknown, but may be linked in different individuals with: infection; allergy; deficiency of vitamin B and certain proteins; or simply nervous stress. Sometimes several causes occur together.
Treatment involves bed rest until the fever has passed; and also careful dietary control, excluding milk and all products derived from milk. Steroids may be used. Relapses are frequent. In extreme cases surgery is needed.

C38 RECTAL PROLAPSE

This is the collapse of the rectal wall. It occurs mostly in young babies and the aged. It is caused by excessive straining during excretion, and (in the old) by weak rectal and anal muscles. In severe cases an entire area of the rectal wall passes through the anal sphincter. Extreme pain from strangulation results.

C39 ABSCESSES

An abscess is caused by bacterial infection. In order to combat the bacteria, body fluid and white blood corpuscles collect in the tissue spaces, and form pus. A painful swelling results that continues to grow until it bursts and discharges its fluid.
To avoid discomfort and the possibility of further complications abscesses are usually drained surgically. Anorectal and perianal abscesses are extremely painful, because of the pressure of the anal sphincter, the passage of feces, and the constant irritation due to their anatomical positioning.

C40 FISSURE-IN-ANO

This is splitting of the walls of the anus. It is usually due to the passing of an exceptionally large stool. An "acute" fissure involves only the outer surface of the wall (the mucous membrane). If it does not disappear after a few days, it develops into a "chronic" fissure, which is deeper. This causes great pain and needs intensive treatment.

C41 THE URINARY SYSTEM

In the male body the urinary and reproductive systems are interconnected. This complexity makes the urinary system a likely and troublesome site for infection.

The system consists of those organs that produce and excrete urine:

a) a pair of kidneys;

b) a pair of tubes called ureters;

c) a muscular bag called the bladder;

d) and another single tube called the urethra.

THE KIDNEYS

The kidneys are located on either side of the spine, in the region of the middle back. The right kidney lies slightly lower than the left. Each kidney is bean shaped, and about 4in long, 2½in wide, and 1½in thick. Each weighs about 5oz.

The kidneys are chemical processing works. In them, waste matter in the blood - both solid and fluid - is filtered off under pressure, through more than two million tiny filtering units. This waste matter is called urine.

THE URETERS

The ureters are muscular tubes, each one about 10in long. One tube leads from each kidney, and down them the urine passes to the bladder, at the rate of a drop every 30 seconds.

THE BLADDER

The bladder is a balloon-like, muscular bag, that acts as a reservoir for the urine. When full it holds about 1.2pt (US) of urine - though the desire to urinate is usually felt when about half that amount is present.

A muscular ring (sphincter) surrounds the exit from the bladder into the urethra. When this is contracted, it prevents leakage of urine out of the bladder. Upon urination the sphincter is relaxed, and the urine passes into the urethra.

THE URETHRA

The urethra is a muscular tube about 8in long in a man, and 1½in in a woman. It leads from the bladder to the exterior, and it is along this tube that urine leaves the body ("urination", also called "micturition").

URINE

Urine consists of 96% water and 4% dissolved solids. Only 60% of the water taken into the body is normally eliminated as urine. The rest passes out in sweat and feces, and through the lungs. Urine is normally straw-colored or amber. In 24 hours an adult usually passes about 2.2pt (US), spread over 4 to 6 occasions (and most do not find it necessary to get up to pass urine at night). However, all these characteristics vary normally with: the amount of fluid drunk, and when; the amount lost in sweat; the size of the bladder; etc.

C42 SYMPTOMS OF DISORDERS

For the physician, the urine and urination are among the most useful signs of disorder - relating sometimes not just to the urinary system, but to the general health of the body.

Characteristics of urination that may interest the physician include: changes in quantity and frequency (including rising at night); slow and weak, or unusually forceful flow; stopping and starting, and dribbling; difficulty in beginning or continuing; inability to restrain (incontinence); sudden stopping; and, of course, pain or other unusual sensation on urinating, or inability to urinate at all.

Characteristics of the urine that may interest him include unusual color, odor, cloudiness, frothiness, and content. Abnormal chemical content can include albumen (which may indicate kidney disorder) or sugar (diabetes). Chemical testing can be carried out very easily, using a treated paper that changes color when moistened with urine. Other abnormal contents can include bacteria, parasites, kidney tube casts, bile fluid, and especially blood or pus.

However, many unusual characteristics of the urine or urination will more usually be due to insignificant causes than to disorder. For example, having to get up from bed to urinate is often due to drinking tea or coffee last thing at night. Strikingly unusual colors can be produced just by certain medicines and foods.

OTHER SYMPTOMS

Other symptoms of disorder include: itching, redness, or stickiness at the tip of the penis;

any discharge of fluid from the tip of the penis;

pain or swelling in the area of the kidneys, or in the ribs in front;

and shivering, temperature, or fever.

C

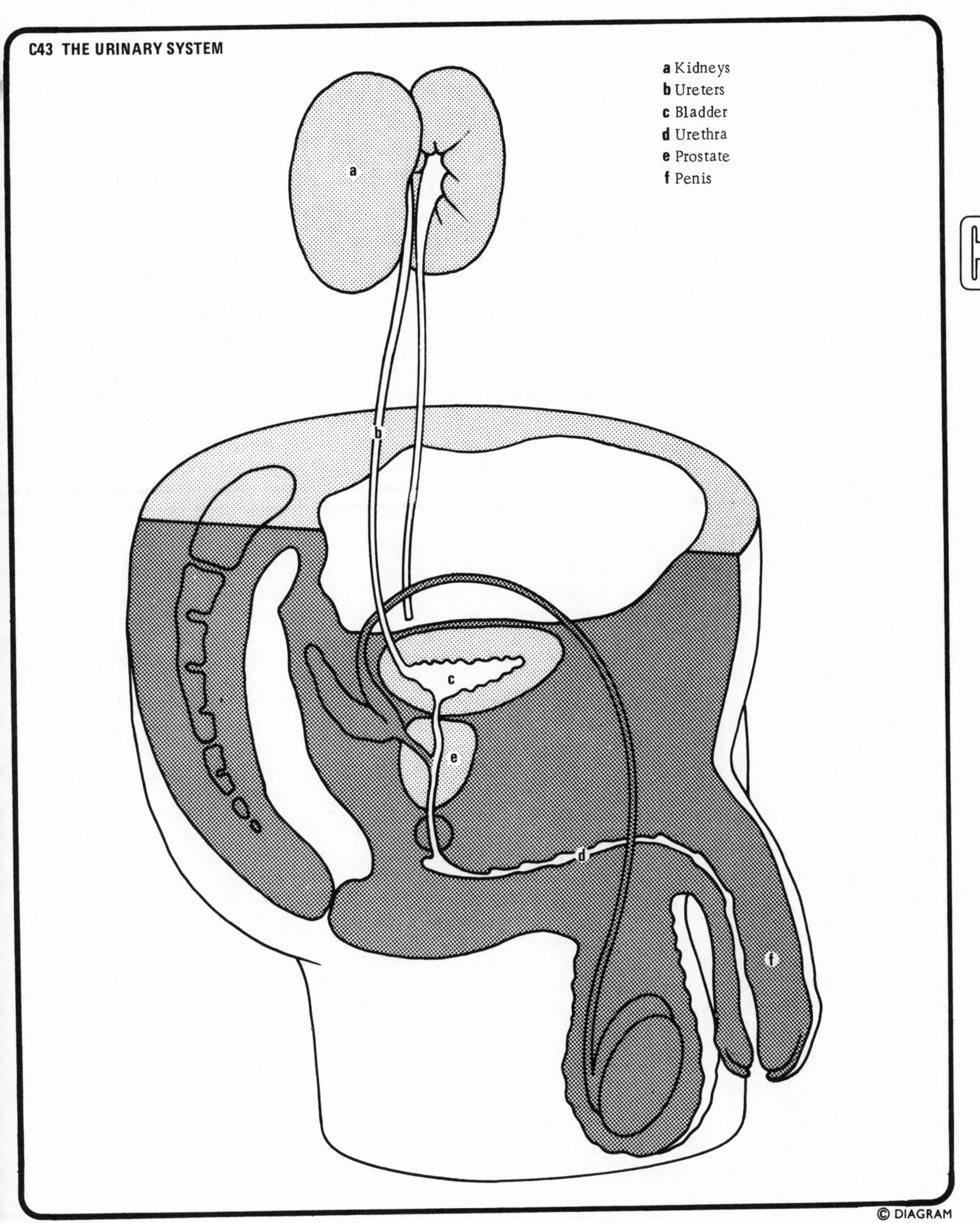
C43 THE URINARY SYSTEM
a Kidneys
b Ureters
c Bladder
d Urethra
e Prostate
f Penis
a
b
c
d
e
f

URINARY AND PROSTATIC DISORDERS 2

C44 URINARY DISORDERS

URETHRITIS

Urethritis is inflammation of the urethra. The most common cause is venereal disease*, but any irritation of the urethra can cause an attack. Sources of irritation can include alcohol consumption, ingredients in the diet, and the passage of instruments along the urethra during surgical examination. The symptoms are: discharge of pus from the penis, pain on urinating, tenderness of the urethra, and possibly inflammation of other organs such as testes, bladder and even kidneys. In women it often leads to cystitis*.

Treatment depends on the cause. Drinking large quantities of fluid usually helps.

RETENTION

Retention refers to the involuntary holding back of urine in the bladder, due to some obstruction of the urethra. The bladder enlarges behind the obstruction as the quantity of urine increases, and may be stretched and weakened. Eventually the ureters and kidneys also dilate, and kidney infection may occur. Rapid surgical treatment is needed, before the kidneys suffer permanent damage.

Retention is most common in elderly men, due to enlargement of the prostate gland. Strictures are another cause.

STRICTURES

A stricture is an abrupt narrowing of the ureters or urethra. In the ureters, it may be congenital, or caused by physical irritation such as the passage of kidney stones or surgical instruments. Treatment is difficult, and surgery is usually necessary.

Strictures of the urethra are more common. They may also be congenital, but are usually "spasmodic" or "organic".

C45 PROSTATIC DISORDERS

The prostate gland* surrounds the junction of the bladder and urethra. It is normally about 1in by $\frac{3}{4}$in by $1\frac{1}{2}$in, and during ejaculation it supplies a fluid without which the sperm is sterile.

However, the prostate can become enlarged, especially in the elderly. There are three possible processes:

a) Benign enlargement, which is the usual form, and occurs when fibrous cells multiply inside the gland. The cause is unknown, but may be due to hormonal imbalance.

b) Cancer of the prostate, which is a common form of cancer* in men.

c) Prostatitis, or inflammation of the prostate, which is usually due to infection in the urinary tract (such as gonorrhea, cystitis or urethritis). Such inflammation may be temporary or chronic.

SYMPTOMS

Enlargement eventually causes retention. In this case the following symptoms occur:

urination is slow to begin, lacks force, and is often interrupted by pauses;

the desire to urinate occurs with increasing frequency, especially at night;

there are further dribbles of urine after urination has stopped;

and, if the stagnant urine retained in the bladder sets up infection, or if infection passes up from the urethra, pain on urination occurs.

Finally, the urethra may be completely blocked, so no urine can pass.

TREATMENT

Prostatitis may be dealt with by antibiotics and prostatic massage, but more serious prostate enlargements require surgical removal of the gland itself. After this operation, a man is usually sterile, and ejaculates his semen backwards into the bladder, rather than externally. However, erection and the experience of orgasm remain as before.

In the case of cancer, hormonal treatment may be an alternative to surgery. Cancer of the prostate may, of course, metastasize* elsewhere.

Other possible disorders of the prostate include tuberculosis and the formation of stones.

Spasmodic strictures are temporary, and due to irritation by cold, excess alcohol, or physical objects. They last only a few hours or days, and cause no permanent discomfort. Organic strictures follow prolonged inflammation or laceration, and if untreated may cause distension and inflammation of bladder and kidneys. Both forms are treated by stretching the urethra with special instruments. In organic strictures this must be repeated regularly.

KIDNEY DISORDERS

These mainly result from infection or kidney stones.

Bacterial infection can reach the kidney through the blood stream, or pass back along the urinary system from a site of stagnant urine or venereal disease. If kidney damage results, waste products left in the blood can cause poisoning, while rising blood pressure can lead to heart failure or brain hemorrhage. The same may occur if back pressure from retention damages the kidneys.

Kidney stones (which generally have unknown causes) may stay in the kidney or pass out without trouble, but they can also cover the entrance to the ureter, or get stuck in ureter or urethra. This can be violently painful, and surgery may be needed.

INCONTINENCE

Incontinence is inability to control the bladder: urination occurs when the person does not want it to. Causes include psychological stress (eg severe fright), disorders of the bladder, and, especially, impairment of the controlling nerves due to injury or disease. Incontinence due to old age is also common.

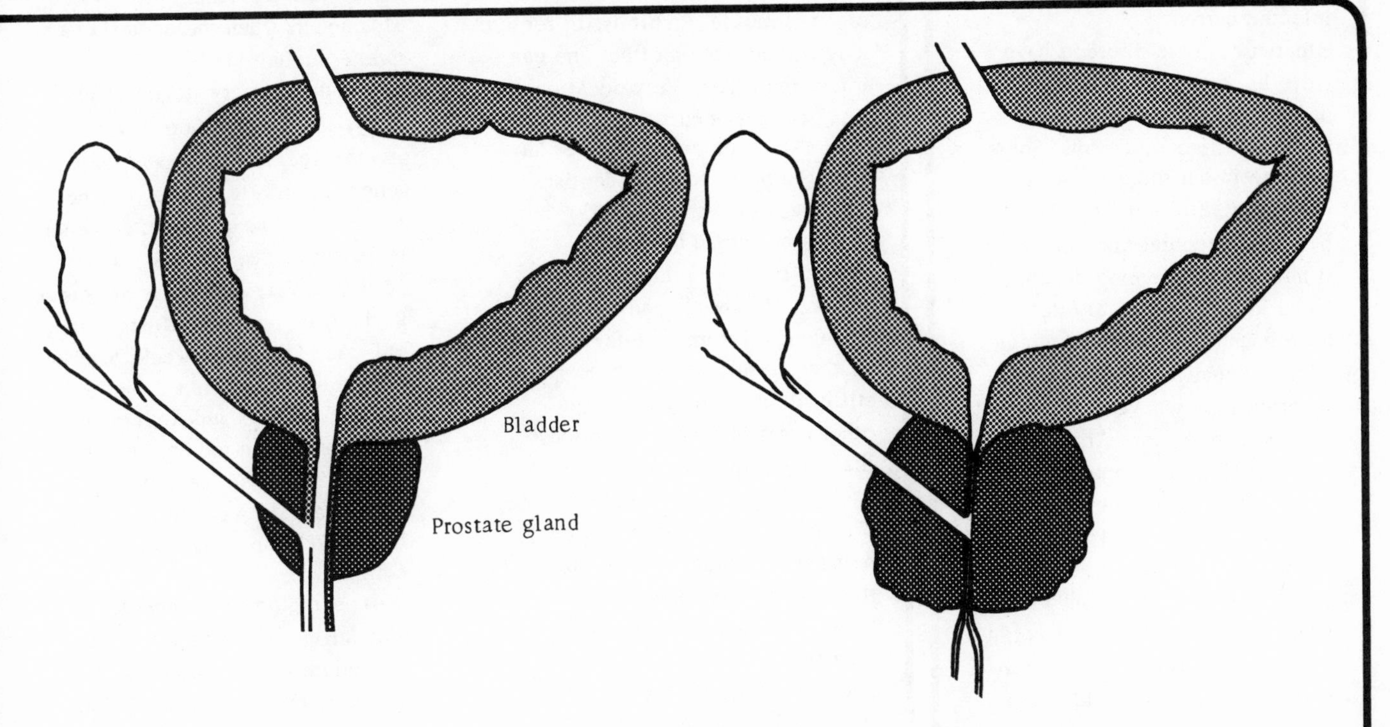

Enlarged prostate constricts urethra, causing retention

SEXUAL INFECTIONS 1

C46 VENEREAL DISEASE

The term venereal disease (VD) is used for certain infections which are almost always passed on by sexual contact. This happens because:

a) the micro-organisms that cause them usually live in the infected person's genitals - or in some other place (such as mouth or anus) where they have been put by sexual activity; and

b) to infect another person, they usually have to enter his body through an orifice (such as the genital opening, anus, or mouth), and sexual activity gives them this chance. The first symptoms of disorder appear on the part of the body that has been in contact with the infected part of the infected person.

Otherwise, these disorders have little in common. Some are caused by bacteria, some by viruses, some by other micro-organisms. Some are rare in our society, others epidemic. And some can be only painful or troublesome, others, if untreated, crippling or fatal. Some kinds of venereal disease have been known since medicine began. Syphilis, the most notorious, may have been brought back to Europe from America as a result of Columbus' expedition in 1492. Cases of VD increased rapidly during World War II, and in the last 20 years cases in many countries have multiplied 3 or 4 times. The frequency of gonorrhea, for example, is now second only to that of the common cold.

C47 SYPHILIS

Syphilis is sometimes nicknamed "the pox" or "scab". It is the most serious of sexual infections. Its prevalence varies. In the USA it is the third most common reportable disease. In the UK, for example, it is comparatively rare. Worldwide, there are about 50 million cases.

CAUSATION

Syphilis is caused by tiny bacteria shaped like corkscrews: "spirochetes". These thrive in the warm, moist linings of the genital passages, rectum, and mouth, but die almost immediately outside the human body. So the infection almost always spreads by sexual contact. Whether the probing organ is penis, tongue, or (perhaps) finger, and whether the receiving organ is mouth, genitals, or rectum, a syphilitic site on either one can infect the other. Very occasionally syphilis does occur from close non-sexual contact (and cases have occurred in doctors and dentists from their professional work); but it cannot be spread by physical objects such as lavatory seats, towels, or cups. It can, however, be inherited from an infected mother, resulting sometimes in stillbirth or deformity, and in other cases in hidden infection that causes trouble later.

INCUBATION

There is an "incubation period", between catching syphilis and showing the first signs - always between 9 days and 3 months, and usually 3 weeks or more. About 1000 germs are typically picked up on infection. After 3 weeks these have multiplied to 100 to 200 million. If the disorder is untreated, they can invade the whole body, eventually causing death.

Syphilis has four stages. Each has typical symptoms, but these can vary or be absent.

PRIMARY STAGE

The first symptom is in the part that has been in contact with the infected person: genitals, rectum, or mouth. A spot appears and grows into a sore that oozes a colorless fluid (but no blood). The sore feels like a button: round or oval, firm, and just under ½in across. A week or so later, the glands in the groin may swell - but they do not usually become tender, so it may not be noticed. There is no feeling of illness, and the sore heals in a few weeks without treatment.

SECONDARY STAGE

This occurs when the bacteria have spread through the body. It can follow the primary stage straight away, but usually there is a gap of several weeks. The person feels generally unwell. There may be headaches, loss of appetite, general aches and pains, sickness, and perhaps fever. Also there are breaks in the skin, and sometimes a dark red rash, lasting for weeks or even months. The rash appears on the back of the legs and front of the arms, and often too on the body, face, hands, and feet. It may be flat or raised, does not itch, and looks like many other skin complaints.

Other symptoms can include: hair falling out in patches; sores in the mouth, nose, throat, or genitals, or in soft folds of skin; and swollen glands throughout the body.

All these symptoms eventually disappear without treatment, after anything from 3 weeks to 9 months.

LATENT STAGE

This may last for anything from a few months to 50 years. There are no symptoms. After about two years, the person ceases to be infectious (though a woman can still sometimes give the disease to a baby she bears). But presence of syphilis can still be shown by blood tests.

TERTIARY STAGE

This occurs in about $\frac{1}{3}$ of those who have not been treated earlier. The disease now shows itself in concentrated and often permanent damage in one part of the body. Common are ulcers in the skin, and lesions on ligaments, joints, or on bones. These are painful, but tertiary syphilis is more serious if it attacks heart, blood vessels, or nervous system. It can then kill, blind, paralyze, cripple, or render insane.

TESTS

Syphilis is not easy to diagnose. Its symptoms are often mild or indistinctive. Testing sores for bacteria or blood for antibodies is necessary. Neither always works, so repeat tests are important.

TREATMENT

This involves antibiotics - usually penicillin. Given in primary or secondary stages, it completely cures most cases. Tests and examination often last more than two years afterwards, to make sure the cure is complete.

In the latent and even tertiary stages, syphilis can still be eradicated and further damage halted; but existing tertiary stage damage often cannot be repaired.

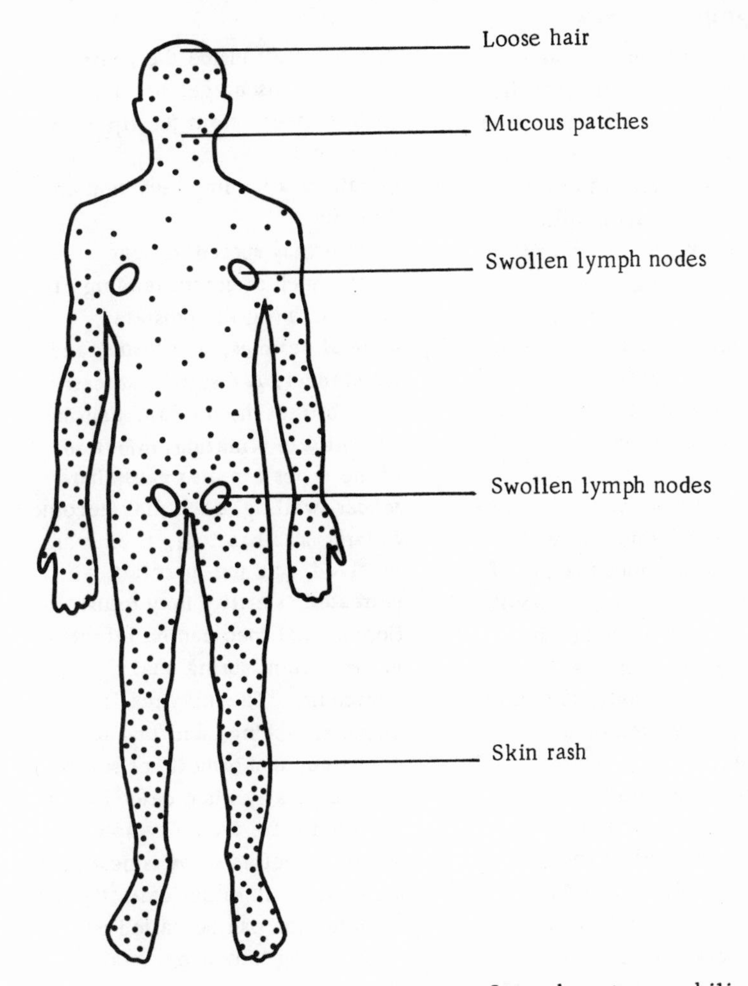

Secondary stage syphilis

C48 GONORRHEA

Gonorrhea (sometimes nicknamed "the clap") has spread very rapidly among young people in recent years - partly because it is so easy for a woman to have it without knowing it. There are over half a million reported cases in the USA every year, and the true figure is probably many times that number. Several infections in one person in a single year are not too uncommon. Worldwide, there are about 150 million cases.

CAUSATION

Like syphilis, gonorrhea:

a) is caused by a bacterium that thrives in the warm moist lining of urethra, vagina, rectum, or mouth;

b) is normally only passed on by sexual contact, but may be sometimes by close body contact or by passage from an infected mother; and

c) cannot be picked up from objects (though it has been suggested that gonorrhea can be carried by pubic lice, and these can be picked up from objects such as lavatory seats).

Unlike syphilis, the form of sexual contact involved is normally only genital or anal intercourse. Oral contact does not often pass on gonorrhea; if it does, it is usually fellatio, rather than cunnilingus that is responsible. (But some scientists even allow the possibility of infection through kissing.)

SYMPTOMS IN MEN

After incubation (usually under a week, but sometimes up to a month), gonorrhea in a man shows itself in marked symptoms:

a) discomfort inside the penis;

b) a thick discharge, usually yellow-green, from the tip of the penis; and

c) pain or a burning sensation on urinating.

Later it may spread to near points, such as glands leading off the urethra (eg the prostate, seminal vesicles, and testes) and the bladder. A resulting abscess may obstruct the urethra, causing difficulty in urinating. Infection of the testes can also cause hard tender swelling: each may become as large as a baseball. If both are involved, and the infection is untreated, sterility may result.

Homosexual men can be infected in the rectum during anal intercourse. This may result in soreness, itching, and/or anal discharge, and sometimes severe pain, espcially when defecating. But often there are no symptoms, or only a feeling of moistness in the rectum. In either case, though, the infection can be passed on again during subsequent anal intercourse.

If oral contact results in infection, it is mainly as a throat disorder that is often not recognized as gonorrhea. It is also unlikely to infect others, because the lymph tissue where the bacteria can survive are deep in the tonsil area.

Unlike syphilis, gonorrhea usually remains fairly localized, but if untreated can finally spread to the blood stream and infect bone joints, causing arthritis.

SYMPTOMS IN WOMEN

In women the incubation period is longer, and the eventual symptoms, if any, much less severe or identifiable. There may be discomfort on urinating, more frequent urination, and a vaginal discharge. The discharge is distinctively yellow, and unpleasant in smell - but this may be unnoticed due to the typically small quantities involved. Seventy to 90% of cases in women occur without the woman being aware of the disease; but she is still just as infectious, even where there are no symptoms.

If untreated, the infection may spread to:

a) glands around the vaginal entrance, making them swell, sometimes as large as a golf-ball;

b) the rectum (because of the closeness of the two openings), causing inflammation and perhaps a discharge; and/or

c) the cervix, uterus, and fallopian tubes. Fallopian infection can result in fever, abdominal pain, backache, sickness, painful or excessive periods, and pain during intercourse. If not treated quickly, sterility can result. It can also kill mother and fetus, by causing any pregnancy to be ectopic*.

Even where gonorrhea does not affect the fallopian tubes, it can result in premature birth, umbilical cord inflammation, maternal fever, and blindness in the child.

TEST AND TREATMENT

Gonorrhea is diagnosed by laboratory analysis of any discharge or of a smear from the affected part.

Treatment is with antibiotics - usually penicillin, though many forms of gonorrhea are becoming more resistant to it. Apart from avoiding infecting others through intercourse, the person being treated should also avoid masturbation and alcohol, since both can irritate the urethra and interfere with cure.

C49 OTHER VENEREAL DISEASES

These are uncommon in temperate climates.

SOFT CHANCRE
Also called chancroid or "soft sore", this is caused by a bacillus (a rod-shaped bacterium) and is contracted sexually (usually by intercourse). After 3 to 5 days incubation, it generally produces an ulcer on the genitals and painful swollen glands (but either sex can carry the infection without symptoms). Treatment is with antibiotics and other drugs.

LYMPHOGRANULOMA VENEREUM
This is caused by a very small bacterium, and can be contracted from infected bedding and clothing as well as (more usually) from sexual intercourse. After 5 to 21 days incubation, it produces a small genital blister or ulcer. Later there can be internal complications. Treatment is with antibiotics.

GRANULOMA INGUINALE
This is caused by a bacillus, and is contracted sexually (usually by intercourse). After 1 to 3 weeks incubation, it produces bright red painless sores around the genitals. Treatment is with antibiotics.

C

C50 NON-SPECIFIC URETHRITIS

NSU is the most common of all sexual disorders in men. In women, the symptoms are often insignificant or hard to diagnose. Well-controlled studies in the past seven years have documented genital strains of *Chlamydia trachomatis* as the etiologic agents of 40 to 50% of non-gonococcal urethritis. It has also been shown to cause the majority of cases of acute epididymitis (inflammation of the epididymis, which is attached to the upper part of each testicle) in young, sexually active men.

SYMPTOMS IN MEN
If NSU develops after a specific intercourse, there is usually 1 to 4 weeks incubation. Symptoms may then include:
a) greenish-yellow discharge from the penis;
b) blockage of the penis tip with dry pus; and
c) discomfort when urinating, and sometimes increased frequency.
Untreated NSU may spread to: the bladder (causing pain on urinating and perhaps blood in the urine); the testes (causing swelling); and/or especially the prostate (causing pains in groin or back or between the legs).

SYMPTOMS IN WOMEN
In women, the endocervix and, to a lesser extent, the urethra are the primary sites of chlamydial infection. The most important manifestation of chlamydial infection in non-pregnant women is acute pelvic inflammatory disease (PID).

Tetracyclines are the current drugs of choice for almost all such infections, except those occurring in children and pregnant women. Dosage is 500mg, four times daily for 7 to 14 days. For pregnant women and children, erythromycin is the recommended alternative to tetracycline.

SEXUAL INFECTIONS 3

C51 THE PENIS AND SEXUAL DISORDERS

Most sexual disorders produce typical symptoms in the penis area, if contracted genitally.

a) Primary syphilis: a single, hard, painless sore; glands often swollen.
b) Gonorrhea: discharge from tip.
c) Chancroid: small painful pimples, breaking down to soft painful ragged ulcers that bleed easily; widely swollen glands.
d) Granuloma: red pimple growing into painless raised area, bright beefy red in color.
e) Pubic lice: the lice appear as bluish-grey dots about the size of a pinhead; the "nits" (eggs) can also be seen, attached to the hairs.

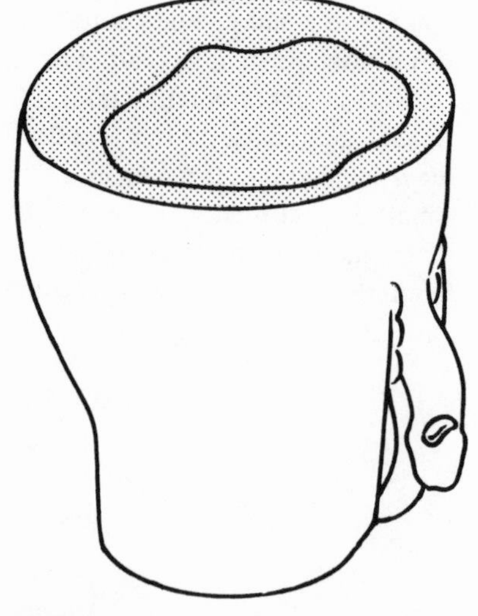
Syphilis

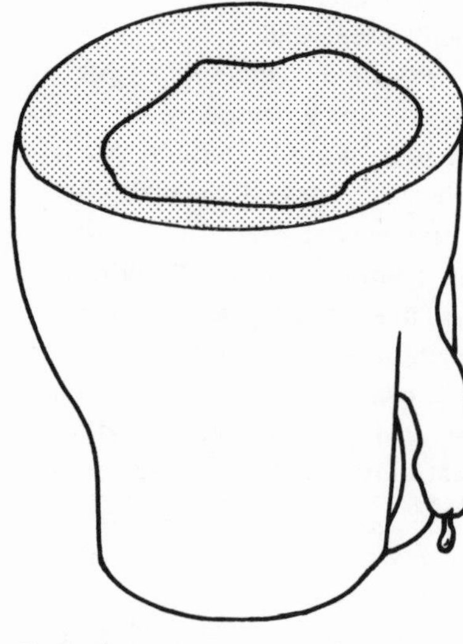
Gonorrhea

C52 OTHER SEXUAL INFECTIONS AND INFESTATIONS

These include:
a) trichomoniasis and candidiasis, which usually develop only in women: see M25.
b) genital versions of two common skin disorders - warts and cold sores; and
c) infestation by certain minute insect parasites, such as pubic lice or the scabies mite.

GENITAL WARTS are fairly common and very contagious. They are spread by sexual contact, perhaps caused by a virus, and appear, after 1 to 6 months' incubation, on, in, or around genitals or anus. They are usually cured by repeated use of a resin application. If this fails, they may have to be burnt off with chemicals or electricity.

GENITAL HERPES are fairly common and contagious.
The virus responsible is thought to lie dormant in the skin for long periods. When activated, it causes a genital sore that weeps colorless fluid and forms a scab.
There is no sure treatment. It usually disappears after about 10 days, but may recur.

INFESTATIONS are passed on by sexual or sometimes other close body contact, and are not especially common.
Scabies, or "the itch", is caused by a tiny mite, which mainly lives on and around the genitals. The female mite burrows beneath the skin to lay her eggs. The symptoms - itchy lumps and tracks - become noticeable after 4 to 6 weeks' incubation. They can occur between the fingers, on buttocks and wrists, and in the armpits, as well as on the genitals. The itching is worse in warm conditions (eg in bed).
Pubic lice, or "crabs", are genital versions of the lice that can also occur in other hairy parts of the body. They feed on blood, and cause itching that can be severe.
Treatment of both parasites involves painting the entire body with appropriate chemicals.
Pubic lice are called by the French "papillons d'amour": the butterflies of love.

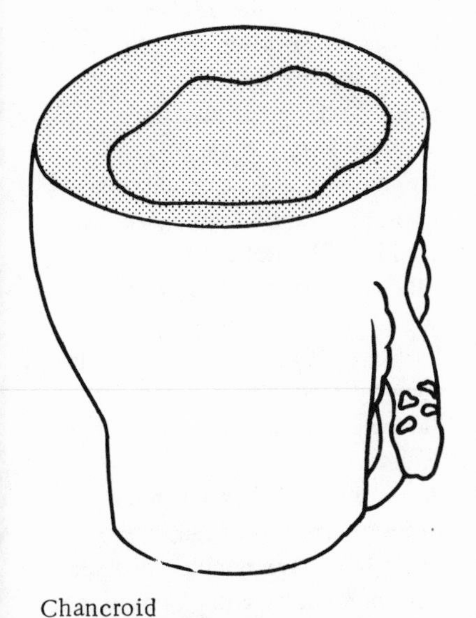
Chancroid

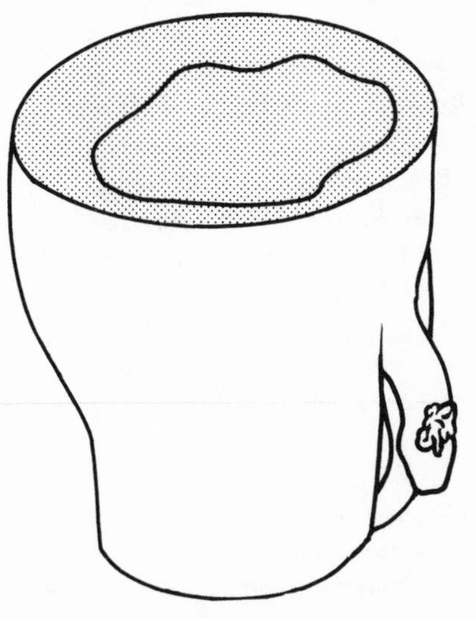
Granuloma

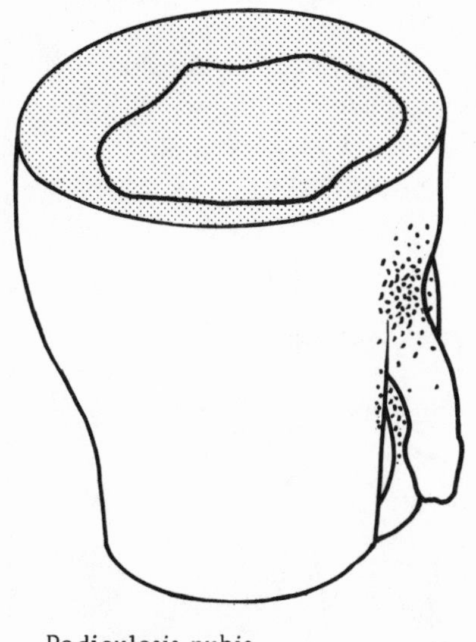
Pediculosis pubis

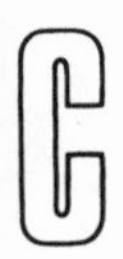

C53 SIGNS AND SYMPTOMS

The following are possible signs of venereal disease (or NSU):

a) a sore, ulcer, or rash, on or around the genitals, anus, or mouth;
b) an unusual discharge from penis or vagina;
c) pain or a burning feeling on urinating;
d) increased frequency of urination;
e) swollen glands in the groin; and
f) itching or soreness of the penis, anus, or vagina.

All these usually have some other cause - not venereal disease.
But do not delay in getting proper medical advice. The disappearance of symptoms may not mean that you were worrying about nothing. It may just mean that the infection has progressed naturally to its next stage. You may still have a venereal disease; and you may still be able to infect others.

C54 PREVENTION

Worrying too much about getting a sexual infection is not a healthy attitude. You may quite sensibly avoid sex with people whose sexual experience seems likely to have been casual and widely indiscriminate.
When having intercourse other than in a stable relationship, two possible "practical" measures are: to wear a condom; and to wash the genitals thoroughly before and after intercourse. But:

a) wearing a condom guards effectively against gonorrhea and NSU, but not against syphilis;
b) for full protection the condom needs to be worn even during sex play beforehand;
c) washing the genitals only reduces the risk slightly; and
d) both these procedures interfere with the naturalness and pleasure of sex.

So - though it is sensible to wear a condom for some chance encounters - it is not sensible to be obsessed with such measures of protection.
What is sensible, in fact, is not so much to guard against getting these infections, as to act carefully to stop it spreading if you do. It is important:

a) to get cured properly, following qualified medical instructions, and returning for prescribed checks and tests even if they seem unnecessary:
b) to avoid sexual contact with anyone until you are sure you are cured; and
c) to make sure that all your recent sexual contacts know what has happened, and that they all get themselves thoroughly tested and, if necessary, treated.

D01 SURFACE AREA

Skin covers the surface of the body. It is the largest organ of the body, accounting for about 16% of total weight. The skin of an average adult man covers an area of about 20 square feet; that of an average woman about 17½ square feet.

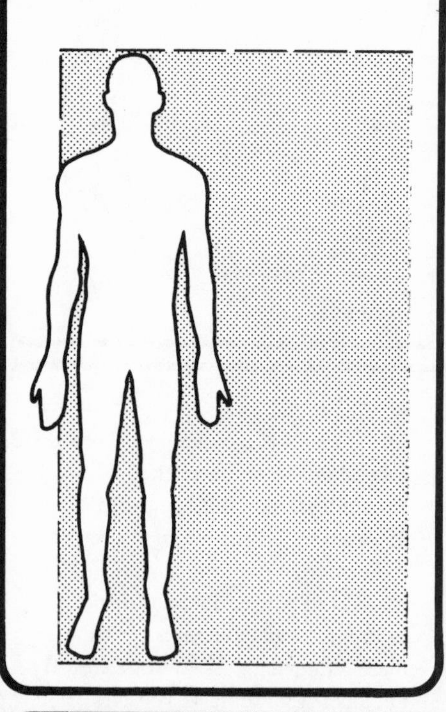

D02 STRUCTURE OF THE SKIN

Skin is made up of several layers of different cells. The top layer is made of dead, flattened cells bound together to form a tough, flexible, and waterproof surface that is constantly being rubbed off and replaced by the living layers below. About 40lb of dead skin is shed by an average adult in his lifetime.

The lower layers contain hair roots ("follicles"); sweat, sebaceous, and apocrine glands; nerves; blood vessels; and fat.

a Epidermis
b Dermis
c Subcutaneous fatty layer
d Sebaceous gland
e Nerve
f Hair follicle
g Sweat gland

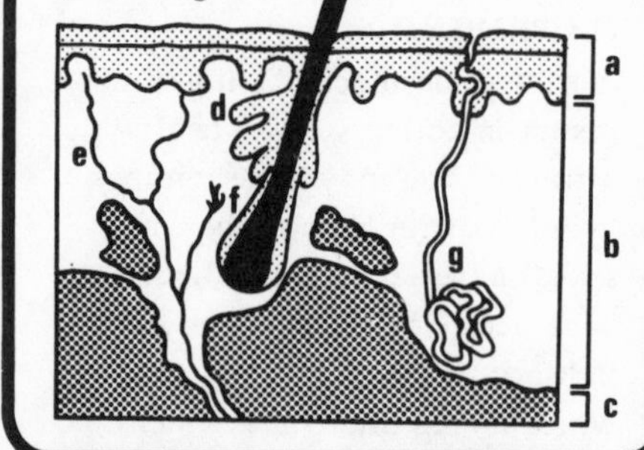

D03 FUNCTION

The skin acts as a protective barrier against the environment. It stops evaporation into the air of the water that makes up 60% of man's body. It also stops bacteria entering the body. Wounds are healed quickly and an antiseptic liquid is secreted from glands in the skin.

The skin also protects the delicate tissues below from the sun's harmful ultraviolet rays. This is done by producing melanin, a dark pigment which forms a layer to absorb the rays.

Races that are exposed to an extreme amount of sun, such as in Africa, have adapted to their environment by being born black. People who have no melanin in their skin and so cannot adapt to sunlight by turning brown are called Albinos and have white hair and skin and very pale eyes.

D04 THICKNESS AND ELASTICITY

The skin is generally about 1-2mm thick, but only 0.5mm on the eyelids and up to 6mm on palms and soles, where it is dense and ridged to increase gripping powers.

Skin is attached to the deeper tissues by elastic fibers, so that it can move about to a certain extent and allow the joints to function.

Skin grows constantly with the body but in old age the body bulk shrinks and the skin loses its elasticity, causing bagginess and wrinkles.

D05 NERVES

The skin is more richly supplied with nerve endings than any other part of the body. Through these nerves we are supplied with a running commentary on our body's surroundings. The skin is sensitive to pain, touch, heat, and cold. Each of these sensations is served by different nerve endings, and messages from them are carried along to the central nervous system, the spinal cord, and the brain.

D06 NAILS

Nails are found at the end of each finger and toe. They are made of hard, flat, transparent keratin, which is also found in the hair. The nail root lies under a fold of skin and grows outward over the nail bed. Fingernails grow quicker than toenails. The average growth rate of nails is 1½ inches a year. Nails protect the tips of the fingers and toes and can also be used as weapons.

D07 SITES OF DISORDER

a Frostbite
b Skin cancer
c Sunburn
d Chilblains

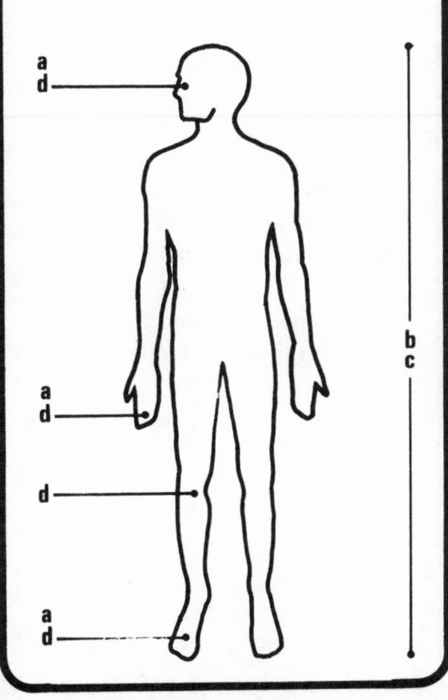

D08 FROSTBITE

Exposure of a part of the body to extreme cold causes the blood vessels to contract. This leaves the surface areas vulnerable to freezing - which is painless, and can happen without the person's knowledge. The lack of blood damages the tissues, while frozen fingers and toes may get broken off.
The aim of treatment is to restore the affected parts to normal body temperature. The patient should be moved to mild (but not warm) surroundings, while thawing occurs. Rapid rewarming, by immersion of the frozen parts in warm water, should only be used when freezing has lasted less than half an hour. Antibiotics are given to prevent infection in the damaged tissues. In severe cases, amputation of parts affected by gangrene may be necessary.

D09 SKIN CANCER

Skin cancers are abnormal growths in the epidermis, that invade other tissues. The cause of most of them is unknown, but one common cause is consistent exposure of an unprotected skin to strong sunlight. A high proportion is found in those engaged in outdoor work or sports, or in white people living in tropical climates. Melanin gives effective protection to a dark skin.
Skin cancers are usually soon noticed and slow to grow, and they can be destroyed in their early stages by careful surgery or radiotherapy. However, if they are neglected, they can spread beneath the skin, or in some cases metastasize* to other parts of the body. Then they are much more dangerous.
Avoidance of excessive exposure to sunlight is the only known preventive technique.

D10 SUNBURN

The extent of damage caused by the sun's ultraviolet rays depends on the intensity and duration of the exposure, and the amount of melanin present in the skin.
Overexposure to sunlight has the same effect as superficial thermal burns, but with some hours delay.
In mild cases of sunburn, lotions can be applied to the affected areas to soothe the pain.
For serious cases hospital treatment may be necessary.
The melanin in fair skins can be built up by gradual exposure to sunlight and so prevent sunburn.

D11 AVOIDING A SUNBURN

To get a suntan without damaging your skin, sunbathe for under half an hour your first few days out. After that, you should be able to stay out for longer periods. Avoid sunbathing at noon when the sun is directly overhead. Always use a lotion or cream that screens out the sun's ultraviolet rays. Choose a product with a high sun-protection factor number (SPF). Doctors believe that exposure to the sun's ultraviolet rays causes wrinkling of the skin and is the leading cause of skin cancer.

D12 CHILBLAINS

These occur on hands, feet, and ears. They are due to poor circulation in cold weather: skin tissue is injured by lack of blood, causing patches of swelling, redness, itchiness, and pain. The best prevention is avoidance of extreme cold; wearing of adequate clothing; and taking exercise to improve the circulation. If the skin does become white and numb through cold, it should be warmed slowly in water or by rubbing, and not by direct heat.

D13 RINGWORM

Ringworm is a fungus infection of the skin characterized by reddish areas. The four communicable diseases caused by fungus growth on the body's surface are ringworm of the feet, ringworm of the nails, ringworm of the body, and ringworm of the scalp. You can prevent ringworm of the skin by observing simple hygiene rules. To prevent athlete's foot and ringworm of the toenails: keep the feet clean and dry, and dust the feet frequently with a fungicidal powder. (See next page for a more detailed discussion of athlete's foot.) Ringworm of the body and of the scalp can be prevented by detection and treatment of infected persons or pets; by going to a barber who sterilizes his tools; by not wearing an infected person's hat, cap, or other clothing; and by not using other people's toilet articles. A doctor should be consulted in all cases of ringworm so that the infection can be eliminated.

Information from the U.S. Department of Health and Human Services, Center for Disease Control.

D14 ACNE

Acne is an infection of the hair follicle and sebaceous gland. It usually develops at puberty, when the sebaceous glands become more active. The disorder is confined to the face, neck, chest, and back, and consists of inflamed boils which produce pus and which scar when they heal.

Little can be done to prevent it, but there are medicines and lotions which can help make the skin peel and unblock the pores. Exposure to sunlight or ultra violet light can also help, because it makes the skin peel and, through tanning, at least helps to hide the spots.

Unlike blackheads, acne does not seem to respond to antiseptic soaps or lotions, or to careful diet.

D15 BOILS

Boils are caused by infected sweat glands or hair follicles, and often occur around sites of friction with clothing, eg on the neck or wrists. They develop as painful lumps, which increase in size and discharge pus.

Boils should never be squeezed or pierced except medically. A single boil should just be given protective dressing. A doctor is needed only if it is very painful, or the patient very young or old. But if a crop of boils occurs all at once or successively, consult a doctor.

Most boils subside spontaneously - antibiotics are not advisable unless the boils are very persistent or inflamed. An antiseptic solution may be applied around each boil to prevent further infection.

D16 DERMATITIS

Dermatitis is a general term for inflammation of the skin - usually resulting from exposure to a particular substance. Some substances normally have an irritating effect on people's skins; others only affect people who are allergic (hypersensitive) to them. An irritant reaction usually develops immediately. In an allergic reaction, there is normally a delay of 7 to 21 days between the first exposure to the offending substance, and the re-exposure which produces dermatitis.

With both types, frequent culprits include cosmetics, dyes, clothing, industrial chemicals, insecticides, detergents, paints, rubber, metal, plastic, and sometimes certain plants and foods. Many are encountered at work.

After contact with the offending substance, the blood vessels dilate and become porous. This allows fluid from the cells to collect in the skin and form blisters, which eventually rupture and expose the skin beneath. Later, the fluid dries out, and the area becomes encrusted. The skin thickens around the sores, and flakes off in scales.

Infection of the sores at any time can complicate the disease and produce pus.

If the cause of the dermatitis is identified, and the patient removed from it, the disease usually subsides and the skin returns to normal.

Recurrence can be prevented by avoiding or protecting against the substance responsible. In work circumstances, this may be done by wearing protective clothing and having special washing facilities.

"Eczema" is a word used for some chronic dermatitis, especially in babies and children. It is often due to a nervous condition or to an inherited food allergy.

D17 HIVES

Hives take the form of painful red swollen areas on the skin, varying in size from small spots to areas as large as a plate. They are an allergic disorder i.e. a sign that the person has an allergic reaction to something he has taken, usually a food or a drug. Hives can also be caused by dust or pollen, or by emotional stress.

An allergy can produce hives because the sensitive tissues of the skin react by releasing a chemical called histamine, which dilates the blood vessels. This increases the amount of fluid leaking to the skin, and results in lumps which itch.

Hives are not very serious, except in the form of "giant hives" - large swellings in the area of mouth and throat, which can interfere with breathing, and should be treated immediately by a doctor. Apart from this, hives are treated by applying soothing lotions, and finding and avoiding the cause of the allergic reactions.

Tranquilizers can be used, when emotional stress is the cause.

D18 ATHLETE'S FOOT

This is a common disorder, best avoided by keeping feet clean, dry, and cool, and avoiding contact with infected people and changing-room floors. It is caused by fungus infection, and first appears in the toe clefts: there may be splits and flaking, or pieces of dead white skin. The soles may also be involved. With some types of fungus it can also spread to legs and hands, forming irritating, white, flaking sores, which extend outwards while the inner part heals. Sweat helps the fungus grow, so the infection is more common in hot weather.

Athlete's foot can be difficult to get rid of. Treatment involves: rubbing away dead skin peelings; applying a mixture of water and medicinal alcohol; and drying the feet and using a dusting powder. A fungicidal ointment may be prescribed by a physician. The feet should be exposed to the air as often as possible, and clean socks of cotton or wool (not nylon) worn each day.

D19 PSORIASIS

Psoriasis usually affects the skin of elbows and knees, forearms, legs and scalp, but can develop in other parts of the body. It appears as red spots and patches, covered with loose, silvery scales. It is not serious, but can be disfiguring. The cause is large-scale production of an abnormal type of keratin. It takes 28 days for normal skin to produce a mature keratin cell, but only 4 days for a person with psoriasis. It is not known why this happens, but there may be a genetic link: psoriasis sometimes runs in families.

Psoriasis usually starts between the ages of 5 and 25, and lasts a lifetime, often appearing and disappearing intermittently. It affects both sexes equally, and is more common in cold climates. But it is not infectious, and does not affect general health; and, though persistant, does not usually spread to new parts of the body. Although there is no cure for psoriasis, it can be treated with crude coal-tar applied locally in conjunction with ultra-violet light. In very bad cases, drugs are used to slow down the growth rate of the epidermis cells, but they also act upon other tissues and so cannot be used as a complete therapy.

D

D20 VIRUS INFECTIONS

WARTS (verrucas) are especially common in childhood and old age. They are most frequent on hands, toes, face, and scalp. Also "plantar warts" grow on the soles of the feet, and "moist warts" on the genitals and anus. Most warts disappear after 3 to 24 months, but very persistent cases can be destroyed by freezing with carbon dioxide snow, or by dissolving in an appropriate solution.

COLD SORES are groups of lumps with red bases - typically around the mouth. The virus can lie dormant for long periods, and then be activated by illness, sunlight, or stress. Soothing lotions ease the irritation; and ointments can soften and shed the crusts.

D21 PERSPIRATION

One of the functions of skin is to regulate body temperature. Chemical activity in the internal organs constantly produces heat, and this must be dispersed or the body temperature will rise to a dangerous level: 85% of body heat is lost through the skin. During exposure to heat, blood vessels near the skin surface dilate. This allows warm blood to flow near the surface, and to lose its heat: by radiation, by convection, and by the evaporation of sweat.

Sweat is a clear fluid containing mostly water but also various chemicals and poisonous wastes that the body needs to get rid of. About ½ pint of sweat is excreted every day, under normal conditions, from the 2 to 5 million pores in the human skin. These are distributed all over the body, but there are more per square inch in the palms and soles than elsewhere. Each pore forms the opening for a sweat gland beneath the skin.

Fluid is also secreted from apocrine glands and sebaceous glands.

Apocrine glands are located at special sites, such as the armpits, the nipples, and around the genitals. They open into the hair follicle, and secrete a milky fluid. This contains fat and dries to form a glue-like substance. They begin to function at puberty. In early man the scent of the apocrine fluid was related to sexual attraction.

Sebaceous glands, in contrast, occur all over the body, except on the palms and soles - though there are more per square inch on the head than elsewhere. They secrete sebum, an oily substance, into each hair follicle, and this gives a waterproof and antiseptic barrier. They become more active at puberty.

D22 BODY ODOR

Body odor is caused by the bacteria which live in the sweat on the skin surface - especially sweat from the armpits and pubic area, which contains proteins and fatty materials favorable to bacterial growth. Odor also results simply from the oxidation of the fat in sweat when it contacts the air. Sweat from most other areas is basically just salt water, so few bacteria flourish - except on the feet, where socks and shoes create warm airless conditions.

Both sweating and body odor can be aggravated by obesity, highly spiced foods, alcohol, and coffee.

Dealing with body odor can involve regular washing and use of anti-bacterial soaps and deodorants or of anti-perspirants.

WASHING

The whole body or offending parts should be washed daily in soap and warm water. This removes bacteria and old perspiration.

ANTIBACTERIAL AGENTS

Chemical agents in deodorants and certain soaps slow the growth of bacteria.

With soaps, any lasting effect comes only from what remains in the pores after washing and rinsing. This may be enough to prevent bacteria on most parts of the body, but not in the armpits or crotch.

Deodorants are more effective, because they dry on the skin as they are applied, and can be concentrated on the relevant areas. The duration of protection depends on the product and the amount of sweat produced. Excess sweat washes away the chemical agent, but under normal conditions a good deodorant last 12 to 24 hours. However, the bacteria may eventually build up immunity to a given chemical. Changing brands fairly often prevents this, providing they contain different ingredients.

ANTI-PERSPIRANTS

These reduce the amount of perspiration. They block the pores, or swell the surrounding areas to shrink the pore size. Good cream, roll-on, or stick anti-perspirants reduce sweat output by 40%, and sprays by 20%. These are also the forms in which deodorants are made - in fact most contain some anti-perspirant, and most anti-perspirants contain some deodorant.

Both deodorants and anti-perspirants can cause skin irritation in some people. Changing the brand or the form of application usually solves this. Neither should be used if the relevant skin is broken.

FEET ODOR

This is a serious problem for a few people. Ordinary levels of foot odor can be dealt with by regular washing, drying thoroughly (especially between the toes), using foot deodorants or anti-perspirants, dusting the feet with anti-bacterial powder, changing socks daily, airing and changing shoes regularly, and going barefoot or wearing sandals whenever possible. Extreme levels of odor may require that socks are disinfected or boiled, and shoes disinfected regularly.

Washing for normal odor should be in warm water, and followed by a cold rinse. Extreme odor requires repeated alternate bathing of the feet in hot water (for 2 minutes) and then cold (for ½ minute).

D23 BLACKHEADS AND WHITEHEADS

A blackhead or whitehead appears when a pore in the skin becomes blocked, either by dust or dirt, or by overproduction of sebum in the sebaceous gland. It usually occurs on the face, neck or shoulders.
The waxy plug that blocks the pore is called a comedo. This forms a blackhead when its contents are open to the air: oxidation turns the head of the comedo black. If it is not open to the air, a whitehead is formed.
The pore may be cleaned by gently pressing out its contents, if this is done soon after the plug is formed. But care should be taken not to damage the skin. An extractor - a small, shaped piece of metal - can be bought from a chemist for the purpose of applying pressure, and the area affected should be washed first in warm soapy water to loosen the plugs and swell the pores.
If a pore is not cleaned, the sebum, unable to reach the surface, ruptures the follicle, and the surrounding dermis becomes inflamed and infected. Touching an infected spot can spread the trouble from one area to another.
Blackhead sufferers should:
wash their faces with antiseptic soap, especially after clearing the pores;
avoid greasy foods and cosmetics;
and get plenty of fresh air and sunlight, and fresh fruits and vegetables.

D24 PLASTIC SURGERY

The main uses of plastic surgery are:
a) to correct congenital defects, such as cleft palate or hare lip;
b) to correct defects due to muscular atrophy, paralysis, and other illness;
c) to restore damaged skin and bones after burns and accidents; and
d) to alter the features of the face and body to make the owner appear younger or more presentable (cosmetic surgery).
Here we are mainly concerned with with the last of these. Cosmetic surgery can remove baggy, wrinkled skin, and change the shape of nose, chin, and ears. It is probably more sensible to be content with the faces we are born with. The product of plastic surgery is hardly likely to be "a mirror of the soul". Still, some people do feel that they suffer from disfigurements that they would be happier without.
FACELIFTS remove deep folds of skin around the jaws and mouth. An incision is made from the temple, down in front of the ear, to the nape of the neck. The flap of skin is pulled taut, the excess trimmed off, and the remainder stitched back in place.
EYELID OPERATIONS remove excess skin and fatty tissue from the upper and lower eyelids. The technique is similar to facelifts.
NOSE SURGERY can correct the bridge line, shorten the nose, build up a depressed nose, straighten a crooked one, or alter the shape of the tip. All involve shaving back or implanting extra bone or cartilage. The incisions are made inside the nose, and the final new shape takes about 6 months to settle.
CHIN SURGERY can correct receding chins by implanting silicone, bone, or cartilage over the jaw to extend it.
EAR SURGERY can correct ears that stick out too far. An ellipse of skin is removed from the back of the ear, and the cartilage beneath is trimmed.
DERMABRASION is removal of skin that has been pock-marked by severe acne, smallpox, etc. The old skin is removed by a high speed rotating brush. Crusts form, and peel after 5 days to 2 weeks, revealing a new layer of pink skin beneath. Success depends on the depth and nature of the problem, and the skin's reaction to treatment.
All plastic surgery requires time for healing and for scars and bruises to disappear. Protective bandages may be needed at first. For some operations, hospitalization is necessary.

D25 HAIR

Hair is found over the whole surface of the human body except the palms, soles, and parts of the genitals.
There are three types of hair - scalp hair, body hair, and sexual hair.
Scalp hair resembles the body hair of other mammals. Human body hair is very fine and usually less pigmented. Sexual hair develops around the genitals, the armpits, and (in men) the face. Its growth is dependent on the male sex hormones produced by both sexes in puberty.
The number of hairs on the body varies between individuals, but on average there are about 100,000 hairs on the head.

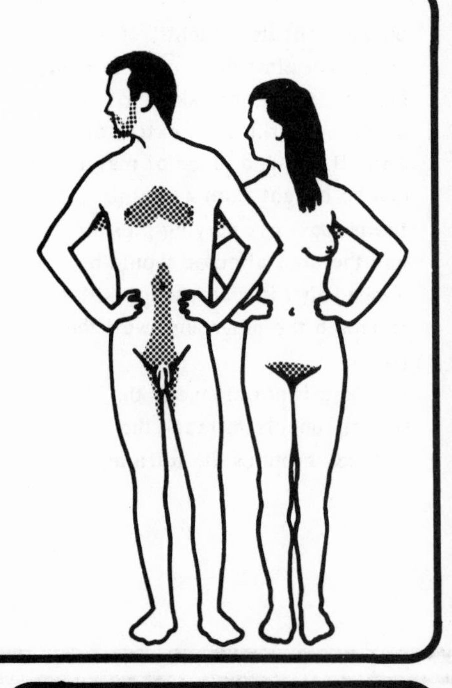

D26 THE HAIR ROOT

a Hair shaft
b Sebaceous gland
c Hair follicle
d Erector muscle

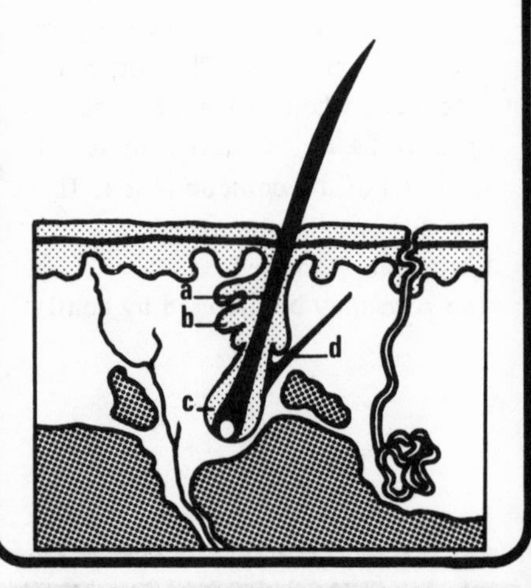

D27 WHAT HAIR DOES

Hair acts as a protective barrier.
The eyelashes protect the eyes and hairs in the nostrils and outer ears trap and prevent the entry of foreign bodies.
The eyebrows prevent sweat dripping into the eyes.
Hair also acts to conserve heat.
Air trapped between hairs insulates the skin and stops heat loss.
The straighter the hair stands the more air can be trapped.
Attached to each hair follicle is a strip of muscle which makes the hair stand on end when it contracts, causing "goose flesh". These muscles are stimulated by cold or emotional stress.

D28 HAIR GROWTH

Hair is made out of keratin, a tough type of protein.
It grows out of follicles in the skin.
All these follicles are established at birth and no new ones are formed later in life.
The root of the hair is the only live part of the hair: it grows and pushes the dead hair shaft out of the skin.
Hair growth is cyclical with a growth phase followed by a rest phase in which the hair is loosened.
A new hair then pushes it out.
30-100 hairs are lost from the scalp each day. In an adult scalp the growth phase is about 3 years and the rest phase is 3 months.
Hair growth is irregular and at different stages all over the body.
Head hair rarely exceeds 3ft in length.

D29 SCALP MASSAGE

Massaging the scalp with the tips of the fingers increases the blood flow to the massaged area. This stimulates the follicles and can aid hair growth. It also means that the scalp is kept more healthy, with a greater supply of nutrients and speedier removal of waste products.
In scalp massage, it is important that the fingers do not slide over the scalp. This exerts pressure on the hair and can damage it.
Massage should move the scalp in relation to the skull - not the hair in relation to the scalp. If possible, the hair should be combed so that the fingers can get into direct contact with the part of the scalp to be massaged.
Massage can go from the neck upwards to the crown, and then again from the temples back to the crown, thus covering the whole scalp.

D30 HAIR COLOR

Pigment production in the hair follicle slows down with age and often ceases, so that the individual hair becomes colorless. A grey hair has colorless sections mixed in with colored; when all the hair is colorless it appears white. The tendency to "go grey" is inherited and some people go grey sooner than others. There is no known way to stimulate pigment production once it has ceased.

D31 HAIR TYPES

The three primary ethnic groups display different hair shapes. Oriental hair is round in cross-section, and therefore straight. Caucasian hair is kidney-shaped in cross-section, and so usually wavy, the degree being dependent on the extent of the curve of the follicle. In negroid hair a highly curved follicle gives the hair a flattened oval shape in cross-section, and causes it to be extremely curly. Interracial breeding has produced many variations on these three basic types. The texture (fine, wiry, etc) and condition of the hair also affects its shape.

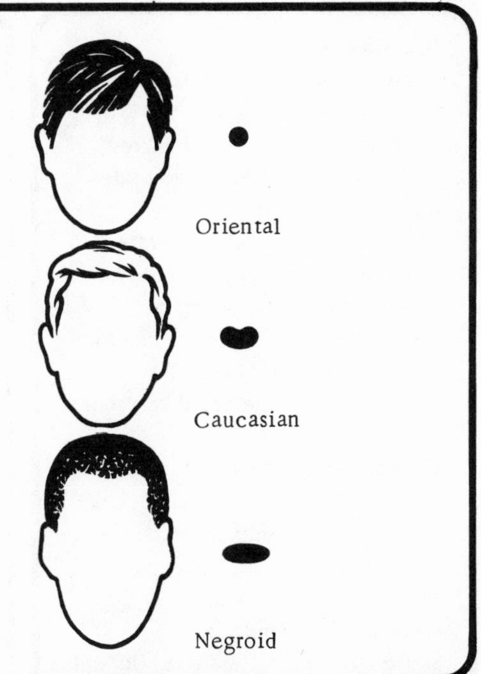

D32 HAIR LICE

Two species of lice affect humans: phthirus pubis, found in the pubic hair (see Sexual infections, C46); and pediculus humanus, found in the hair on the head. The latter can be acquired not only by contact with an infected person, but also via objects such as combs and hats.

The infestation causes severe itching. It is most easily diagnosed by examining the scalp for the tiny eggs ("nits"), attached to the hair shafts. The lice themselves are more difficult to find. Suitable treatment should be obtained from a physician or pharmacist: it will include a shampoo and often also a scalp emulsion. The eggs are hard to kill, and treatment should be repeated at intervals until completely successful.

D33 HAIR CARE

DO

(a) Keep the hair clean. Oily hair should be washed every 2-3 days, dry hair every 5-6 days. Choose the shampoo according to type and condition of your hair.

(b) Ensure that the comb is clean and well made. Unclean combs spread bacteria and infection. Sharp edges damage the structure of the hair.

(c) Take care when the hair is wet: it is more vulnerable and prone to pulling and splitting in this state. Comb gently.

(d) Check the condition of the scalp, looking for itching, inflammation, scaling, dandruff, or degeneration. Visit a general practitioner or dermatologist if worried. Also avoid mental stress if possible, as this can damage the hair.

(e) Remain as healthy as possible, physically and emotionally.

DON'T

(a) Choose your shampoo for superficial reasons. A too strong shampoo can damage the hair and leave the scalp dry and itchy. If too weak, it will not clean the hair properly.

(b) Brush your hair unless you have to. Brushing pulls and twists hair, damaging its structure and splitting its ends.

(c) Tug at tangles, especially when wet. If hair gets tangled, start from the ends of the hair and comb gently, eliminating the tangles as you near the roots.

(d) Worry about the few hairs left on the comb or in the shower. Hair is constantly being shed and replaced.

(e) Cultivate diet fads, thinking they will benefit your hair. A normal healthy diet* provides all the nourishment necessary.

D34 DANDRUFF

There are two kinds of dandruff. The first, affecting about 60% of the population to a mild degree, takes the form of fine, dry scales which fall from the scalp.
The second kind, which is rarer, takes the form of thick, greasy scales adhering to the scalp.
The cause of both types is unknown and there is no real cure for dandruff, but there are things that can be done to control it.
Washing with ordinary shampoo may not be enough, in which case a medicated shampoo can be used. These shampoos are designed to remove the scales and delay the recurrence of dandruff.
Some have a simple antiseptic and others contain stronger chemicals. If none of these succeed in controlling the dandruff, it may be caused by a skin disorder or some other condition that a doctor can treat.

D35 HAIR LOSS CLINICS

There are a large number of clinics suggesting various kinds of treatment, which can include creams, lotions, massage, shampoos, and ultra-violet and infra-red radiation.
Courses of these treatments are expensive; but there are no known medical grounds for them. In fact, there is a risk of being wrongly diagnosed, and being given inappropriate treatment for a condition that could be dealt with by a physician.

D36 BALDNESS

If the hairs lost every day from the scalp are not replaced by normal hairs but by fine, downy hair, then baldness will result. This happens in varying degrees to nearly all men and women.
Hair can be lost for various reasons.
Physical ailments that cause hair loss include:
scars or burns that destroy the hair follicles;
skin disturbances, such as dermatitis, psoriasis, or allergic reactions;
general bodily ailments, such as serious anemia;
and chemical pollution of the body (as in mercury poisoning).
Hair loss can also be caused by mental stress. This is because hair growth is linked with hormonal production, which in turn is closely linked to one's emotional state. The hair grows back when the period of stress is over.
In the above cases, by treating the illness, hair will usually be restored. But the commonest type of hair loss is male-pattern baldness. This is caused by a male hormone influenced by hereditary ageing factors. Nothing, short of castration, can be done about this condition! Not only can it not be reversed but it cannot be stopped or even slowed down by any means so far discovered.

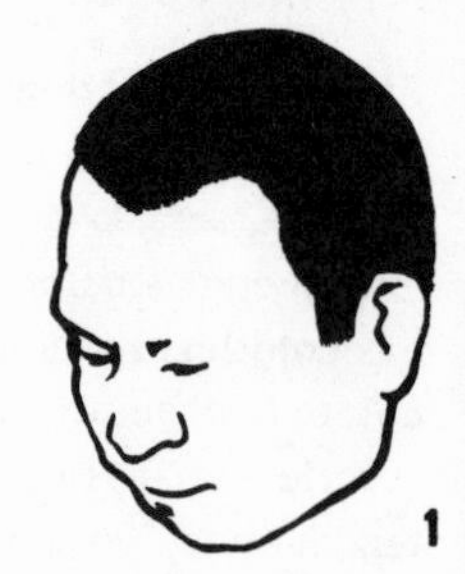
1

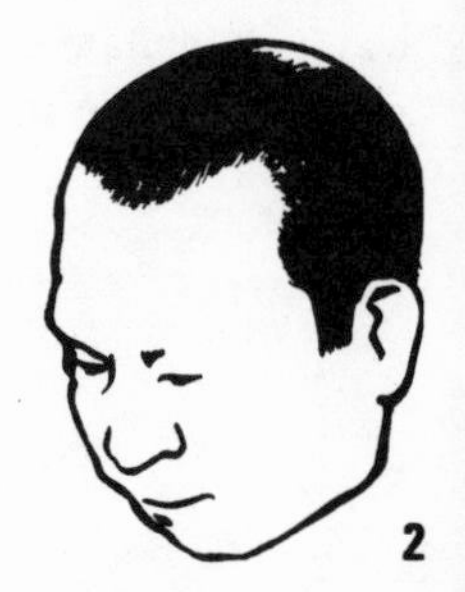
2

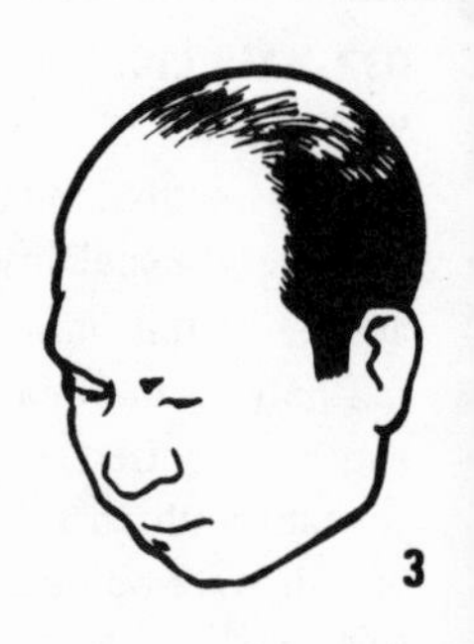
3

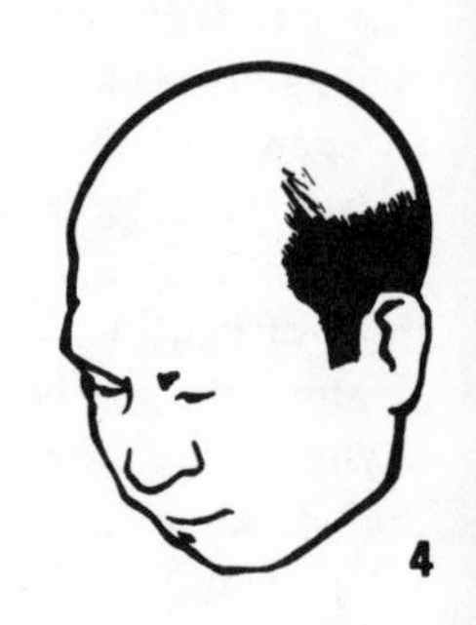
4

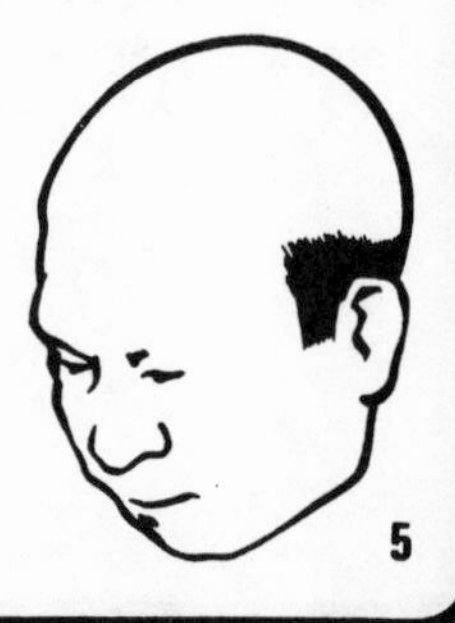
5

D37 TOUPEES

This is the traditional way of concealing hair loss.
The hairpiece is built from a base shaped to the bald area. Hair is attached to this base and cut to match the rest of the hair. The base can be hard or soft. The hard type is made from fiberglass or plastic. The soft type is made out of silk, cotton, Terylene, or nylon netting.
Human hair is usually used but animal hair can be added to give a special color or texture.
The hairpiece is fixed onto the scalp with strips of double-sided sticky tape. This makes it unlikely to move accidentally.
Two hairpieces are usually needed: one to wear when the other needs to be cleaned or repaired. This adds considerably to the cost.
The main advantages of wearing a hairpiece are - hopefully - a more youthful appearance and a gain in confidence. Hairpieces also serve some of the true functions of hair: keeping the scalp warm and protecting it from the sun.
The disadvantages of wearing a hairpiece are:
discomfort from perspiration;
fear of the hairpiece getting unstuck, or being disarranged by the wind - and embarrassment if it does;
having to protect the hairpiece from strong sunlight, in case it fades or changes color;
and the time and expense involved in its care.
A good hairpiece has to match the color and texture of the surrounding hair, fit the scalp perfectly, look natural, stand up to sunlight and rain, stick firmly to the head, be easy to clean, and last for several years. A bad hairpiece reveals itself to observers by a bad color match, unnatural parting, or hard front hairline.

D38 HAIR WEAVING

This is another way of covering up baldness. It is also known as hair linking, hair extension, and hair replacement.
There are two methods. In the first, a hairpiece is made in the normal way, and then attached to the scalp by stitching the sides of it to the normal hair.
In the second, threads are strung across the bald area, from one side to the other, and pieces of hair, sewn together in clumps, are woven directly into this.
In both cases, around the edge of the area to be concealed, the existing hair is gathered and woven into a strengthened line, to take the strain of the hairweave.
The fitting takes from 2 to 4 hours. In addition, as the existing hair grows, the hairweave gets looser, and so about every 6 weeks - sometimes more often - it has to be taken off and refitted.
The basic cost, and the need for frequent return visits, make the process expensive. Also the continual pulling of the hairweave on the natural hair can help speed up hair loss. Washing of the hairweave can be a lengthy business, as it tends to get tangled and cannot be combed hard.
Because of this difficulty, the hair is often not washed enough, which means that the scalp is irritated by dirt, dead skin, and soap not washed out.

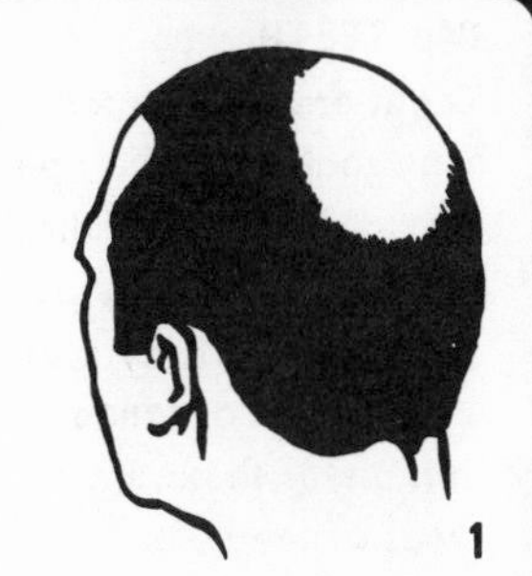
1

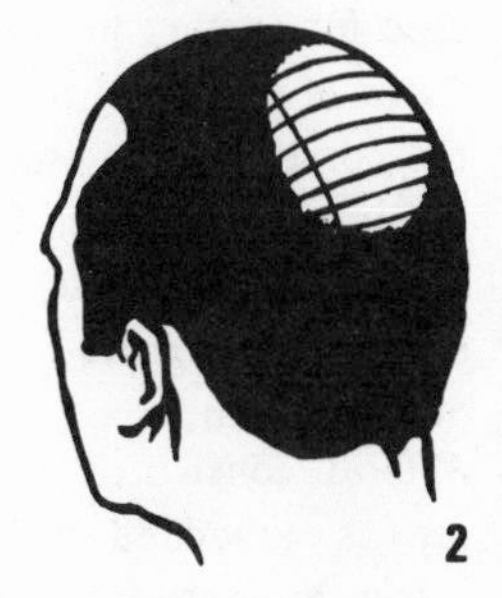
2

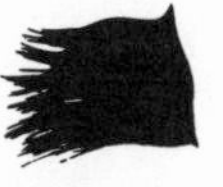
weft

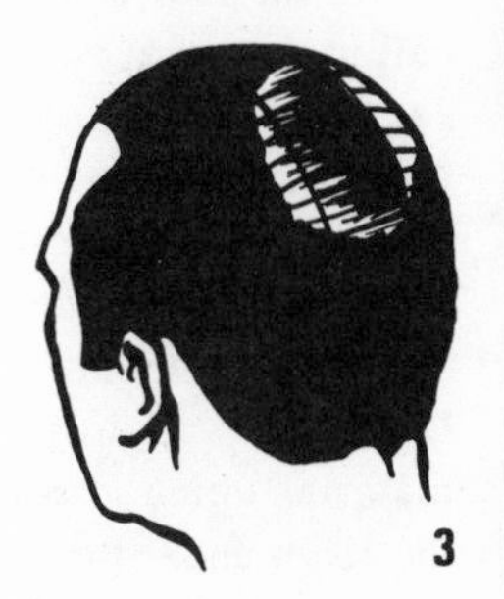
3

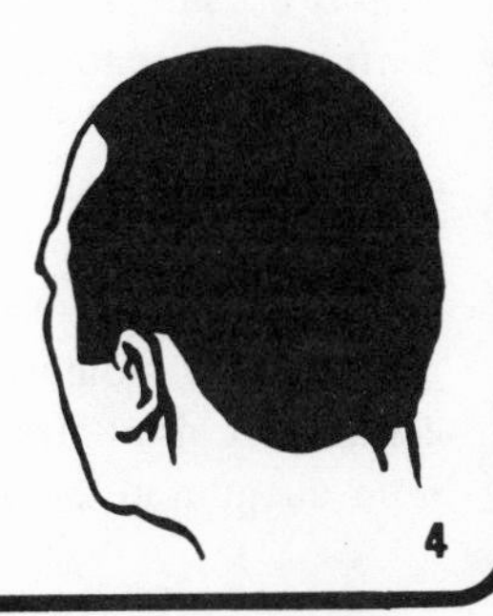
4

D39 HAIR TRANSPLANT

This is a recent technique. Hair follicles are surgically removed from parts where there is abundant hair, and implanted into the bald areas. But there is no guarantee that they will grow in their new location.

a Recipient site
b Donor site

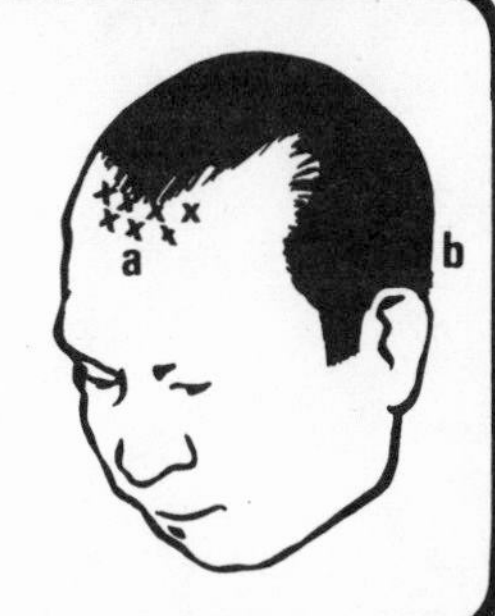

TEETH 1

D40 TEETH

Teeth are hard structures set in bony sockets in the upper and lower jaws. Their main function is to chew and prepare food for swallowing. They also help in the articulation of sounds in speech.
In humans there are three main types of teeth.
Incisors are sharp, chisel-like teeth at the front of the mouth, used for cutting into food.
Canines are round pointed teeth at the corners of the mouth, used for tearing and gripping food.
Molars are square teeth with small cusps, which grind food at the back of the mouth.
A tooth consists of two parts: the root is embedded in the jaw; the crown projects out of the jaw.
Where the root and crown meet is called the neck.
Each tooth is made up of enamel, dentine, pulp, and cementum.
Enamel is the hardest tissue in the body, and it protects the sensitive crown of the tooth.
Dentine is a slightly elastic material which forms the bulk of the tooth under the enamel. It is sensitive to heat and chemicals.
Pulp is the soft tissue inside the dentine, and contains nerves and blood vessels, which enter the root of the tooth by a small canal.
Cementum is a thin layer of material which covers the root of the tooth and protects the underlying dentine. It also helps attach fibers from the gum to the tooth.

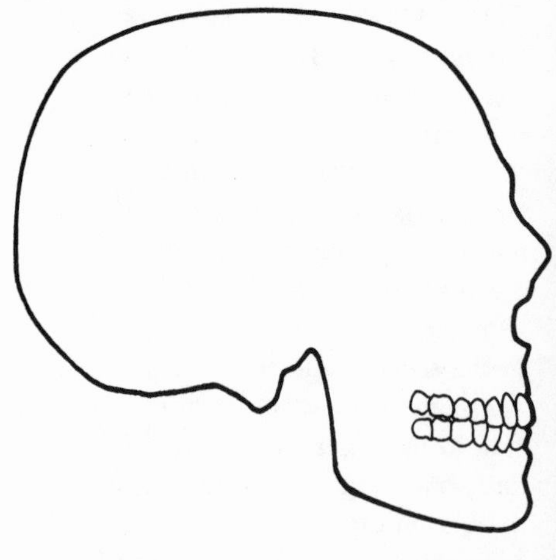

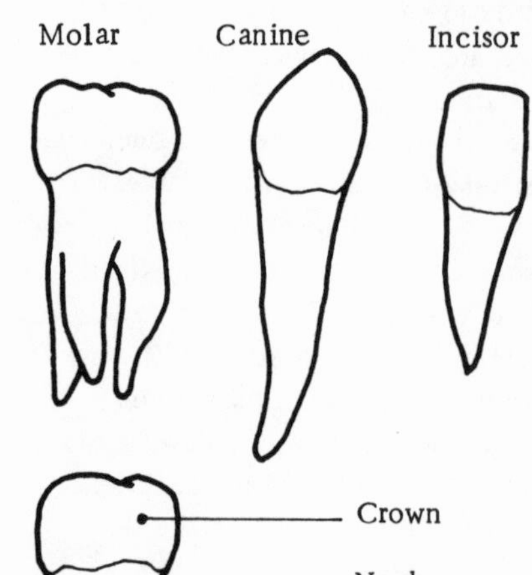

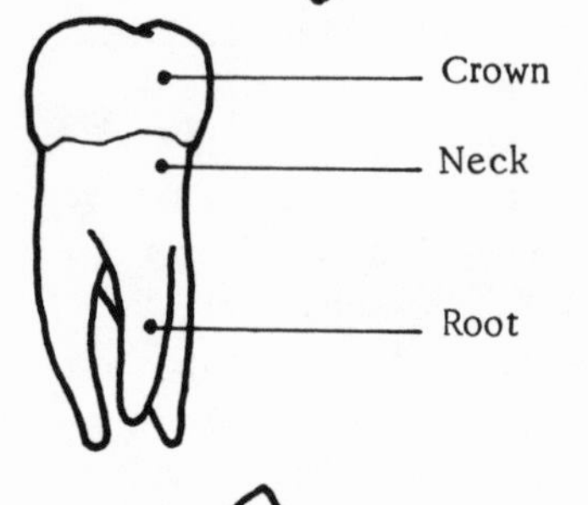

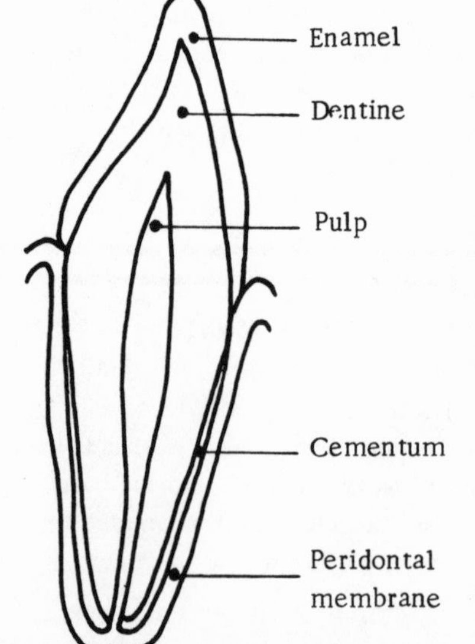

D41 THE TEETH WE'RE GIVEN

In humans there are two successive sets of teeth. The primary or "milk" set arrive 6 to 24 months after birth. Later they gradually fall out, from the age of 6 on, as the permanent teeth appear. Most of these are out by the age of 13, but the 3rd molar or "wisdom tooth" can erupt as late as the age of 25, or never.
Human teeth do not keep growing, but reach a certain size and then stop. Also, when the permanent teeth fall out, they are not replaced by a new set. But in some animals, such as the rabbit, the incisors keep growing, as they are worn down by use, while the shark grows set after set of teeth - to its great advantage!

AGE OF APPEARANCE

These are average figures only: actual dates vary greatly from child to child.

PRIMARY TEETH		
Central incisors	6 to 8 months	**1**
Lateral incisors	9 to 11 months	**2**
Eye teeth	18 to 20 months	**4**
First molars	14 to 17 months	**3**
Second molars	24 to 26 months	**5**
ADULT TEETH		
Central incisors	7 to 8 years	**2**
Lateral incisors	8 to 9 years	**3**
Canines	12 to 14 years	**6**
First premolars	10 to 12 years	**4**
Second premolars	10 to 12 years	**5**
First molars	6 to 7 years	**1**
Second molars	12 to 16 years	**7**
Third molars	17 to 21 years	**8**

The key numbers give the typical order of appearance.

Primary teeth

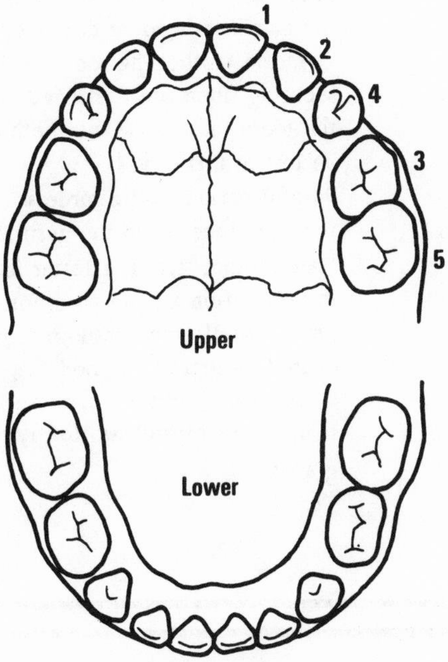

1
2
4
3
5

Upper

Lower

Looking into the mouth

Right

Left

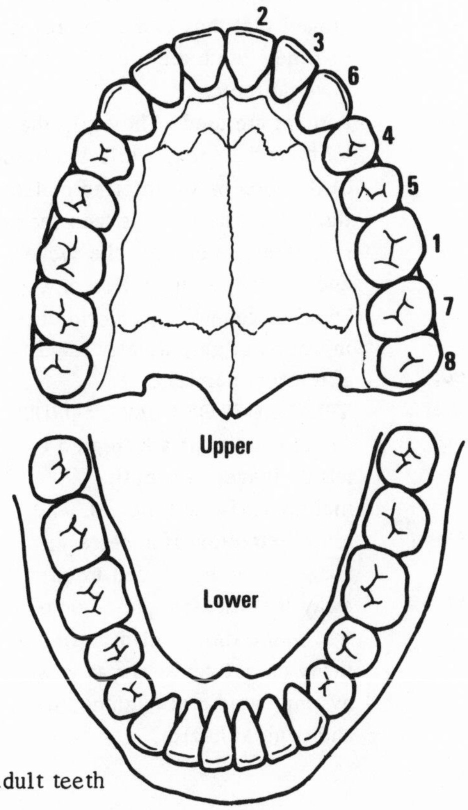

2
3
6
4
5
1
7
8

Upper

Lower

Adult teeth

Sequence of appearance (upper jaw)

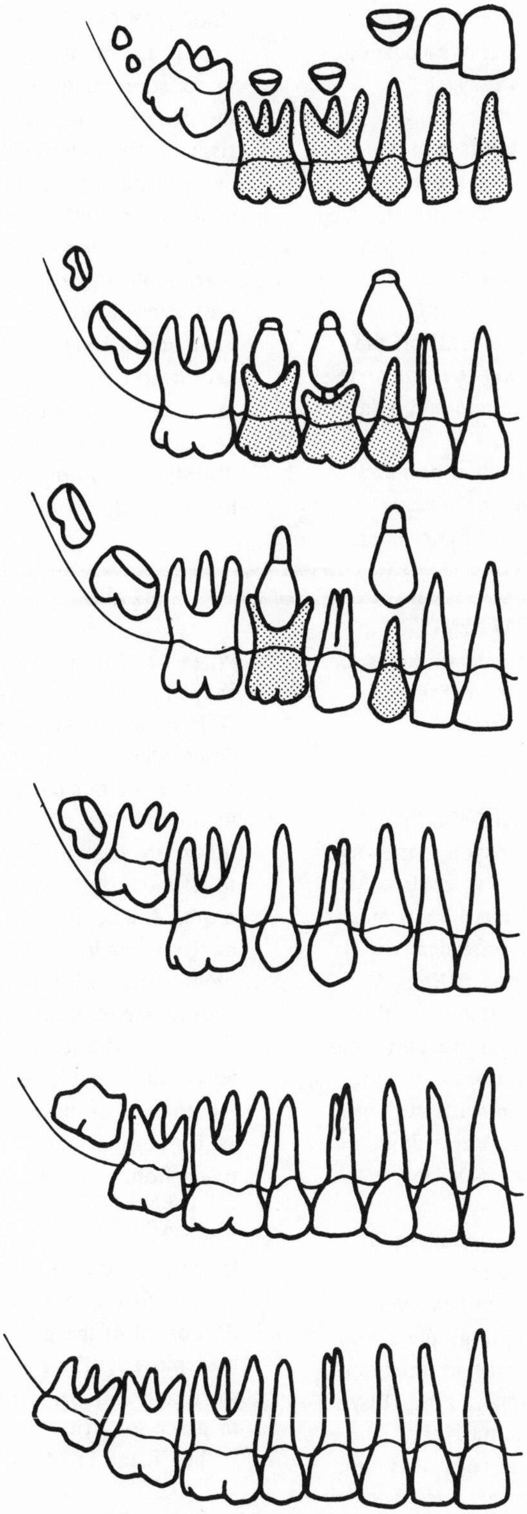

5 years

8 years

9 years

11 years

13 years

Adult

D42 DENTAL DISORDERS

Tooth decay is the most universal of human diseases. It especially afflicts those who eat a highly refined diet which is overcooked, soft, sweet, and sticky.

Bacteria in the mouth change carbohydrates in the food into acids strong enough to attack tooth enamel. Gradually the enamel is broken down and bacteria invades the dentine, forming a "cavity."

The pulp reacts by forming secondary dentine to wall off the bacteria, but without treatment the pulp becomes inflamed and painful (toothache).

The infection may then pass down the root and cause an "abscess" - a painful collection of pus under pressure, affecting the gum and face tissues.

PERIODONTAL DISEASE

This is a general term for disorders in the supporting structures of teeth: the gums, cementum, and other tissues. The commonest cause is overconsumption of soft food, which cannot stimulate and harden the gums. Other causes include sharp food which scratches the gums, inefficient brushing, badly-contoured fillings, ill-fitting dentures, irregular teeth, and teeth deposits. General factors such as vitamin deficiencies, blood disorders, and drug use may also be involved.

Periodontal diseases may be painless, but, if allowed to progress, the gum can become detached from the tooth. The socket enlarges, securing fibers are destroyed, and the tooth loosens. Many teeth can be lost in this way.

Painful periodontal disorders include abscesses in the gum and "periocoronitis." The latter is inflammation around an erupting tooth (usually the "wisdom tooth"), caused by irritation, food stagnation, pressure, or infection. It may accompany swollen lymph glands.

D43 DENTAL TREATMENT

The dentist's intricate work has to be carried out in the confined, dark, wet, and sensitive environment of the mouth.

FILLING CAVITIES

Tooth decay is dealt with by drilling out the decayed matter and filling up the resulting cavity. All decayed and weakened areas must be removed, otherwise decay will continue beneath the filling. Also the cavity must be shaped so that the filling will stay in securely and withstand pressure from chewing.

High speed electric drills are now usual, and so is the use of injected local anesthetic to make the procedure painless.

A lining of chemical cement is put in the prepared cavity to protect the pulp from heat and chemicals. The filling, placed on top of this, is usually an amalgam of silver, tin, copper, zinc alloy, and mercury. Alternatively, translucent silicate cement is used, for its natural appearance - but, since it can wear away, this cannot be used on grinding surfaces.

When the filling has hardened, it is shaped, and any excess trimmed off.

OTHER RESTORATIVE WORK

Some other replacement work can be prepared outside the mouth, and then cemented into place.

Inlays are cast gold fillings, shaped to fit a cavity in the crown of a tooth. A wax impression of the cavity is made, and the resulting mould filled with molten gold.

Crowns are extensive coverings to the crown of a tooth, made of porcelain or gold. The whole of the enamel of the tooth is removed, an impression made, and the crown made from a model.

PULP AND ROOT CANAL TREATMENT

If the pulp or root canal is decayed, normal fillings are complicated. Part or all of the pulp may have to be removed. The root canal is sterilized and a silver pin sealed in place to fill it. The pulp cavity is then filled in.

EXTRACTION

Teeth need to be removed if they are irretrievably decayed, or so broken that they cannot be repaired, or if new teeth are erupting and have no room.

Forceps are used. They grip the tooth at the neck, while the blades of the forceps are inserted under the gum. The tooth is then moved repeatedly to enlarge the socket, and finally can be pulled out.

Local or general anesthetic, by injection or gas, usually makes extraction painless.

TREATMENT OF GUM DISORDERS

Acute conditions are treated by pus drainage, antiseptic mouthwashes, antibiotics, and tooth extraction if necessary.

Surgery may be needed to cut away the diseased gum. Long-term treatment aims at eliminating as many causative factors as possible, by improving oral hygiene, diet, and general health.

D44 THE TEETH WE LOSE

Here we show the average fate of western teeth. For example, upper right 3 is sound in over 60% of adults, treated in over 10%, decayed in about 5%, and missing in the remainder. Upper right 6, in contrast, is missing in about 55%.

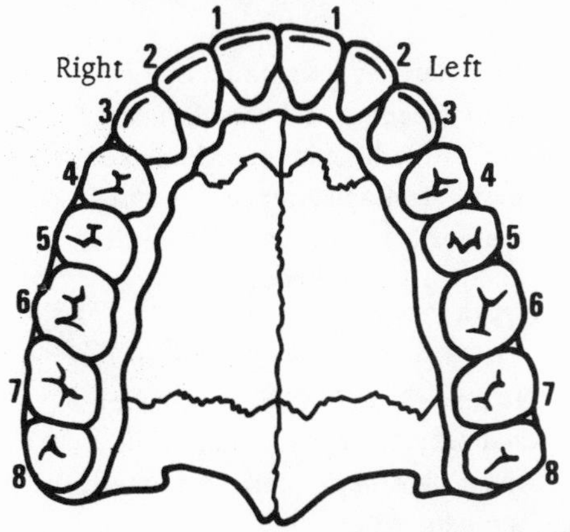

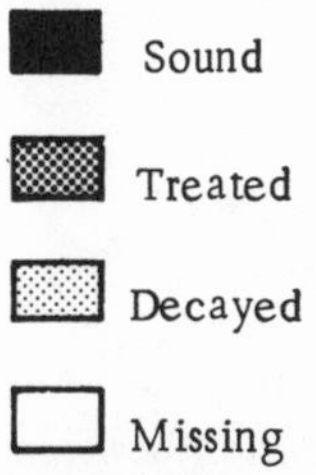

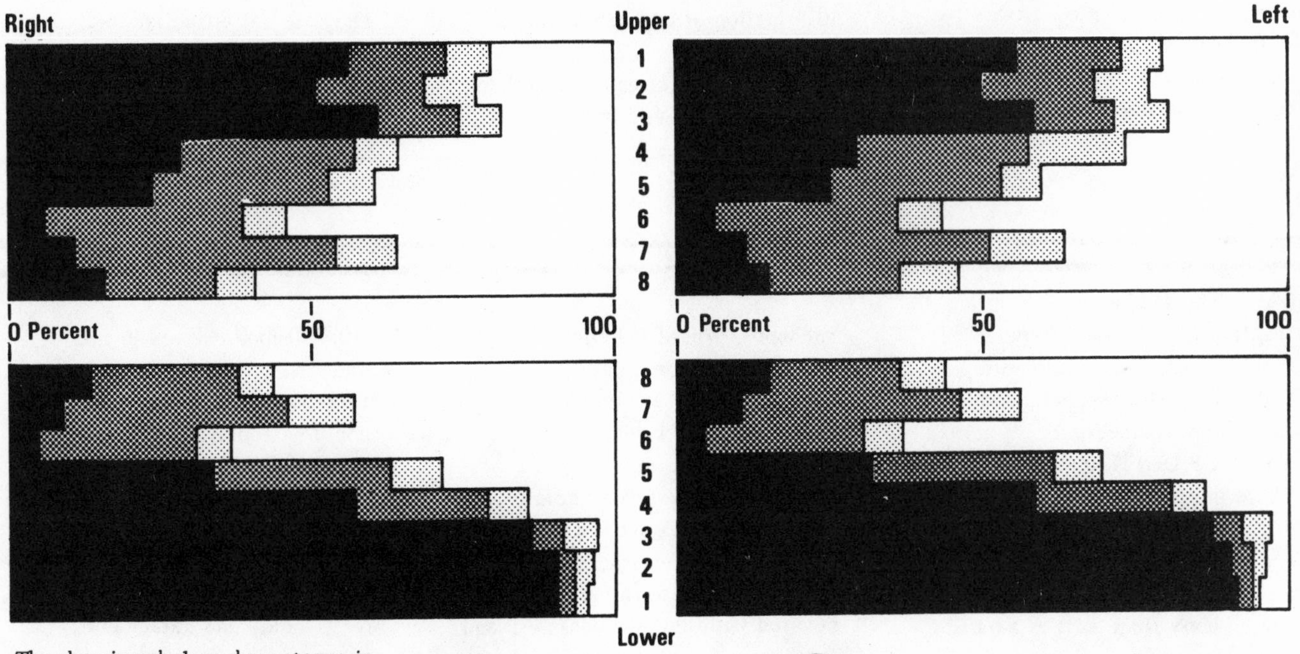

The drawings below show stages in the progress of dental disorder. Different stages are shown in different teeth. For example, tooth decay (below right) is only a spot in the incisor on the left of the row. In the center tooth (a molar), it has reached the dentine; in the next, the pulp; and in the last, the roots.

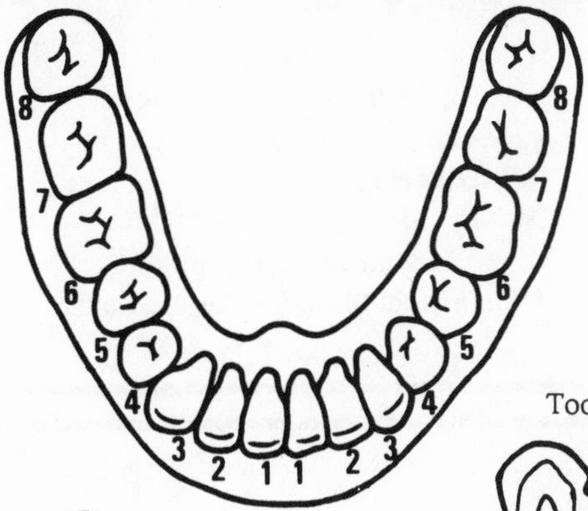

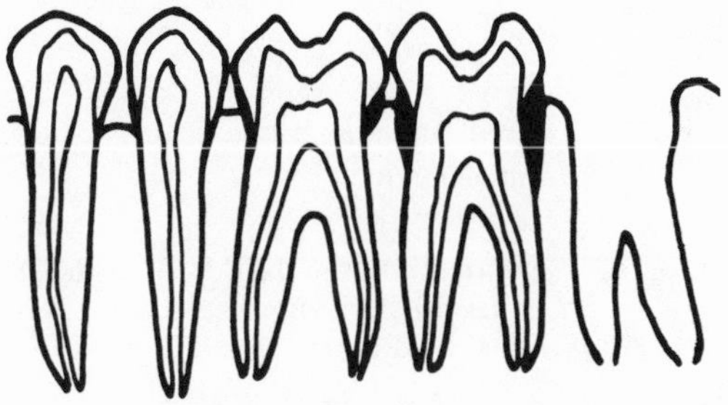

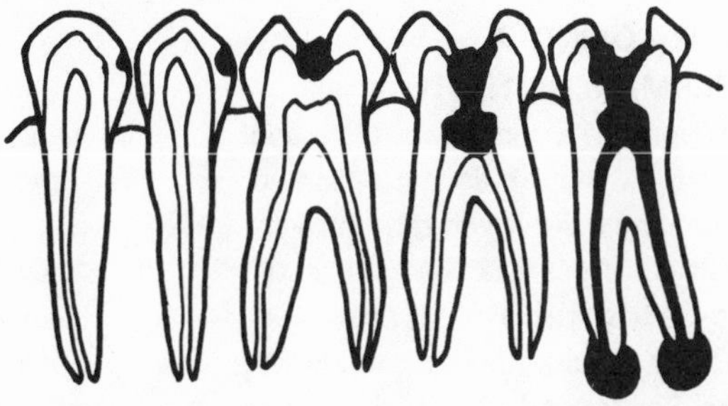

D45 ORTHODONTICS

This is the branch of dentistry concerned with preventing and correcting irregularities of the teeth, eg variations in the number of teeth and abnormalities in their shape, size, position, and spacing. All these can cause defects in eating, swallowing, speech, and breathing.

Malocclusion is the typical example. This means that the teeth are not in the normal position when the jaws are closed, relative to those in the opposite jaw. Teeth may stick out or in, or there may be spaces between the biting surfaces due to uneven growth of teeth or jaws.

Irregularities may be caused by: bottle feeding and thumb sucking; loss of teeth, non-appearance of teeth, and appearance of extra teeth; birth injuries and heredity; and disease and poor health.

TREATMENT

Treatment may be long-term, but it is needed if the health, function, and esthetic appearance of the mouth are to be preserved. Methods include:

elimination of bad habits such as thumb-sucking;

practice of exercises to strengthen certain muscles and improve mouth movements;

relief of overcrowded teeth by extraction;

surgery on the soft tissues or bones to recontour the jaws.

But the commonest technique is to attach "braces" or similar appliances to the teeth, to apply continual pressure and so make them shift position. The braces, made of steel bands, wires, springs, or bands of elastic, may have to be worn for up to two years or more. They are not attractive and, if cemented in position, can make cleaning the teeth difficult. They are also more effective in the young than in older people.

D46 FALSE TEETH

Ideally, false teeth ("dentures") should preserve normal chewing and biting, clear speech, and facial appearance.

TYPES OF DENTURES

These include full sets, partial dentures, and immediate dentures.

For the construction of a full set, all the teeth are removed, and the healed bony ridge acts as a base. Impressions of both jaws are made in warm wax, and these give the basic patterns from which the dentures are made up.

With partial dentures, the new teeth are attached to surviving natural ones to keep them anchored. Where the anchoring teeth are not immediately alongside, they are linked to the false teeth by a bridge.

With immediate dentures, the false teeth are prepared before the teeth being lost have been removed. After extraction the empty sockets are immediately covered with the new dentures, and healing takes place beneath. A new set is then needed after about 6 months, as the ridge where teeth have been extracted shrinks.

USING DENTURES

Dentures can be uncomfortable. To avoid gum soreness, new dentures should at first be used only, with soft food chewed in small amounts.

If soreness does occur, the dentist should be consulted. The dentures should not be left out of the mouth for more than a day or two, or the remaining natural teeth may begin to shift position.

False teeth should be brushed after every meal, and detachable dentures should be soaked overnight in water containing salt or a denture cleaner.

The wearer can regain his usual articulacy by practicing reading aloud.

D47 LOSING A PERMANENT TOOTH

If you lose a permanent tooth and its root, you can have it replanted in many cases if you take quick action. If possible, have the tooth replanted within a half hour by a dentist. Rinse the tooth well with cold water and wipe it with a clean moist handkerchief or linen. Be careful to preserve gum fibers. Place back in the socket. Make an emergency appointment with a dentist.

Or you can place the tooth in a glass of cold water with ½ teaspoon of salt and take it to a dentist immediately.

Information from the U.S. Department of Health and Human Services, National Institutes of Health.

D48 PREVENTING DENTAL TROUBLE

DIET

At any age, the ideal diet for dental health should be:
well balanced and adequate, so general health is maintained;
chewable enough to stimulate the gums; and
low in sugar content.

The balance and adequacy of the diet is especially important in the case of expectant mothers and growing children, so strong teeth form.

ORAL HYGIENE

Teeth should be cleaned at least twice a day: after breakfast, and last thing at night. But it is better if they are cleaned after every meal. Cleaning polishes the teeth and removes stains and food debris.

Methods of cleaning vary from culture to culture. The toothbrush can be used ineffectively, and even cause damage (electric toothbrushes tend to be better). The value of toothpaste is doubtful, and it can give a misleading "clean feeling". Brushing with salt stimulates the gums and cleans just as effectively. "Dental floss", or toothpicks of soft wood, are valuable for dislodging food between the teeth. Highly effective techniques used elsewhere include the fibrous chewing stick used in Africa, and the Moslem tradition of rubbing teeth and gums with a towel.

DENTAL INSPECTIONS

Regular visits to the dentist about every 6 months catch disease in its early stages and so avoid drastic measures in the future.

FLUORIDE

Fluoride is a tasteless, odorless, colorless chemical, which, if added to the drinking water in small amounts, reduces decay in children by 60%. (Excessive amounts can cause the enamel to become mottled.) In the USA, 60 million people now drink water with fluoride added, and 7 million others drink it naturally. Some toothpastes contain fluoride, and tablets can be bought to add to unfluoridated water. So far, no ill effects of the use of fluoride in these quantities have been established, but it only benefits the teeth of children under 14.

D

D49 CLEANING OUR TEETH

HOW TO BRUSH

Most people use scrubbing motions, backward and forward and up and down.

Backward and forward strokes with the brush length are good for the tops of the molars (a), and the back of the front teeth (b).

But on the side teeth, use the brush sideways in a repeated stroke in one direction - upward on the bottom teeth (c), and downward on the top ones (d).

HOW TO FLOSS

By flossing in the morning after breakfast and in the evening after dinner, you keep your teeth and gums in good shape. Take a long piece of dental floss or dental tape. Wind it around a finger of each hand (see right). Then work floss up and down between all teeth, being sure to clean below the gumlines (see drawing far right). Use new floss when necessary. Afterward, gargle with water.

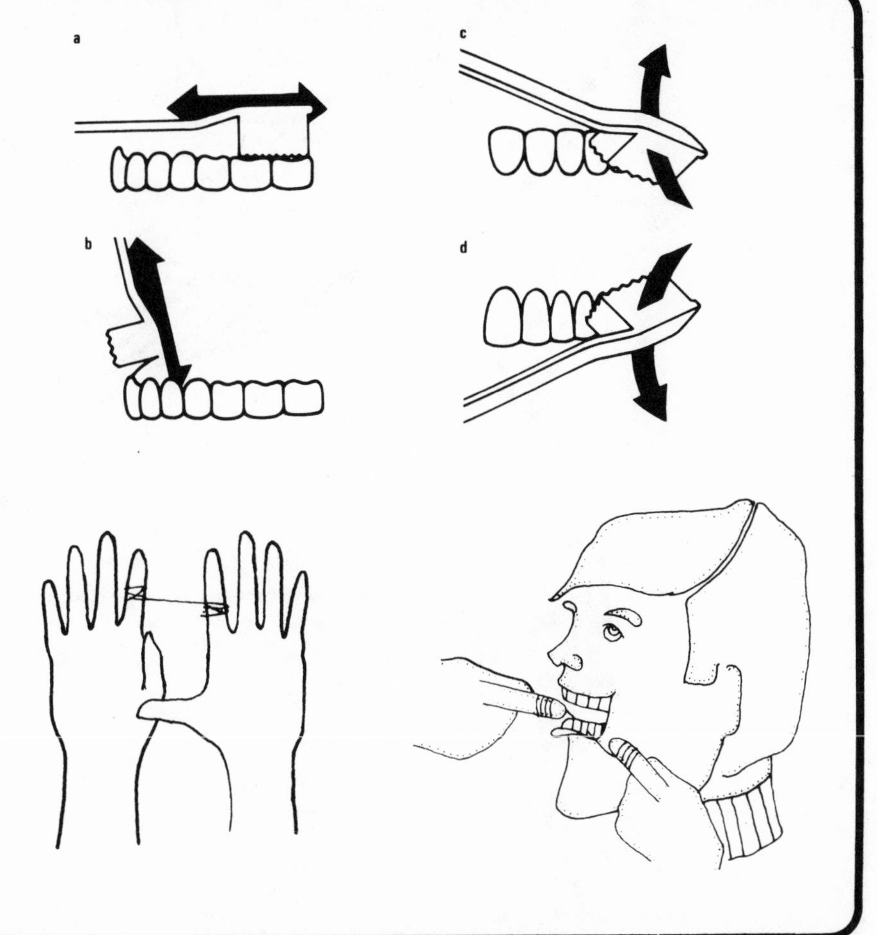

E01 THE BRAIN

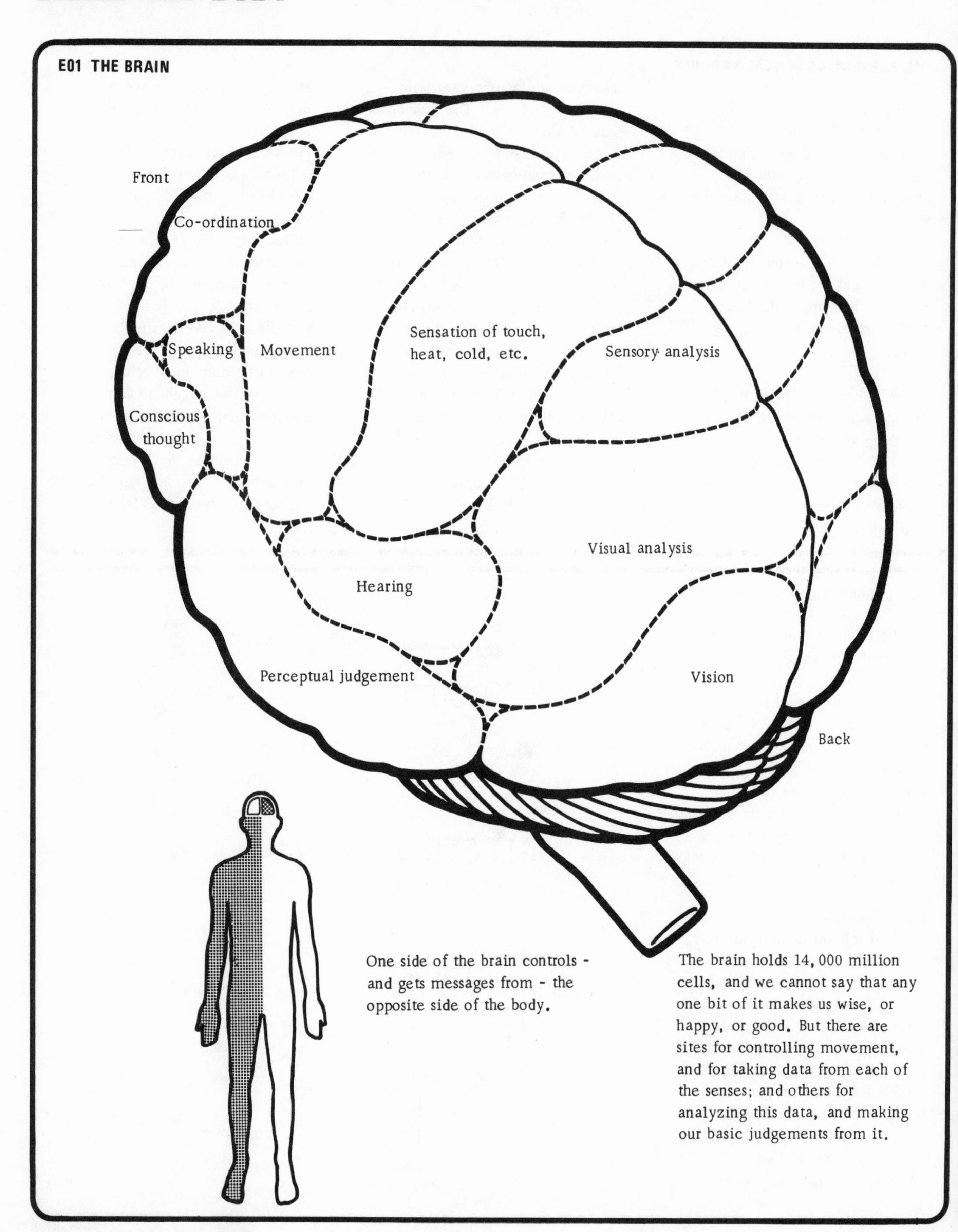

One side of the brain controls - and gets messages from - the opposite side of the body.

The brain holds 14,000 million cells, and we cannot say that any one bit of it makes us wise, or happy, or good. But there are sites for controlling movement, and for taking data from each of the senses; and others for analyzing this data, and making our basic judgements from it.

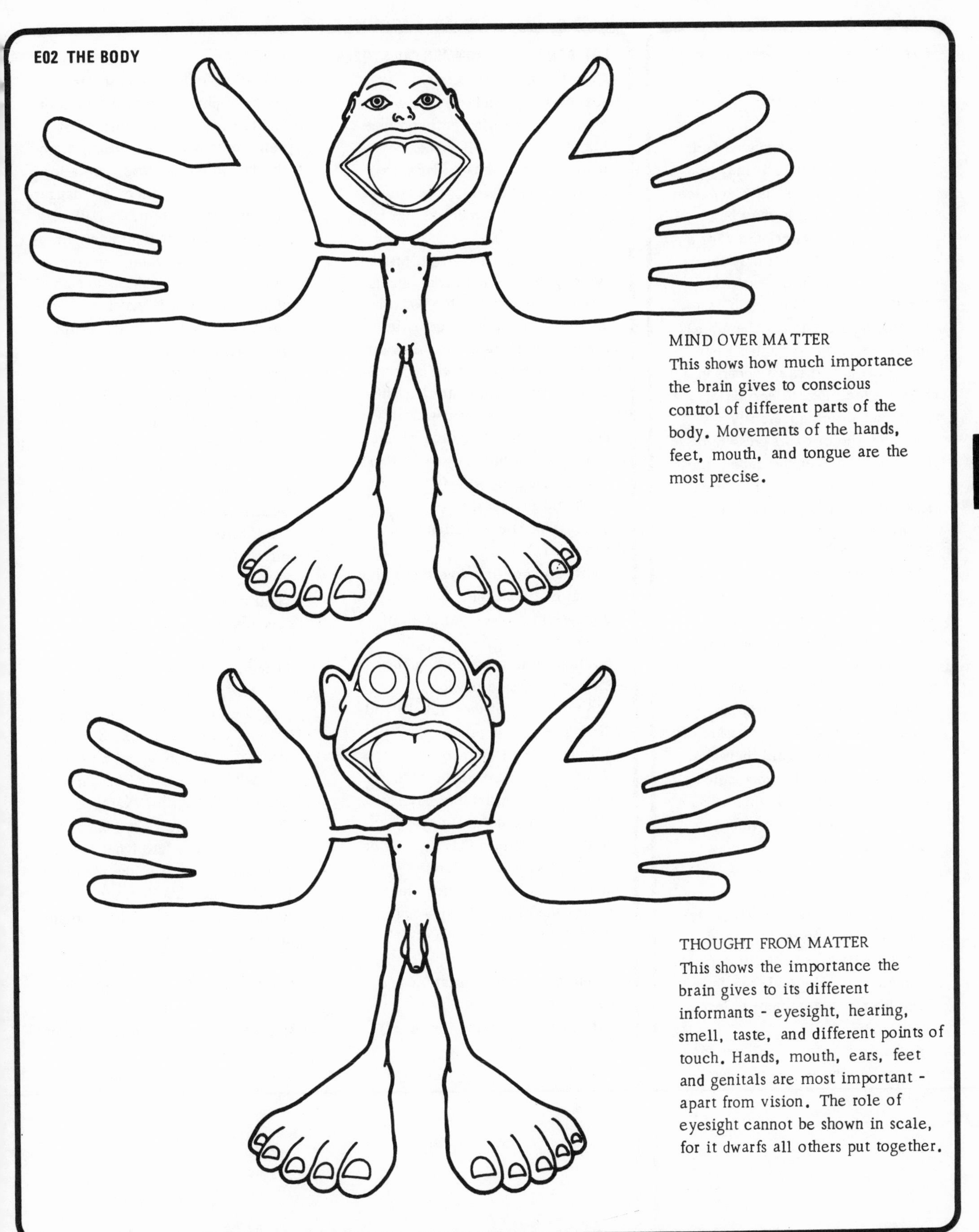

MIND OVER MATTER
This shows how much importance the brain gives to conscious control of different parts of the body. Movements of the hands, feet, mouth, and tongue are the most precise.

THOUGHT FROM MATTER
This shows the importance the brain gives to its different informants - eyesight, hearing, smell, taste, and different points of touch. Hands, mouth, ears, feet and genitals are most important - apart from vision. The role of eyesight cannot be shown in scale, for it dwarfs all others put together.

E03 STRESS

WHAT IS STRESS?

Stress is nervous tension. It may be conscious or unconscious - that is, the person may know he feels tense or he may not. It may be "environmental" or "psychological" - that is, the person may be reacting to a physical threat or a mental threat. And it may be "acute" or "chronic" - that is, the threat may be an event or a continuing situation. (These are just some of the variables.) But the result is that stress occurs in a person's reactions to certain situations which apparently threaten him or exert pressure on him. So whatever the cause, stress in the end depends on the person's reaction - not on the outside event.

STRESS AND HEALTH

The distinction between types of stress is important, though. It is commonplace to talk vaguely about the impact of stress on the body. But such talk usually confuses these different types, when their relationship with the body may differ considerably. It is especially important to distinguish between environmental and psychological stress, and acute and chronic. Combining these two criteria, examples of stressful situations might be:

a) acute environmental: being nearly run over by an automobile;

b) chronic environmental: working in extremely noisy conditions;

c) acute psychological: ranging from losing an argument to losing a wife; and

d) chronic psychological: unhappy at work, living in an unhappy marriage, etc.

E04 ACUTE ENVIRONMENTAL STRESS

I am going slowly across the street, feeling tired. Suddenly I see an automobile bearing down on me: I leap to the sidewalk. Then my body begins to shake, and I start panting breathlessly. The "fight or flight" reaction syndrome has taken over.

FIGHT OR FLIGHT SYNDROME

When a threatening event occurs in the environment, the body has a specific reaction. Signals from the brain stimulate the autonomic nervous system (over which we have no conscious control). This causes the release of powerful hormones (including epinephrine), which key up the body for action. The resulting fight or flight syndrome includes:

increase in rate and strength of heartbeat;

constriction of blood vessels and rise in blood pressure;

increase in blood sugar and fatty acids;

dilation of nostrils and bronchi;

increased muscle tension;

and retraction of the eyeballs and dilation of the pupils.

All these speed the person's reactions and make him more capable of any supreme physical effort that the danger may demand - whether it is fighting or running away. Also blood coagulation time shortens, to reduce the effect of any wounds.

INAPPROPRIATE REACTION

In primitive man the fight or flight syndrome was appropriate to the dangers he faced.

But (apart from being run over!) few of our modern threats are ones we have physically to run from or fight. Imagine that, instead of being a harassed pedestrian, I am driving an automobile, and a lorry swerves in front of me. My danger may be just as great, and all the body processes of fight or flight instantly start working. But the only action I can take is to step on the brake. Even if that is successful, my body is left ready for a struggle that never happens.

DAMAGING EFFECTS

In fight or flight, the epinephrine has prompted the release into the blood stream of fatty acids - needed to fuel the muscles and make the blood clot more quickly if a wound occurs. When there is no struggle, these fatty acids are left circulating through the blood vessels, and may convert into cholesterol deposits. Moreover, repeated incidents may result in a constant high blood pressure.

In fact, research suggests that repeated environmental stress situations can be a major cause of atherosclerosis and related troubles - if no physical movement is possible to "use up" the fatty acids produced. For example, English bus drivers have been found to have a far higher incidence of heart disease than the men who go round the same buses selling the tickets - experiencing perhaps no less stress, but getting more exercise. (But of course there may have been different susceptibility to disease in the types of people who came to choose these different jobs.)

E05 ACUTE PSYCHOLOGICAL STRESS

This refers to the psychological effect of particular incidents (though their impact may last over a long period of time). There are two main sources of such stress: conflict, and change.

CONFLICT

Acute conflict may be with a person, or with an abstract such as time. It produces emotions of either anger or anxiety, and both these are often accompanied by the physical changes of the fight or flight syndrome. The link is an automatic one, over which we can have little conscious control. Again, the reaction is usually physically inappropriate, and so the same physically damaging effects can occur.

CHANGE

Here no fight or flight syndrome is involved. But being faced with change and having to adapt to it does create psychological stress - and recent research has also shown that it consistently results in physical illness, even though the process is not understood. People who have experienced a high degree of stressful change in their lives in a limited period of time (whether one large source of stress or a number of small ones) typically develop some form of physical illness in the next few months. One researcher scored people on their recent experience of typical stressful events (ranging, for example, from changing one's eating habits to suffering the death of husband or wife). The top 10% of scorers suffered twice as much physical illness in the next four months as those in the bottom 10%.

E06 CHRONIC STRESS

ENVIRONMENTAL

Every day a city bus driver may face several incidents of acute stress, when a traffic accident threatens. But he is also working under constant conditions of chronic environmental stress, even if no such incidents occur. This is due to:

a) the physical conditions of his work setting (unpleasantly cramped and noisy); and

b) the need for constant alertness and readiness, in case incidents of acute stress do occur.

In these circumstances the body reacts with what has been named the General Adaptation Syndrome: a long term adaptation to the presence of stress. One of the above causes alone is sufficient: for example, noise polluted work conditions tend to set up permanently high blood pressure (and perhaps also high blood cholesterol levels). Eventually the person feels exhausted, mentally and/or physically. Resistance to disease, or simply the desire to go on, break down, and physical, mental, or psychosomatic illness occurs.

PSYCHOLOGICAL

Chronic psychological stress depends much more on the person than on what happens to him. Someone promoted above his abilities will probably be under such constant stress - but some personalities may not be aware of the pressure, or of not being up to the job. On the other hand, someone in a position well within his abilities may carry it out with constant drive and tension. Perhaps it is because he does not realize he can do it easily; or because he wants to win promotion; or simply because that is his way of going about things.

Some heart researchers, in fact, have contrasted two personality types. Type A has intense ambition, competitive drive, and a sense of urgency. Type B, in contrast, has a content, unhurried personality. These researchers have also suggested that Type A is far more likely to get heart disease. But so far there has been no satisfactory proof of this. The high correlation between supposed "Type A" people and heart disease can equally be explained by higher cholesterol and blood pressure levels occurring for other reasons.

Nevertheless, chronic psychological stress does often end in some form of illness. In cases where the constant tension is felt to be unpleasant, exhaustion may again lead to physical, mental, or psychosomatic symptoms. In other cases, the person is often trying to escape deep psychic conflicts by rushing through life. Here the process itself is less likely to end in illness. But what is likely is that the person's psychic balance eventually collapses, as outside events force the hidden conflicts to the surface. The conflicts (such as social or sexual fears) then expose themselves in neuroses and other mental illnesses.

PSYCHOSOMATIC ILLNESS

This is the name for illness that has its underlying cause in psychological stress. Illnesses sometimes brought about in this way include alcoholism, arthritis, asthma, constipation and indigestion, dermatitis, hair loss, migraine, ulcers, and stress symptoms in specific organs (such as heart pains and heartbeat irregularities).

E

SLEEP 1

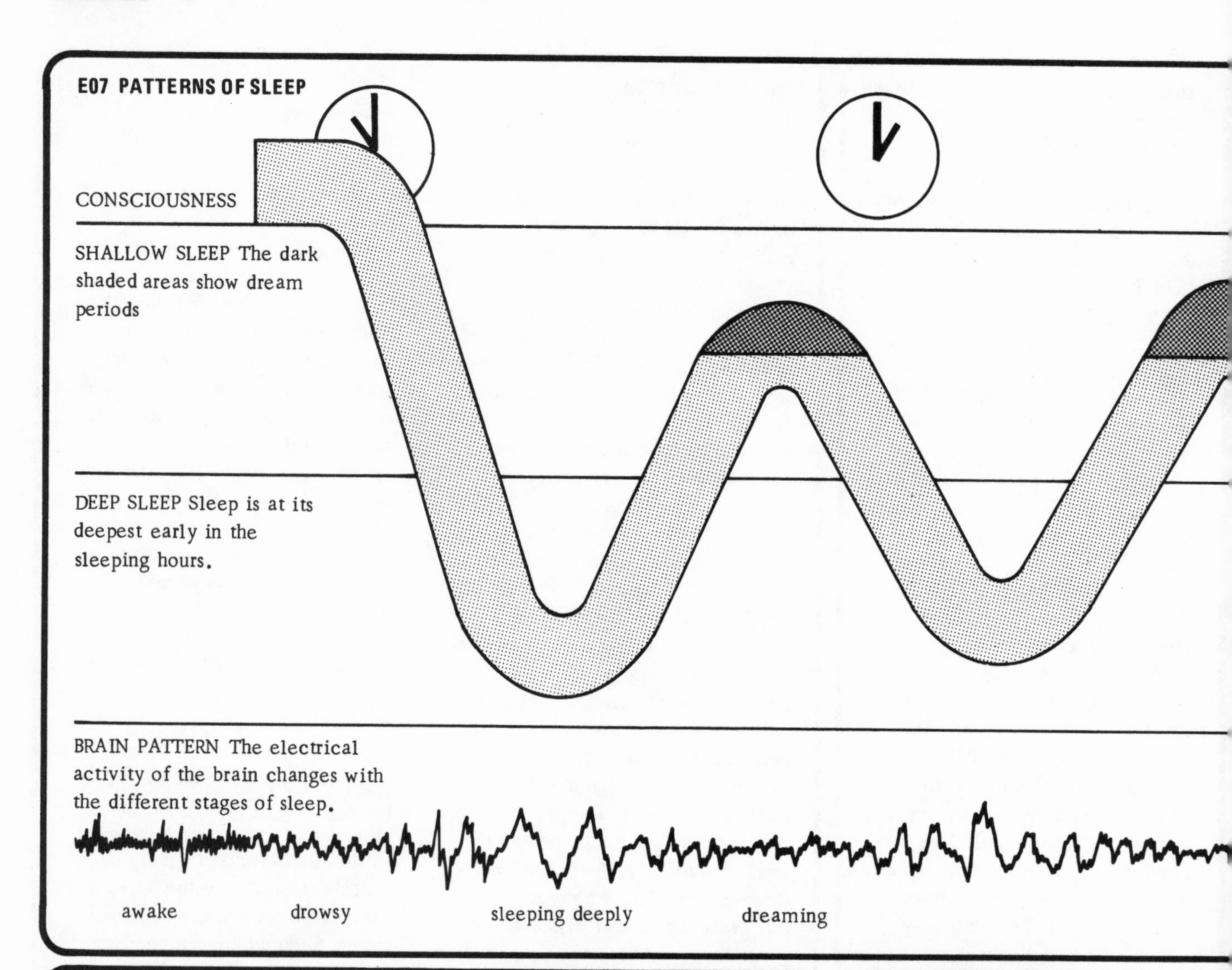

E08 SLEEP

Every person has a natural rhythm of sleeping and waking, that is based on his daily rhythm cycle. About one-third of a person's life is spent in this state of near unconsciousness. However, a sleeper is still aware of aspects of his surroundings, such as noises, and some parts of his brain and body are less affected than others. It is not known what mechanism triggers off sleep. Different theories suggest that it is due to:
a reduction in the amount of oxygen reaching the brain;
a reduction in the number of impulses reaching the conscious centers;
a chemical process in the brain;
or the repeated promptings of a conditioned response.
It is also known that there are certain cell groups throughout the brain which bring about sleep when stimulated, and others that cause a sleeper to wake.

E09 STAGES OF SLEEP

Sleep falls into two stages.
ORTHODOX SLEEP is characterized by a fall in the heart rate, the blood pressure, and the metabolic rate. Breathing is regular but slow. In light orthodox sleep, movement may occur, up to 40 changes of position a night. But in deep orthodox sleep both muscles and brain are at their most relaxed and there is no movement; the electrical activity of the brain becomes markedly different from the waking state. It is during this deep stage that there is a rise in

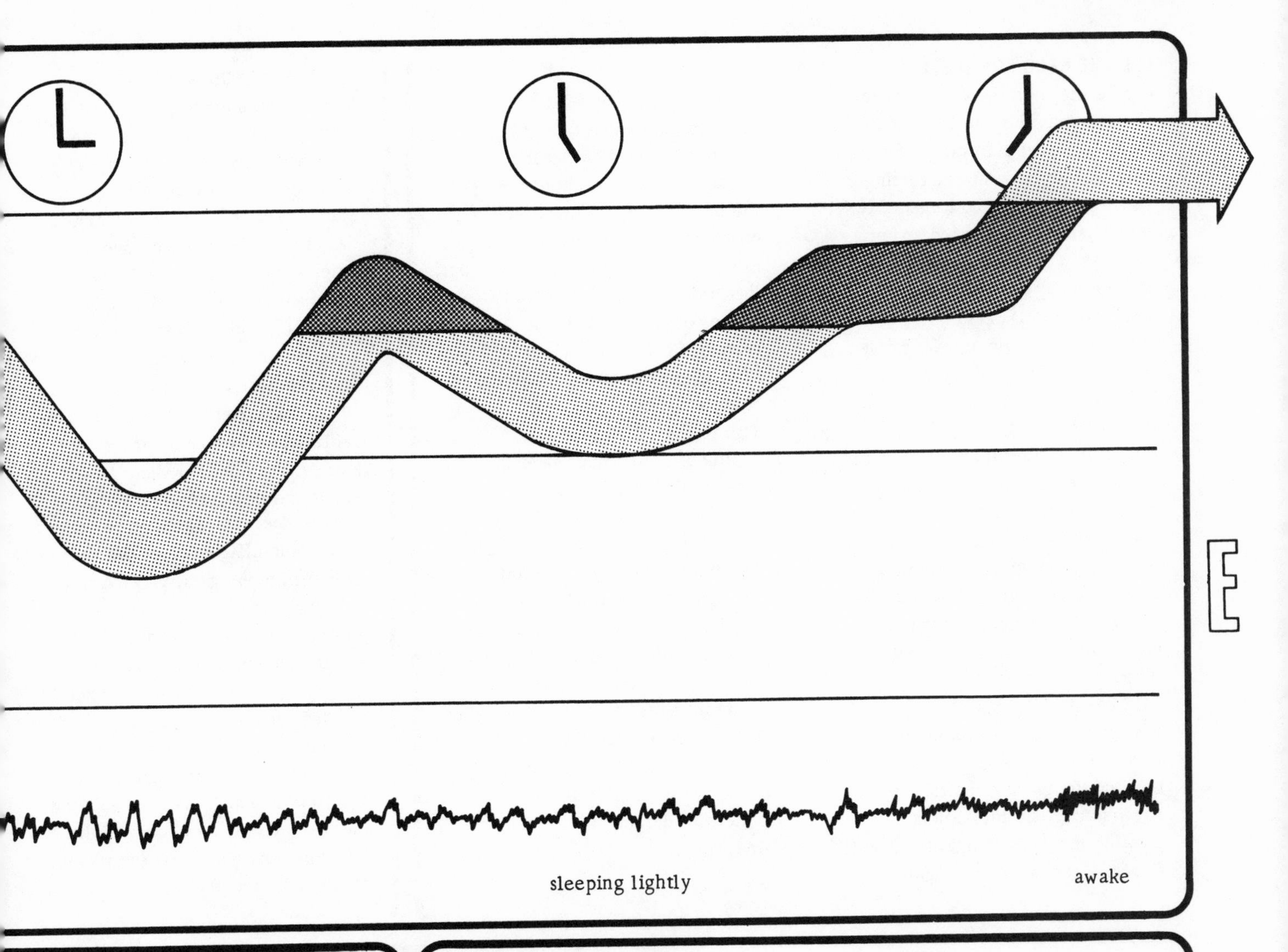

the output of the growth hormone, and protein production is stepped up; the body repairs itself, and dead cells are replaced. PARADOXICAL SLEEP (REM) is the stage in which dreams occur. Breathing and heartbeat become irregular, and there is rapid eye movement (REM) behind the closed eyelids. The electrical activity of the brain resembles that of the waking state. Although movement may occur, the muscles are often as relaxed as in orthodox sleep, and the sleeper is just as difficult to wake.

E10 THE PATTERN OF SLEEP

The sleeper begins with light orthodox sleep, until after about 20 minutes he enters into deep orthodox sleep. This first period of deep sleep is the longest of the night, lasting about an hour. The sleeper then moves through light sleep to the first period of paradoxical sleep, about $1\frac{1}{2}$ hours after falling asleep. During a typical night's sleep of 7 to 8 hours this cycle recurs about five times. However, as the night progresses, the periods of deep sleep become shorter, until after about three hours the stage is not reached at all. The periods of light and paradoxical sleep become correspondingly longer: from 10 to 30 minutes in the early part of the night, to up to an hour at the end of it. Normally, paradoxical sleep takes up about 20% of an adult's sleeping time (and 50% or more of a baby's).

E11 THE NEED FOR SLEEP

People die more quickly from lack of sleep than they do from lack of food. A person kept awake for long periods becomes increasingly disorientated, and both mentally and physically exhausted. After ten days of total sleep deprivation, death usually occurs.

THE BODY AND SLEEP

But it seems we do not sleep just because the body needs to rest. Lying down would be adequate for that. In fact, the body shifts regularly during sleep, to prevent its muscles seizing up; and if we do have to do without sleep for several days, our automatic body processes can go on functioning in a fairly steady way. The body does get rest during sleep - but it does not seem to be sleep's special purpose.

THE BRAIN AND SLEEP

What cannot go on in a normal way, without sleep, is the brain. Lack of sleep brings irritability, irrationality, hallucinations, growing mental derangement, and finally insanity, before death occurs. This, and the steady way body processes carry on, suggest that our feelings of physical exhaustion are also produced by the brain in its unwillingness to go on controlling the body.

Sleep, then, "rests" the brain. But the brain's electrical activity carries on during sleep: it certainly does not "switch off". So what special needs of the brain are being satisfied?

THE NEED TO DREAM

A famous experiment gave the answer. One group of sleepers was woken whenever their REM sleep began, so preventing them from dreaming. They soon showed all the signs of mental disturbance. Another group, woken equally but only in other stages of sleep, hardly suffered. So sleep occurs because the brain needs to dream (and when sleep is prevented, the hallucinations which eventually occur are in roughly the same pattern as dreams would occur in sleep).

E12 SLEEP REQUIREMENTS

Most of the unborn child's day is spent sleeping. After birth, the amount of sleep needed gradually declines with growth. A newborn baby sleeps on average 16 hours a day (though he may be deceptively quiet at other times); a 6 year old, 10 hours; a 12 year old, 9 hours; an adult, 7 hours 20 minutes.

But there are wide variations around these figures: some babies sleep 10½ hours, others 23 hours; some adults sleep 14 hours, others only 2 or 3. The need for sleep is highly personal, and it is not known why: it does not match one's sex, or one's intelligence, or the amount of exercise one gets. However, it is thought many people try to get too much sleep: they have insomnia or use sleeping tablets, because they fail to realize that their need for sleep is relatively low.

Whether adult needs decline with advancing age is uncertain. The tradition is that those over 65 need on average only 5½ hours a night. But recent evidence has suggested that needs are constant from 30 on.

E14 DREAMS

Everyone dreams every night - even if they do not remember it. Dreams total two hours of an average night's sleep. If the sleeper is woken in the middle of an REM period, he will remember a vivid dream. But if woken 5 minutes after REM, he will have only a hazy recollection of a dream, and if woken 10 minutes or more afterwards he will have no memory of it.

Dreams have always intrigued and puzzled humanity. They have been used to prophesy the future and comment on the present and past. But it is only in this century that any theories have suggested why the brain needs dreams so badly.

FREUDIAN THEORY

The psychologist Freud suggested that dreams symbolize the unconscious needs and anxieties of the dreamer. Civilization, he argued, requires us to suppress many of our urges. We cannot act on them, and even have to hide them from ourselves. So they reappear as dreams, which form a "gateway to the subconscious" - to the fears and anxieties that make us psychologically unhealthy. This is almost certainly one function of dreams - though the repressed urges may be less purely sexual than Freud supposed. But there are probably other functions, even psychologically, of dreams: Jung, for example, thought they symbolized ideal images. And - though from this we would expect someone deprived of dreams to become psychologically disturbed - none of it explains why lack of sleep drives us insane quite so rapidly and dependably as it does.

THE COMPUTER ANALOGY

A recent theory about sleep and dreams compares the brain with a computer. A computer carries out various tasks according to the instructions ("programs") it has been given. From time to time

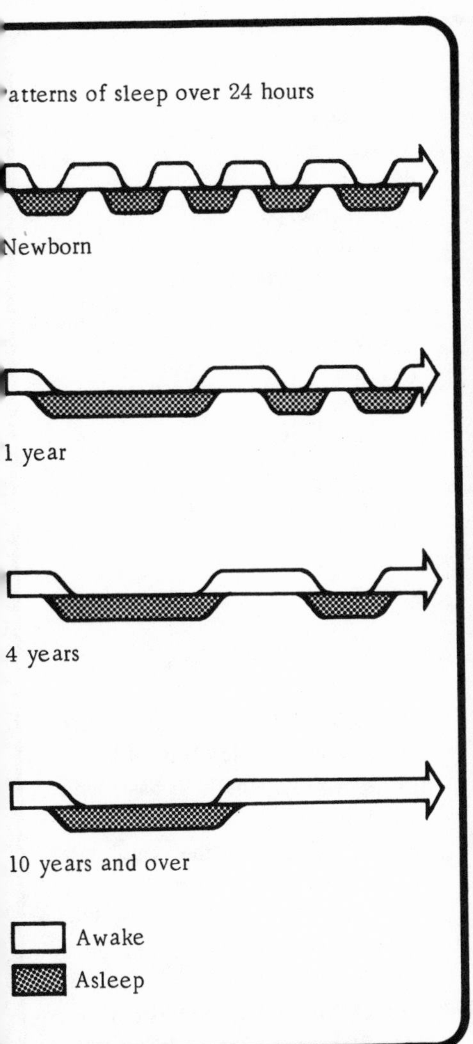

E13 SLEEP DISORDERS

SOMNAMBULISM ("sleep walking") is sleep in which the parts of the brain that control the muscles have stayed awake. The person may speak, sit up, and even get out of bed and walk about. The senses are partly awake, for objects are avoided, but the experience is not remembered on waking.

PARALYZED WAKEFULNESS is the opposite condition: the person wakes intellectually, but for a time cannot move. The experience is frightening but harmless.

INSOMNIA ("sleeplessness") may be occasional or chronic. Sometimes it is not really sleeplessness at all; the person has slept, but not realized it, because it was so restless and unrefreshing. Causes of occasional insomnia include: feeling cold or using too-light bedclothing; indigestion; excessive fatigue; excitement, nervousness, or worry; and pain or illness. Causes of regular insomnia include: difficulty in breathing when lying down (as in heart and lung disorder); bad food habits, especially eating, or drinking tea or coffee, too late in the evening; a need to urinate during the night; a noisy, airless, or overheated bedroom; lack of exercise during the day; trying to sleep more than you need; and, especially, psychological factors - overwork and worry about work, anxiety, emotional upset, and depression. But the main cause of any insomnia, whether occasional or regular, is simply the fear that one is not going to sleep.

Sufferers from insomnia should remove any external causes, and cultivate a relaxed attitude to sleep. A warm bath, a warm drink, quiet reading or talking, and a gentle routine of preparing for bed, can be useful in re-educating the mind to the idea of a good night's sleep. Sleeping pills are best used only when there are serious and fairly temporary outside emotional disturbances, eg acute grief at a death.

E

these instructions have to be changed - but this can only be done when the computer is not trying to carry out its usual tasks i.e. it must be "off duty". Similarly, the brain carries out many tasks required by the body - sorting out, analyzing, interpreting, understanding, and acting on the information it receives from the senses. But in sleep the number of these tasks is greatly reduced, and the influx of new information almost ceases. So it may be that sleep is the time when the brain goes over again the information it has received during the day, modifies or rejects existing programs - and establishes new ones - in the light of this, and stores some information in a more permanent way. For, of course, in contrast to a computer, the brain is self-modifying: it gives itself its own new programs.

If this is so, paradoxical sleep may be the time when these processes are going on. But such processing of data will follow the brain's own rules, and may not correspond with outside reality at all. When a sleeper wakes up while the process is going on (during REM), his consciousness is suddenly presented with a jumbled mass of unconnected images. He will then try to understand them by imposing a meaning - with the result that he seems to have experienced a dream. If the theory is correct, the amount of sleep needed depends on the amount of new information being received that makes program changes necessary. So babies - for whom everything is new - need most, and the old - whose lives often contain little change - may need least. The theory may also explain differences between species: the amount of sleep taken coinciding very roughly with brain complexity.

E15 THE EYEBALL

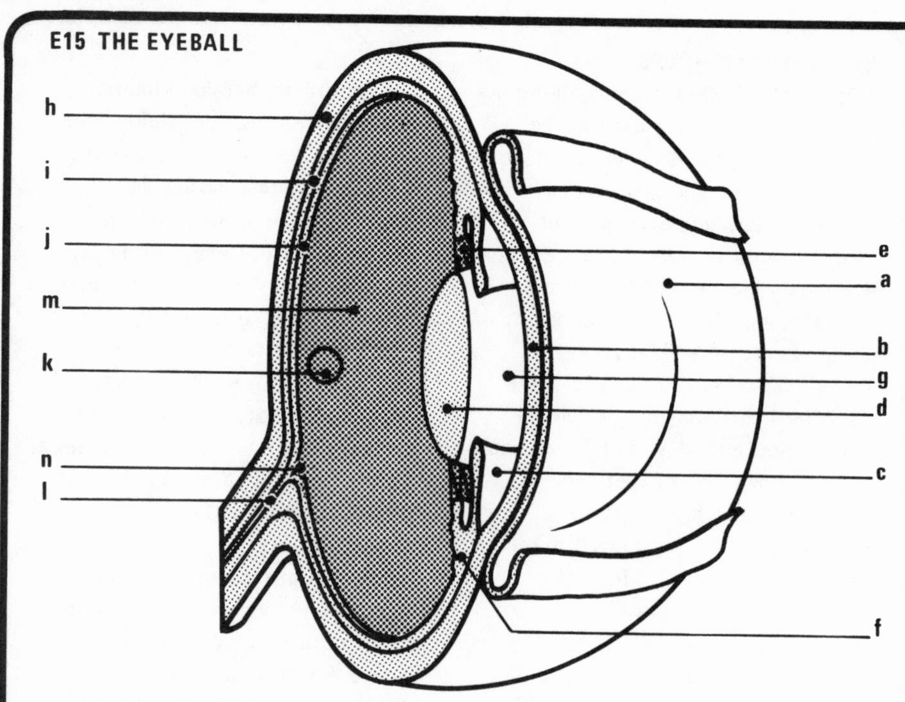

a Conjunctiva
b Cornea
c Iris
d Lens
e Suspensory ligaments
f Ciliary body
g Anterior chamber
h Sclera
i Choroid
j Retina
k Fovea
l Optic nerve
m Vitreous body
n Blind spot

THE CONJUNCTIVA is the membrane covering the front of the eyeball and the inside of the eyelids. It has a rich supply of blood vessels and is extremely sensitive.

THE CORNEA is the clear part of the eyeball which lets in the light.

THE IRIS controls the amount of light entering the eyeball. By contracting, it reduces the size of the pupil (the hole through which the light enters). It is the iris which gives the eye its "color".

THE LENS has a firm center, surrounded by a softer substance contained in a fibrous capsule. By being stretched or thickened, it focuses light on the back of the eyeball.

THE SUSPENSORY LIGAMENTS are attached at one end to the lens and at the other to the ciliary body. They hold the lens in place.

THE CILIARY BODY. The muscles of the ciliary body control the shape of the lens. If they contract the lens is stretched and light rays from long distances are focused on the retina (are "accommodated"). If they relax the lens thickens, and close objects are accommodated. Both the lens and the iris are under the control of the autonomic nervous system, and cannot be controlled at will.

THE ANTERIOR CHAMBER lies in front of the lens and is filled with a watery fluid called the aqueous humor.

THE SCLERA or sclerotic coat is a layer of dense white tissue. It completely surrounds the eyeball, except where the optic nerve enters at the rear, and where it is modified at the front to form the transparent cornea. The sclera forms the "whites" of the eyes.

THE CHOROID tissue lies beneath more than two-thirds of the sclera. It is colored brown or black, and contains blood vessels. The ciliary body and the retina are formed from the choroid. Its color absorbs excess light within the eyeball, making for clearer vision.

THE RETINA is a thin layer of light sensitive cells which lines the inside of the eyeball. It has a rich blood supply.

THE FOVEA lies on the visual axis of the eyeball. It is a small depression in the retina, at which vision is sharpest. It contains only "cone" cells (see E20).

THE OPTIC NERVE is a direct extension of the brain. It enters the eyeball at the rear. The head of the optic nerve is called the optic disc. It forms a blind spot in the vision, as there are no light-sensitive cells there. We are sometimes aware of this blind spot as a black dot at one corner of our vision.

THE VITREOUS BODY occupies the space behind the lens. It is a transparent jelly-like substance that fills out the eyeball, giving it its shape. It contains small specks which are often seen when looking at white surfaces.

E16 PROTECTIVE STRUCTURES

The eyes - the organs of sight - lie in deep hollows in the skull, on either side of the nose, and are protected in various ways.

THE EYEBROWS prevent moisture and solid particles from running down into the eye from above.

THE EYELIDS are folds of skin which, when closed, cover and protect the eyes. The inner membrane of each eyelid is a continuation of the "conjunctiva" which covers the front of the eyeball.

THE EYELASHES are hairs that protrude from the eyelids. They prevent foreign bodies from entering the eye, and trigger off the protective blinking mechanism when touched unexpectedly.

THE LACRIMAL GLANDS produce a watery, salty fluid that cleans the front of the eyeball. It also lubricates the movement of the eyelid over the eyeball. When stimulated by strong emotion or irritants, the glands produce excess fluid.

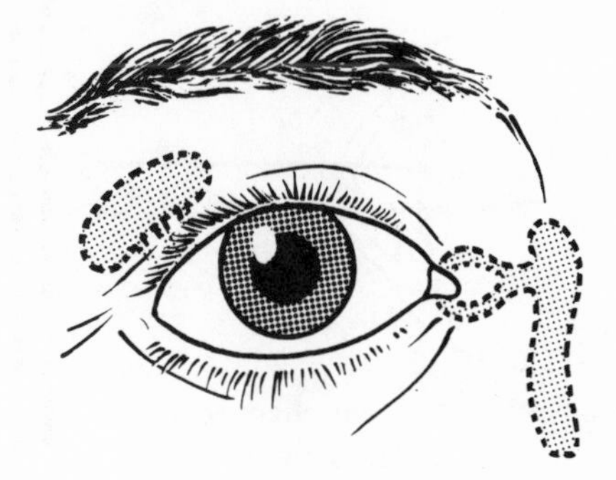

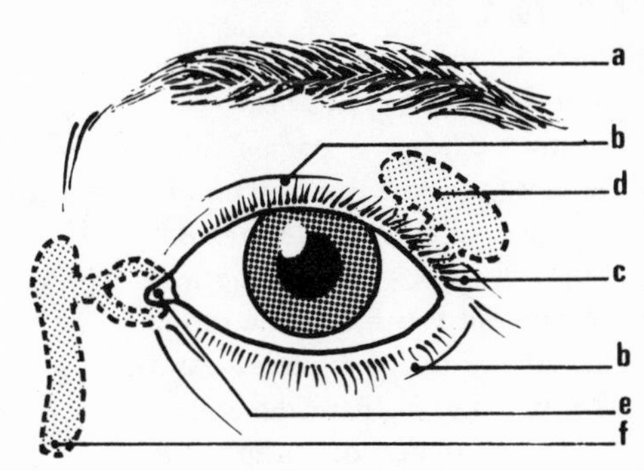

a Eyebrows
b Eyelids
c Eyelashes
d Lacrimal glands
e Lacrimal ducts
f Lacrimal sacs

THE LACRIMAL DUCTS drain the fluid from the eyeballs into the lacrimal sacs which lead into the nasal passage. When the ducts cannot clear the fluid fast enough it overflows and falls down the face as tears.

BLINKING is a protective action of the eyelids which spreads the lacrimal fluid over, and cleans, the front of the eyeball. Blinking is controlled by the brain. It occurs every 2 to 10 seconds, and the rate increases under stress, in dusty surroundings, or when tired, and decreases during periods of concentration.

E17 EYE MOVEMENT

MOVEMENT OF THE EYEBALL is controlled by six muscles attached to the outside of the sclera*.

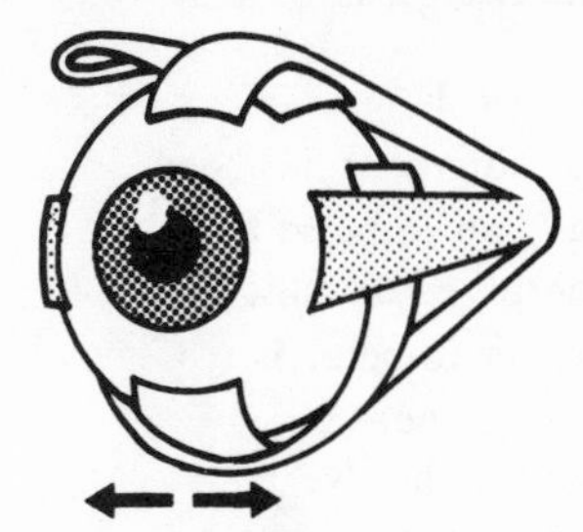

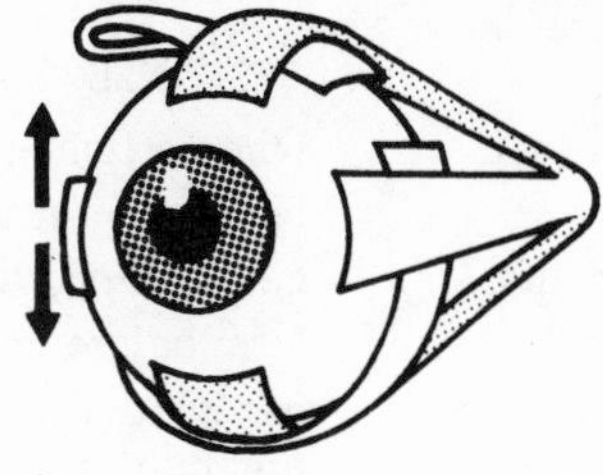

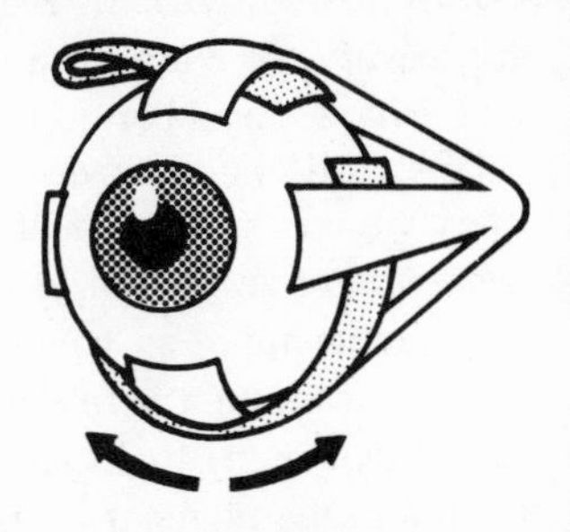

E18 THE BLIND SPOT

How to find your blind spot. Hold the book at arms length, and shut your left eye. Then look at the cross with your right eye, while slowly moving the book towards you. At one point the dot will disappear.

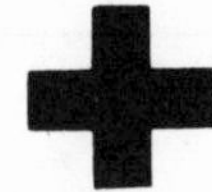

EYESIGHT 2

E19 SIGHT

When the light rays from an object enter the eye they are bent ("refracted") by the cornea and the lens (and to a lesser extent by the aqueous humor and vitreous body). Because of this refraction the rays are focused on the retina (though the image is upside down). The action of light on the cells of the retina triggers off an impulse which travels down the optic nerve to the visual centers of the brain. Here the impulses are interpreted and "seen" as colors and shapes the right way up.

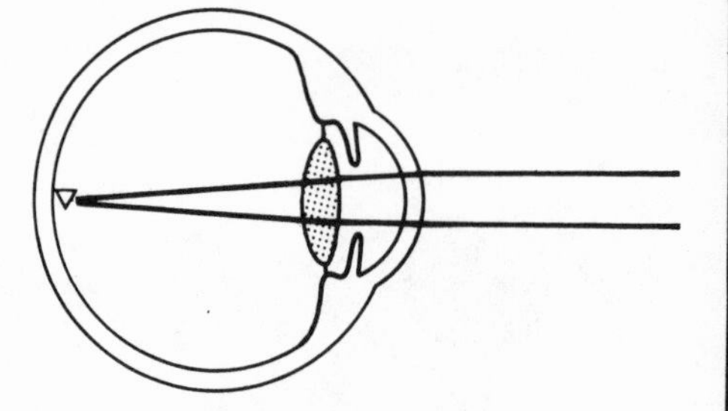

Refraction: the lens changes shape to focus on objects at different distances

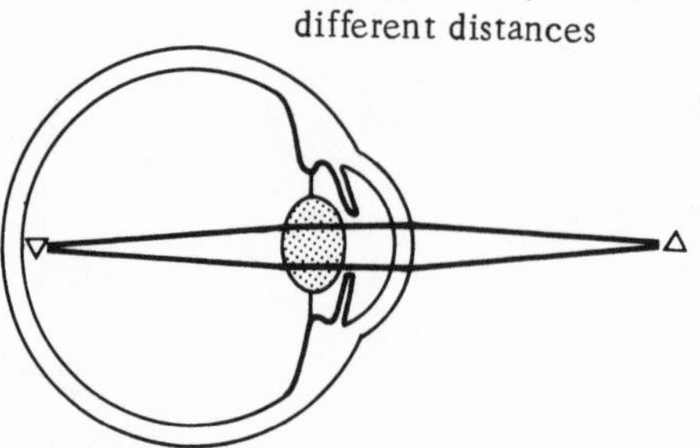

E21 THE OPTIC NERVE

The nerves from the left sides of the two retinas travel to one side of the brain, those from the right sides to the other side of the brain. The images received in the two visual centers (at the rear of the cerebral hemispheres) are composite images from both eyes, mixed 50:50.

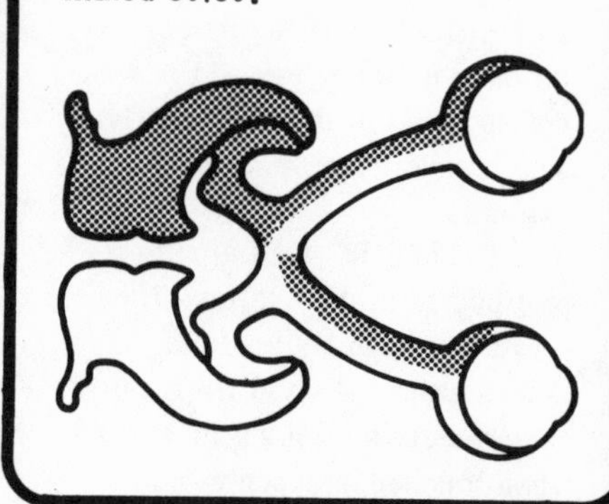

E20 THE RETINA

There are two types of light sensitive cells in the retina. They are classified by shape: rods and cones. They are connected by nerve fibers to the optic nerve.

RODS

There are about 125 million rods in each eyeball. They are sensitive to low intensity light, and are used mainly in night vision. They are not sensitive to color, and therefore give only a monochrome image (black, white, and shades of grey). They are less than one four-hundredth of an inch in length and one-thousandth of an inch thick. The rods contain a purple pigment called rhodopsin. Light bleaches the rod as the pigment breaks down. This sets off electrical charges in the rods, which are transmitted down the optic nerve to the brain in the form of nervous impulses.

CONES

These are shorter and thicker, for most of their length, than the rods. They are used for high intensity light, such as daylight, and give color vision.

The actual process of color vision is not known, but it is thought that there are three different classes of cones, each containing a different pigment. Each pigment would be sensitive to a different color: blue, green, or red. Other colors would be combinations of these. It is thought that the nerve messages are produced by bleaching, as in the rods.

RESPONSE TO LIGHT

When a light-cell pigment has been broken down, and an impulse has been passed, the pigment must re-form before another impulse is possible. This takes about one-eighth of a second. The eye is therefore like a cinema screen. It does not give a continual picture, but successive "stills" at intervals of one-eighth of a second. These seem continuous because run together.

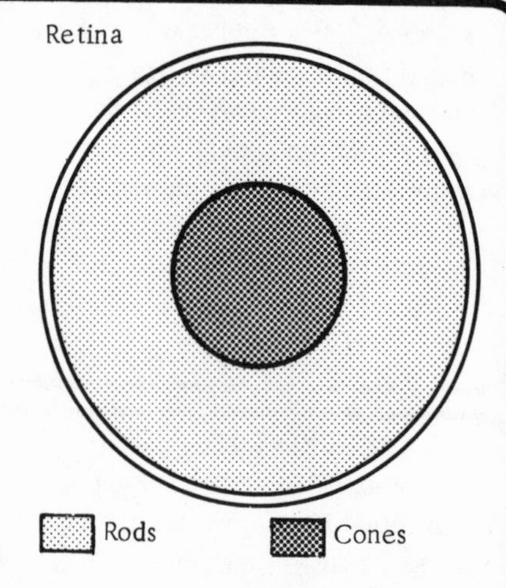

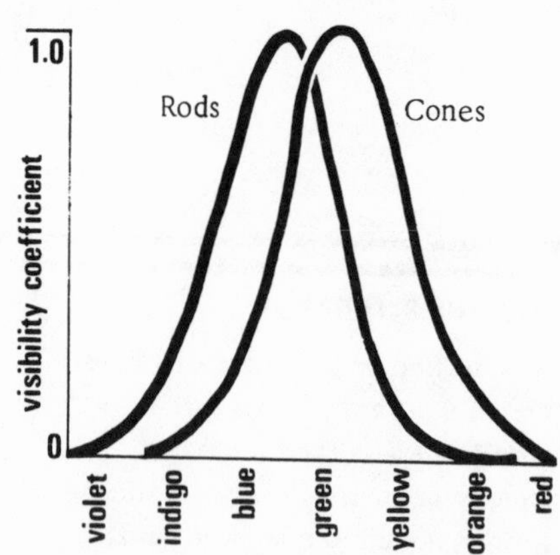

Sensitivity of rods and cones

E22 PERCEPTION

The ability to perceive objects, colors, and distances is learnt by experience. To the newborn child, the images he receives are meaningless and confused. It takes time for him to learn to use his eyes and correlate past with present information to bring about recognition.

This dependence of perception on the brain's judgements can be shown by presenting the eye with trick pictures: ones that allow alternative interpretations, or that give evidence that seems contradictory. Perception will then shift or struggle between the alternative interpretations.

The same process can be observed naturally, in unfamiliar surroundings or moments of confusion - such as waking up in a strange room. A series of alternative pictures then flash through the brain, as it tries to make familiar sense of the data it is receiving.

Each eye sees a slightly different view of the same object. The further away the object is, the less the discrepancy between the two views. This, plus the amount of tension needed to focus and the amount of blurring, forms the basis of judgement of distance.

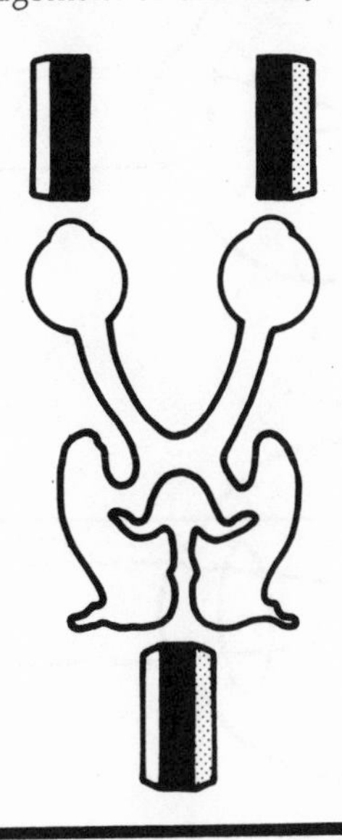

E23 VISUAL SCOPE

THE FIELD OF VISION is the area that can be seen by an eye without moving it. The size of the field varies with different colors. White has the largest, then yellow, blue, red, and green.

THE RANGE OF MOVEMENT of the eyeball with the head still is also limited. The human eyeball can tilt 35° up, 50° down, 50° in (i.e. towards the other eye), and 45° out. The greater angle available when turning in allows an eye to focus on an object that is just within the other eye's outer range.

THE AREA OF VISION is the total range through which a creature can see without moving head or body. It is determined by:

the position of the eyes in the head;

the shape of the head;

the eyes' range of movement;

and, at the edge, by the eyes' field of vision.

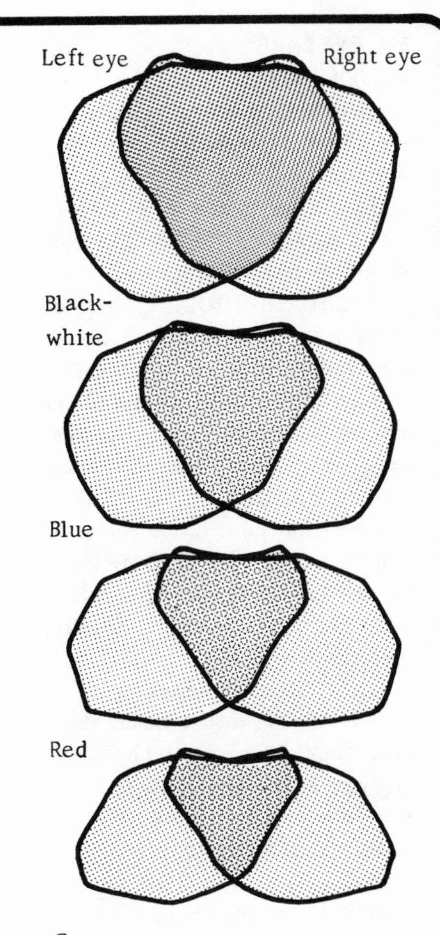

Field of vision

Area of vision

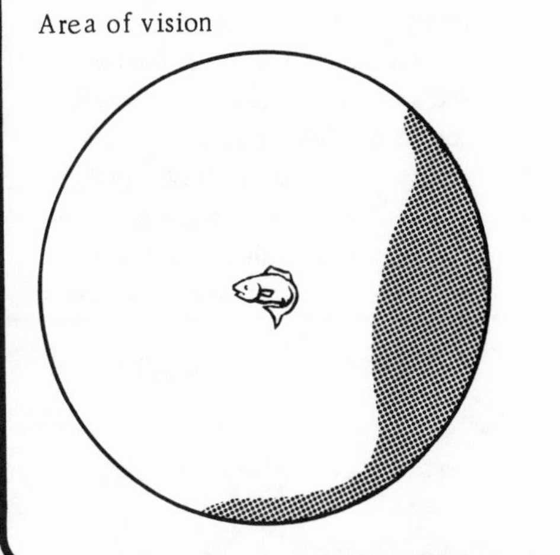

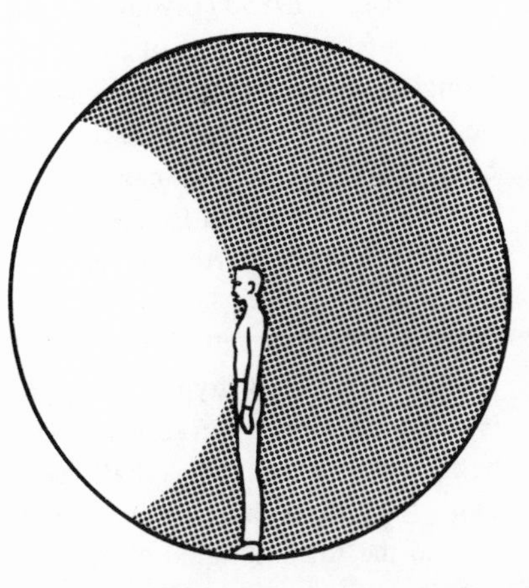

E24 EYE CARE

INJURIES to the eye and the immediately surrounding area should receive expert medical attention. Infection is a danger even if there is no significant damage. The eyes are tough but vital, and should be treated with care.
SMALL FOREIGN BODIES that get stuck in the eye can usually be removed by blinking. If this fails, then pull the upper lid outward and downward over the lower lid. When the upper lid is released the particle may be dislodged. A particle can also be removed with the corner of a handkerchief or by blowing it towards the edge. If none of this succeeds, get help and if necessary medical attention.
BLACK EYES are bruises of the eyelids and the tissues around the eye. They can be treated by applying a cold compress. If a black eye appears after a blow elsewhere on the head, see a doctor.
A STYE is an inflammation of the sebaceous gland* around an eyelash, and is caused by bacterial infection. It is found most often in young people. A large part of the eyelid may become affected. To treat a stye, remove the relevant eyelash and bathe the eye with hot water. Antibiotics should be used only in extreme cases.
CONJUNCTIVITIS is inflammation of the conjunctiva. It can be caused by infection or irritation. If due to bacterial or viral infection, it needs the appropriate antibiotic eyedrops; if due to irritation, the irritant (eg an ingrowing eyelash) is removed. Bathing the eye with warm water and lotions is soothing and is all that is needed in mild cases. Bandages or pads encourage the growth of bacteria, but dark glasses or eyeshades protect the eye from light and wind.
Conjunctivitis is not very serious in itself (except for the trachoma form found in the tropics), but can sometimes cause serious complications such as ulceration of the cornea.

E26 CONTACT LENSES

Contact lenses are thin round discs of plastic, that rest directly on the surface of the eye. They often give better vision, and counteract many year to year changes in the eyesight. However, not everyone can wear contact lenses successfully.
They also require more care.
They need to be cleaned and stored in special fluid when out of the eye, and it is wise to insure them.
TYPES OF LENS
Contact lenses can be "hard" or "soft". Hard lenses are either "scleral" lenses - covering the whole of the visible part of the eye - or "corneal" lenses, which rest on the center of the eye, floating on a film of tear fluid. Corneal lenses are the most popular of all contact lenses, but scleral lenses are useful for very active sports.
Soft lenses differ because they absorb water from the tear fluid. Soft lenses are immediately more comfortable, easier to get used to, can generally be worn for longer periods, can be left off for several days and then worn again without

E25 CORRECTIVE LENSES

Spectacles (or contact lenses) are used because of faulty focusing the eye. The artificial lens corrects the work of the defective part of the eye.
NEARSIGHTEDNESS (myopia) is due to the refractive power of the eye being too strong (eg the lens may be too thick) or to the eyeball being too long. In both cases, the light rays are focused in front of the retina, giving a blurred image. Concave corrective lenses are needed to focus on distant objects.
FARSIGHTEDNESS (hypermetropia) is due to the eye's refractive power being too weak or the eyeball too short. The light rays are focused behind the retina, again giving a blurred image. Convex corrective lenses are needed for close work such as reading.
ASTIGMATISM means that the cornea does not curve correctly, and the person cannot focus on both vertical and horizontal objects at the same time. A special spectacle lens is needed, that only affects the light rays on one of these planes. Alternatively, a hard contact lens can be used, as the fluid layer between eye and lens compensates for the cornea.
PRESBYOPIA* occurs in old age.

Nearsightedness

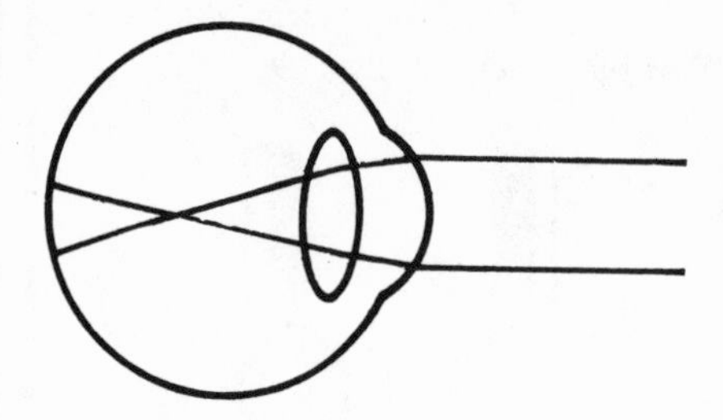

Farsightedness

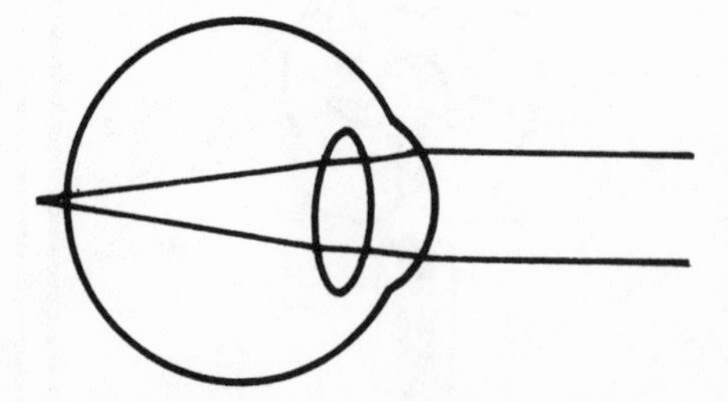

discomfort, can be alternated more easily with the use of spectacles, and can be worn with less discomfort in dirty atmospheres. Hard lenses are much less easy to damage, much cheaper, last perhaps 6 to 8 years (compared with 2 to 3 years for soft lenses with routine wear-and-tear, and often under a year as damage occurs), are more suitable for the majority of eye prescriptions, often give clearer vision, are easier to keep free from bacteria, and are much easier for the eye care practitioner to adjust if difficulty arises.

EXTENDED-WEAR LENSES

These lenses, approved by the Food and Drug Administration for aphakic individuals (those having no crystalline lens in the eye), are still under investigation by an advisory panel of the FDA for general or cosmetic use. The period of wear is determined by the patient and practitioner, up to 30 days or longer. Follow-up care is essential.

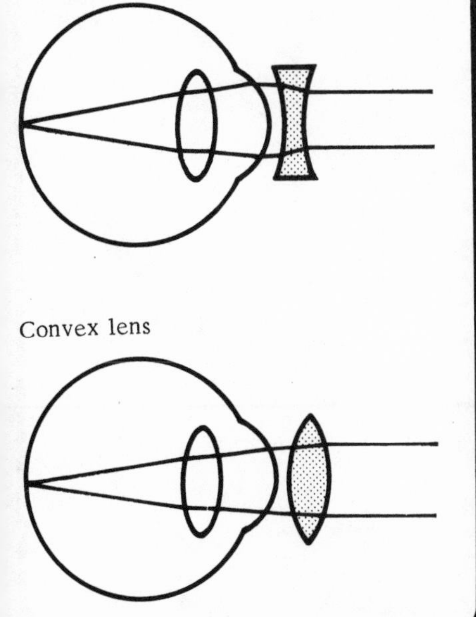

E27 BLINDNESS

Blindness has many causes, and is seldom total. Those who are legally "blind" usually have some vision; and even the totally blind can lead useful lives.

OBSTRUCTION OF LIGHT

If transparent parts of the eye become opaque, light rays are prevented from entering the retina. Opacity of the cornea can be due to ulcers or inflammation (keratitis). Opacity of the lens (cataract*) usually occurs with ageing, but can be due to injury.

DISEASES AFFECTING THE RETINA

These are often caused by diseases elsewhere in the body, especially those involving the blood supply.

a) Retinitis is inflammation of the retina with consequent loss of vision. It is associated with diabetes, leukemia, kidney disorders, and syphilis.

b) Retinopathy covers any disease of the retina that is not inflammatory. It is usually caused by degeneration of the blood vessels, impairing the retina's structure and function. It can be due to high blood pressure, diabetes, kidney disorders, and athersclerosis.

c) Detachment of the retina. Primary detachment occurs if damage to the retina allows fluid from the vitreous body to leak through and lift the retina from the choroid. Treatment is possible. Secondary detachment occurs if the retina is pushed away from the choroid and damaged by underlying tumors, bleeding, or retinal disease. No treatment is possible.

d) Glaucoma* can occur with age.

e) Choroiditis is inflammation of the choroid due to infection or allergy (especially syphilis). The effects depend on the size and position of the inflammation: the nearer the fovea, the greater the vision loss. The inflammation can be treated, but damaged vision is seldom improved.

Stages in a progressive blindness

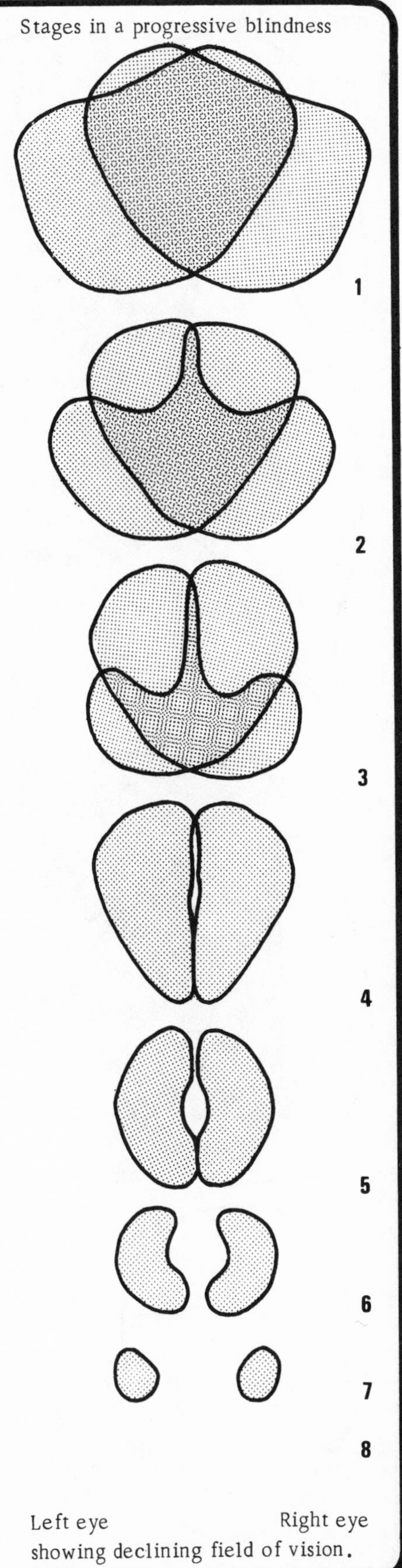

Left eye Right eye showing declining field of vision.

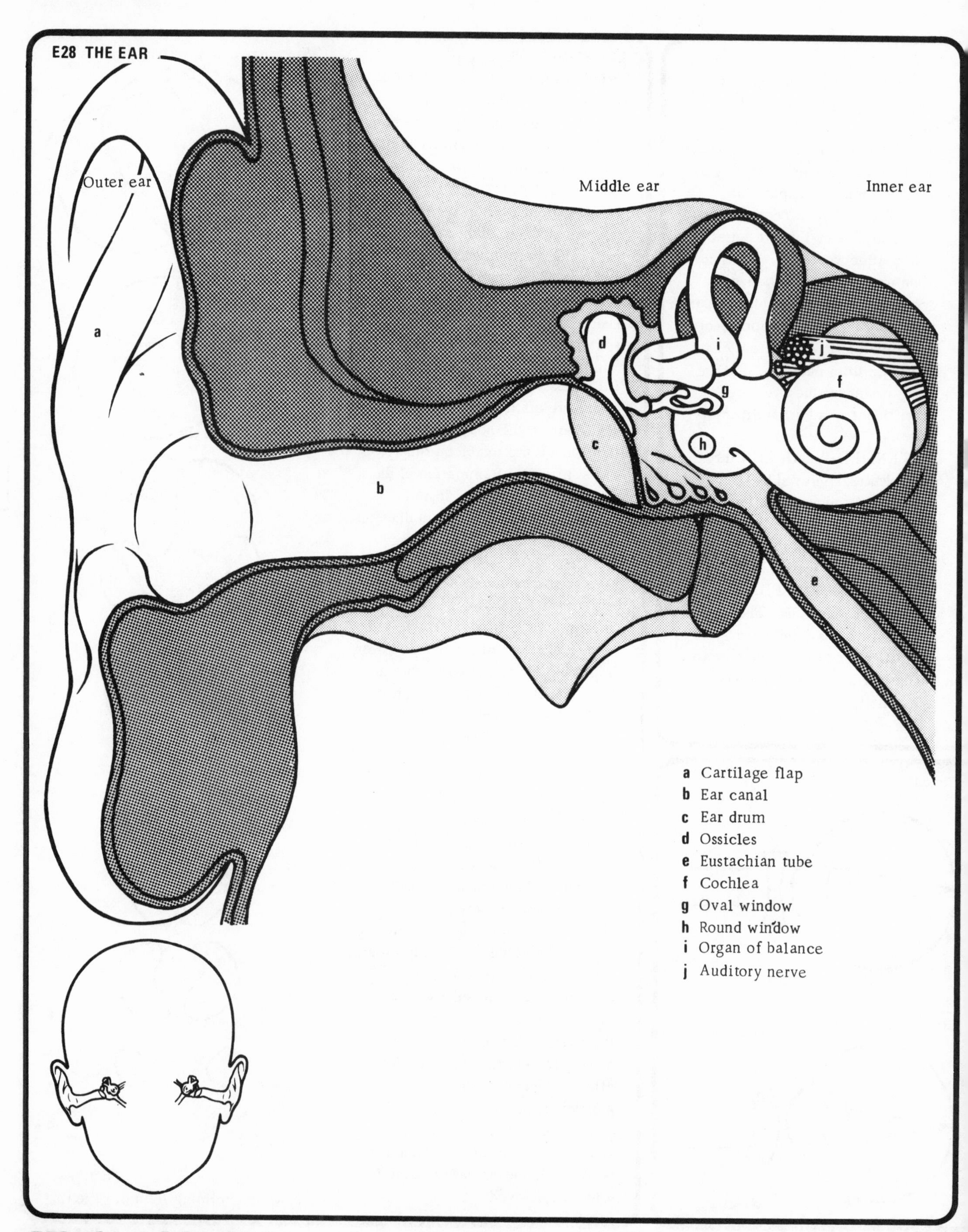
E28 THE EAR
Outer ear
Middle ear
Inner ear
a
b
c
d
e
f
g
h
i
j
a Cartilage flap
b Ear canal
c Ear drum
d Ossicles
e Eustachian tube
f Cochlea
g Oval window
h Round window
i Organ of balance
j Auditory nerve

E29 THE EAR
The structures of the ear fall into three groups.
THE OUTER EAR includes:
the external flap of cartilage (the "pinna" or "auricle");
and the ear canal (the "meatus");
THE MIDDLE EAR includes:
the eardrum (the "tympanic membrane");
three small bones called the "ossicles", and known individually as the hammer ("malleus"), anvil ("incus"), and stirrup ("stapes");
and the eustachian tube, which opens into the back of the throat, and keeps the air pressure in the middle ear equal to that outside.
THE INNER EAR includes:
the cochlea, a spiral filled with fluid and containing the "organ of corti",
the oval window;
the round window;
and the organs of balance.

E30 SOUND
When a solid object vibrates in air, it passes on this vibration to the surrounding air molecules. Sound waves are the vibration of air molecules.
Sound has three qualities:
PITCH, which is the sharpness of a sound, depends on the "frequency" of the sound waves i.e. the number of vibrations per second.
High pitched (piercing) sounds have a high frequency. Low pitched (deep) sounds have a low frequency.
INTENSITY is the loudness of a sound, and depends on the amount of energy in the sound waves i.e. how widely they vibrate. Intensity is measured in "decibels".
TIMBRE is the quality of a sound. Sounds with the same pitch and intensity can be distinguished by their timbre. Timbre is created by the subordinate notes that accompany the main pitch.

E31 HEARING
THE OUTER EAR Sound waves are collected by the pinna and funnelled into the ear canal.
THE MIDDLE EAR The ear drum vibrates in time with the sound waves. This vibration is passed on along the three ossicles to the oval window. The lever action of the ossicles increases the strength of the vibration. This allows the vibration to be passed from the air of the outer and middle ear to the fluid of the inner ear.
THE INNER EAR The vibration of the oval window makes the fluid in the cochlea vibrate. The pressure changes in the fluid are picked up by specialized cells in the organ of corti. This organ converts the vibrations into nerve impulses, which pass along the auditory nerve to the brain. Meanwhile, the vibrations pass on through the cochlea and back to the round window, where they are lost in the air of the middle ear and eustachian tube.

E32 SENSITIVITY
LOUDNESS The human ear can hear sounds ranging in loudness from 10 decibels to 140 decibels (though the loudness becomes painful after 100 decibels). On the decibel scale, a ten unit increase means 10 times the loudness. Therefore the quietest sound the human ear can hear is 10 million millionth the loudness of the loudest.
PITCH Different frequencies stimulate different parts of the organ of corti. That is why we can distinguish one sound from another. The human ear can hear sounds ranging in pitch from 20 cycles per second (low) to 20,000 cycles per second (high). Frequencies above this are called ultrasounds, and can be heard by some animals but not by man.
DIRECTION The slight distance between the ears means that there are minute differences in their perception of a given sound. The brain interprets these differences to tell from which direction the sound came. But if a sound comes from directly behind or in front of the listener, both ears receive the same message, and the listener must turn his head before he can pinpoint the location.
DECLINE in hearing progresses with age.

E33 BALANCE
The organ of balance is in the inner ear next to the cochlea. It consists of three U-shaped tubes ("semi-circular canals"), at right angles to each other. They are filled with fluid, which is set in motion when the person moves. Hairs at the base of each canal sense this movement and send messages to the brain, which are interpreted and used to maintain the person's balance. The organ also contains two other structures, the saccule and the utricle. These have specialized cells which are sensitive to gravity, and so keep a check on the body's position.

E34 EAR CARE

THE OUTER EAR should be kept clean at all times, to prevent wax and bacteria from collecting in the ear canal and damaging the ear drum.
To examine the outer ear, a beam of light from a flashlight is shone down the ear canal.
THE INNER EAR is tested by using a tuning fork. The fork should be heard clearly when it is held in front of the ear.
If the tuning fork is heard more clearly when placed on the bone behind the ear, then:
either the outer ear is blocked with wax;
or, if not, the middle ear is faulty, since sound vibrations are being heard better through the skull.
If hearing is still poor when the fork is placed on the bone behind the ear, it is the inner ear or the auditory nerves that are at fault.
SYRINGING of the outer ear cleans it, and washes out obstructions such as wax or foreign bodies. A large glass or metal syringe is used - one with a blunt point not more than 1in long, so it cannot hurt the eardrum.
The syringe is filled with warmish water, containing, if necessary, an antiseptic and/or a wax dissolving agent. The fluid is directed along the upper wall of the canal, and flows out along the lower.

E35 SYMPTOMS OF DISORDER

DEAFNESS can be temporary or permanent, caused by obstruction or disease.
EARACHE is usually caused by infection and inflammation in the ear. In the outer ear this can occur through physical damage, boils, or eczema. Large wax deposits can also cause earaches. Individuals with respiratory distress, such as severe asthma or a bad cold, or a fever of 101° F or more should consider delaying airplane flights. If the pressure of the cabin is reduced or if the cabin is unpressurized, an infection can spread from the nose and pharynx to the middle ear or directly into the nasal sinuses and perhaps in

E37 EAR DISEASES

OTITIS EXTERNA is infection and inflammation of the outer ear, due to physical damage, allergy, boils, or spread of inflammation from the middle ear. There is itching and often a discharge, which may cause temporary deafness if it blocks the ear canal. Treatment is by antiseptic syringing and use of soothing lotions. Hot poultices and asprin may relieve the pain.
OTITIS MEDIA is middle ear infection, usually due to bacteria arriving via the eustachian tube. The eardrum becomes red and swollen, and may perforate. Pressure and pain increase as pus fills the middle ear. There is often temporary deafness and ringing, and sometimes fever. Treatment is with antibiotics.
A form of otitis in which a sticky substance is discharged in the middle ear is common in children. The ossicles cannot function, and in severe cases permanent deafness results.
MASTOIDITIS Middle ear infections can spread to the mastoid bone - the part of the skull just behind the ear. Infection swells the bone painfully, and the patient is feverish. Treatment is by antibiotics. If those fail, surgical removal of the infected bone (mastoidectomy) may be needed.
MENIERE'S DISEASE affects the inner ear, and results in too much fluid in the labyrinths. Its cause is not known. It tends to occur in middle age, usually affecting more men than women. The symptoms are attacks of giddiness and sickness, followed by deafness with accompanying tinnitus.
Treatment is with drugs and control of fluid intake (not more than 2½ pints a day). In extreme cases the labyrinths or their nervous connections are destroyed.
FUNGUS INFECTIONS can occur in the outer ear. They are more common in tropical climates. There is persistent irritation and discharge, which is treated with antibiotics and antiseptic cleansing of the ear canal.

E38 DEAFNESS

TYPES OF DEAFNESS
"Conductive deafness" refers to any failure in those parts of the ear which gather and pass on sound waves eg blockage of the ear canal, eardrum damage, ossicle damage, etc.
"Perceptive deafness" refers to any failure in: that part of the ear which translates the sound waves into nerve impulses (the cochlea); or in the auditory nerves which transmit the impulses to the brain; or in the auditory centers of the brain which receive the message.
Perceptive deafness may not mean that the person can perceive no sound. It may be that sound is received, but so scrambled as to be unintelligible.
CAUSES OF DEAFNESS
a) Disease. Some disorders can end in deafness. See E37.
b) Noise-induced. Any exposure to extremely loud noise, or continued exposure to moderately loud noise, can damage the eardrum and middle ear, causing hearing decline and eventually deafness.

rare cases even to the brain.
Earache can also arise without any ear disorder, because of disturbances affecting the nerves it shares with other parts of the head. Tonsilitis, bad teeth, swollen glands, and neuralgia can all cause earache in this way.
RINGING in the ears ("tinnitus") is usually associated with earache in the middle ear and/or high blood pressure. It is also caused by certain ear diseases.
GIDDINESS or vertigo can be caused by infections of the inner ear that affect the organs of balance.
DISCHARGES can come from boils or other infections.

E36 SITES OF DISORDER

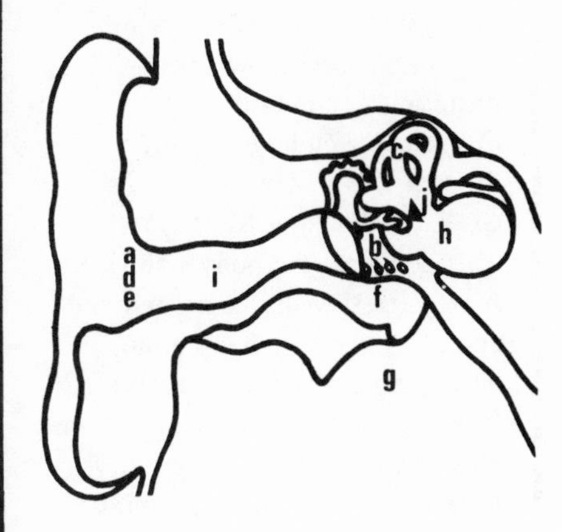

a Blockage
b Ringing
c Vertigo
d Discharge
e Otitis externa
f Otitis media
g Mastoiditis
h Meniere's disease
i Fungus
j Otosclerosis

The main victims are those who work in very noisy surroundings, and also the fans - and performers - of loud popular music.
c) Congenital deafness.
Deformities at birth range from complete absence of the ears, to minute mistakes in the internal structure. The latter can often be cured surgically. Congenital deafness can be due to heredity (genetic defects). It can also result from certain infections in the mother in the first few months of pregnancy, including german measles, flu, and syphilis. If there is anything in your child's response to sounds that gives rise to worry, consult your doctor.
d) Otosclerosis. This is a condition in which the stirrup becomes fixed within the oval window, due to deposits of new bone. About one person in every 250 suffers from this, and it is more common in men than in women. Surgical treatment can give improvement, but there is no way of halting the process responsible (though it may stop spontaneously).

E39 HEARING AIDS

Hearing aids work by amplifying sound. If the amplification is loud enough, it can overcome the blockage or damage that causes conductive deafness, and allow the sound to reach the inner ear.
Amplification also seems to help in many cases of perceptive deafness. However, sometimes the aid does not allow speech to be distinguished: it only makes the person more aware of unintelligible noise.
The performance of a hearing aid depends on:
a) The frequency response. Normal speech usually lies between 500 and 2000 cycles per second.
b) The degree of amplification.
c) The maximum amount of sound that the aid can deliver. Too much sound can make speech unintelligible, and/or damage the ear mechanisms.
INSERT RECEIVERS are the most common type of aid. They are molded to fit into the ear canal and form a perfect seal. No sound escapes, there is little or no acoustic feedback, and background noise is at a minimum. They can also be very small and, if transistorized, need no wires or attachments. A high degree of amplification is possible.
One problem with hearing aids is "acoustic feedback". This is the re-amplification of sound vibrations that have already passed into the ear but have partly leaked out again.
FLAT RECEIVERS fit against the external ear cartilage, and are kept in place by a metal band. They are usually used only if there is a continuous discharge from the ear, or if there has been a serious mastoid operation. Because of the bad contact, many sounds escape, and acoustic feedback produces much background noise.
BONE CONDUCTORS amplify the sound waves and send them through the bone of the head, not the air passages of the ear. They are uncomfortable and not very efficient, and are usually only used where some ear condition rules out an insert receiver.

F01 WHAT IS FITNESS?

In the most general sense, a person's fitness is his ability to cope with his environment and the pressure it puts on his mental and physical system.

But in a more usual, and useful, sense, fitness refers to the body's physical capabilities, as measured by tests of strength, speed, and endurance.

Notice that, though fitness is usually associated with health, it is not the same thing. An olympic athlete can be ill, and someone free of diagnosable illness may still be extremely unfit.

In the absence of planned exercise, work and transport effort (such as walking or climbing stairs) are the main determinants of a person's actual physical capabilities.

In modern society, as the element of physical activity in work and transport declines for most of us, we are increasingly dependent on planned exercise if we are to hold on to fitness and its benefits.

F02 COMPONENTS OF FITNESS

There are four basic components of physical fitness:

a) general work capacity;
b) muscular strength;
c) muscular endurance; and
d) joint flexibility.

GENERAL WORK CAPACITY

This concerns the body's ability to supply itself with the oxygen and energy it needs to keep going during general physical activity.

It depends on the efficiency of the cardio-vascular and respiratory systems, and is therefore usually called "circulo-respiratory fitness" (CR fitness). In general, CR fitness is called on in those activities that involve a good proportion of the body's muscles over an extended period of time, eg hard walking, running, jogging, swimming, cycling. The limit of CR endurance is marked by labored breathing and a pounding heart, rather than by failure of a particular muscle group to respond any more.

MUSCULAR STRENGTH

This concerns the maximum force a particular muscle group can apply in one action. There are two types.

a) Isometric strength is force applied against a fixed resistance.
b) Isotonic strength is force applied through the full range of movement available to a certain muscle or muscle group (as set by the joint or joints acted upon).

An example involving both types of strength is arm-wrestling. The beginning, when the participants arms first lock motionless against each other, involves isometric strength. The latter part, in which one participant's arm forces the other's down to the table, involves isotonic strength. The two types are at least partly independent of each other.

MUSCULAR ENDURANCE

This concerns the ability of particular muscle groups to go on functioning over a period of time.

F04 FACTORS AFFECTING FITNESS

POTENTIAL FITNESS

Even if all people were as fit as possible, their physical abilities in terms of strength, speed, and endurance would not be equal. Three main factors limit someone's potential fitness.

a) Age. The natural atrophy of age affects the efficiency of the whole body. But different aspects of fitness reach peak potential at different times. Speed is at its best at the beginning of adulthood, strength in the late 20s, while endurance can improve up to middle age.

b) Sex. Women are constitutionally more fit than men. For example, they are better able to withstand extremes of temperature, and have a longer life expectancy. Men are specifically more fit - they have a greater potential for strength and speed.

c) Somatotype*. The shape of a person's body limits the degree of fitness that can be obtained. Most athletes have a high mesomorphic rating, and many also have a high ectomorphic one. People with a high endomorphic rating do not have the same capabilities.

ACTUAL FITNESS

Similarly, several factors determine actual fitness.

a) Medical health. A person cannot become or remain fit if his body is not in good health.

b) Nutrition. A healthy diet is essential in attaining and maintaining fitness and health (see G20).

c) Weight. If someone is above his desirable weight*, his body is always functioning under the burden of an extra load. If someone is too far below optimum weight, his tissues will lack the ability to function at maximum efficiency.

d) Physical activity. With lack of activity, the body atrophies. This is shown by the muscular weakness that follows confinement to bed,

Again, there is both isometric and isotonic endurance. Isometric endurance involves the ability to maintain force as long as possible against a fixed resistance or in a fixed position (as when the opening lock of arm wrestling continues over a period of time). Isotonic endurance involves the ability to repeat a muscular movement against resistance as many times as possible (as with push-ups or repetitive weight-lifting).
In both cases, the limit is marked by inability of the muscle group to respond any more.

FLEXIBILITY
This concerns the range through which a joint will move. Except in the case of certain bone disorders, it depends more on the nearby muscles than on the structure of the joint itself.

INTER-RELATION
a) Localization. Levels of muscular strength, muscular endurance, and joint flexibility are all localized i.e. development of one part of the body does not necessarily imply the development of any other part. CR fitness, in contrast, usually develops as a single entity.
b) Inter-dependence. Muscular strength and endurance in any one muscle or muscle group are inter-related. For example (taking isotonic strength), a muscle capable of a maximum 200 lb force through its whole range of movement will be able to go on moving 50 lb through that range longer than one with an 80 lb maximum. Otherwise the components of fitness are fairly independent of each other.

MOTOR ABILITIES
An individual's physical capabilities are limited not only by his fitness, but also by his motor abilities: coordination, balance, agility, reaction time, speed, movement time (i.e. speed of moving a part of the body), and power (i.e. ability for explosive movement).

F03 HUMAN EFFICIENCY
The efficiency of any system is measured by how much energy output (work) it gives, for a set amount of energy input (fuel). Its efficiency will vary, depending on how near to its limits it is working. The nearer it is to maximum energy output, the more units input are needed for each unit gain in output. But all systems are more or less inefficient over all their output range i.e. all give less than 100% return.
The average human body is between 16 and 27% efficient - which compares badly with several products of the human mind. But by regular exercise the body's efficiency can be raised to 56%, which is better than many machines.

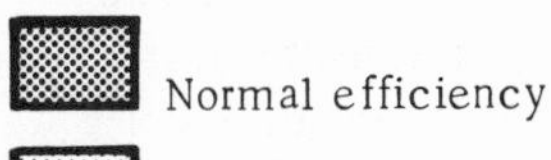

Normal efficiency
Normal variation
Efficiency with fitness

a Electric motor
b Steam turbine
c Petrol motor
d Steam engine
e Human body

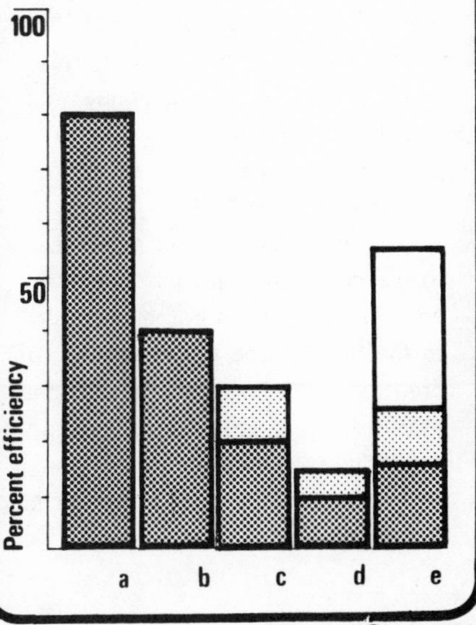

and by the way limbs change shape when encased in plaster casts.
e) Sleep. In order to function at optimum efficiency, the body and mind must have adequate rest (see E07-E14).

Muscle strength, by sex and age

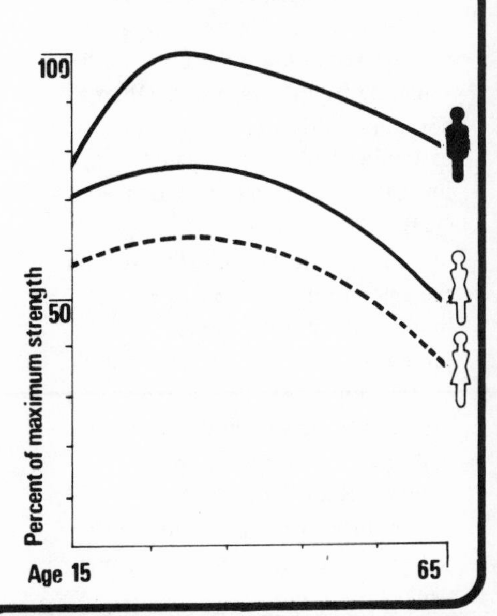

This graph shows how strength varies with age in men and in women. The dotted line shows actual average strengths for women. The other line for women shows what their strength would be if they were the same size as men.

F05 BODY DURING ACTIVITY

Any muscular effort requires some energy, and puts some demand on the rest of the body to supply that energy. When a large proportion of the body's muscles are involved over a period of time, the effects of this become noticeable.

CARDIO-VASCULAR SYSTEM
The blood network supplies the cells of the body with the oxygen and other nutrients (glucose, fat, etc) that they need for activity, and takes away the resulting waste products (carbon dioxide, lactic acid, etc). The heart is the pump that drives blood around the system. During exertion, more nutrient and waste transportation is needed. This is mainly supplied by increased heart activity. The total rate of blood flow may rise by up to 600% due to increase both in the rate of heart beat and in the amount pumped at each stroke. Systolic blood pressure may rise up to 70%. At the same time, levels of nutrients build up in the blood, as physical need increases, and levels of waste products as usage exceeds disposal.
Constriction of capillaries in uninvolved areas (such as stomach and skin) reduces their blood supply, while dilation of others increases the supply to involved areas (involved muscles, lungs, and heart). Later, as body heat builds up, dilation of capillaries near the skin surface allows blood flow to give radiation heat loss.

RESPIRATORY SYSTEM
This steps up activity in response to the cells demand for oxygen and the build up of carbon dioxide in the blood. The depth and rate of breathing increases, so ventilation may rise up to 12 times the resting rate. Overall oxygen consumption may rise from $\frac{3}{4}$pt (US) a minute to $10\frac{1}{2}$pt (US).

ANAEROBIC ENERGY SUPPLY
If oxygen supply does not equal need, the muscles can still go on working for a time, because they have some ability to function "anaerobically", i.e. without oxygen. Some forms of exercise can be completely anaerobic, because they occur in short concentrated bursts of up to 10 seconds (eg sprinting). But an "oxygen debt" is built up - i.e. large quantities of oxygen are then needed to clear the accumulated waste products.
Other forms must be chiefly aerobic, because of the length of time they last (eg long-distance running). So they have to be at a lower level of exertion, so oxygen supply can more nearly keep up.

LIVER
During physical exertion, the liver is important for its ability to convert waste lactic acid into useful glycogen or glucose (providing oxygen is present). This maintains glucose levels, slows the build up of oxygen debt, and increases the blood's ability to carry carbon dioxide.

ENDOCRINE SYSTEM
The main short-term hormonal response to physical exertion is release of adrenalin by the adrenal glands, stimulating the body to the "fight or flight" response*. Other hormonal activity controls, for example, body water, and aids increased energy mobilization

OTHER RESPONSES
a) It is possible that during exertion the spleen releases reserve red blood cells into the blood, increasing its gas carrying capacity.
b) The skin's heat loss by sweat and radiation is determined not only by body mechanisms but also by external conditions. High environmental temperatures limit radiation loss; high humidity limits sweat loss.

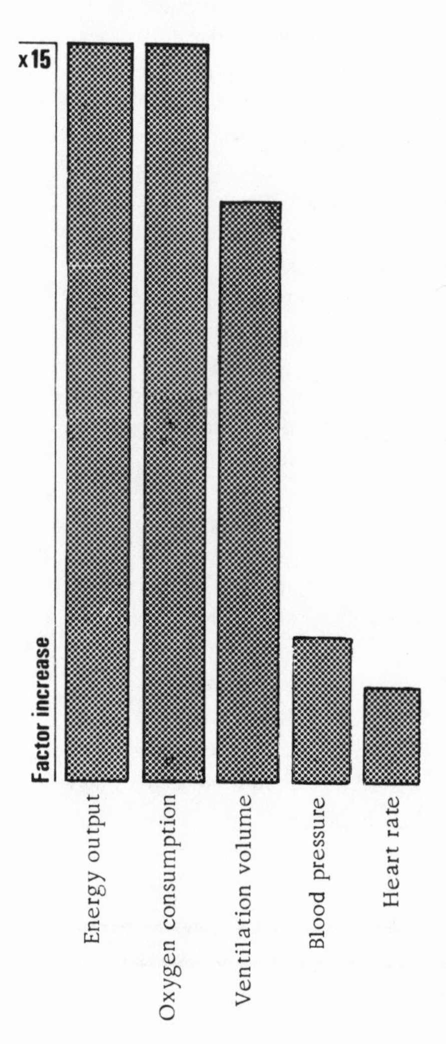

F06 INACTIVE MAN

In a mechanical system, use produces wear and deterioration. In the human body, the changes during strenuous activity are drastic - but it is chiefly disuse that causes deterioration. Once growth has ceased, there is no physical improvement without increased physical demand. This is true not only of muscular strength and cardio-vascular and respiratory response, but also of motor abilities such as co-ordination and reaction time. Moreover, inactivity not only fails to develop latent capacity, but also results in a general deterioration of many body systems, through disuse.

The effects on the muscular system are the most obvious. There are 639 muscles in the body, accounting on average for 45% of body weight. Loss of muscle tone results, for example, in:

a) general physical weakness and tiredness;
b) a weak and sagging abdomen;
c) back pain due to weak back muscles; and
d) a weak and lethargic heart.

Degeneration of the abdomen and heart have, in particular, general effects throughout the system. Abdominal weakness favours digestive trouble, while sluggish blood flow encourages blockage of arteries and capillaries.

In general terms, the effects of inactivity show themselves in reduced vitality, lowered resistance to infection, and perhaps in such mental conditions as lack of enthusiasm, inability to concentrate, nervousness, irritability, and insomnia. Physical inactivity also increases food intake (see G27), often producing excess weight with all its harmful consequences. When inactive man does have to undergo physical stress, his heart cannot greatly increase its stroke volume. A pounding heart results, as it tries to keep up with demand just by beating faster.

F07 HARMFUL EFFECTS?

Despite the benefits of activity for the body, some harmful effects can occur from ill-judged exercise.

HEALTH AND AGE

Sudden violent exertion after a period of inactivity or ill health is to be avoided. Any fast or vigorous physical activity should never be attempted without a gradual development of fitness first - especially over the age of 30. The older one is, the more unhealthy, or the lower the existing level of fitness, the more careful one should be about the rate of progress - and the more sensible it is to check with a physician first, especially if more than one of these factors is involved. In fact, any inactive person aged 35 or over should check with a physician before starting a serious exercise program. And no one should suddenly begin doing activities that exhaust them or make their heart pound.

THE HEART

Appropriate exercise will usually benefit even a seriously diseased heart (see F08). Severely inappropriate exercise can damage even a healthy one. Anyone, of any age, who suspects he has something wrong with his heart, or his blood pressure, should, again, check with a physician. A heart already weakened by disease or congenital deformity will suffer rather than gain from any sudden extra burden.

BODY HEAT

a) Always precede vigorous localized muscle activities with general warm up movements - especially when exercising in cold conditions. Sudden activity in a few muscles when the rest of the body is cold can send the blood pressure soaring. Isometrics, in particular, should be preceded by warming up movements.
b) Never wear sweat clothing or rubber suits during exercise, in the belief that this will help you "lose weight". The resulting dehydration could even kill you.
c) Don't stop suddenly after violent exertion, especially if suddenly changing to a warm environment. Slow down gradually.

SORENESS AND PAIN

Normal soreness or stiffness after exercise is simply due to the build-up of waste products, and will go as these are cleared. But during exercise sudden unaccustomed movements can wrench muscles and joints. You should get accustomed to new movements gradually, so your body can learn what positions and efforts it can safely allow. Take any feelings of pain or strain seriously, and ease off. Within a session of exercise (and within each exercise, where appropriate), work up gradually from gentle movements to forceful. Where some jolting against the ground in inevitable, use shock absorbing footwear or a suitable surface. Treat any muscle injuries that occur (whether impact or wrenching) with ice or cold water, elastic pressure dressing, elevation, and rest, rather than with heat.

F08 THE GAIN FROM ACTIVITY

MOTOR ABILITIES When the same activity is repeated, learning allows control of movement to become involuntary and so freed from the retarding influence of thought. Co-ordination and skill improve, and wasted motions become fewer.

MUSCLES Depending on the degree of exertion and the type of exercise, there may be increase in the size, strength, hardness, endurance, and flexibility of muscles used.

a) Size changes with growth in muscle mass due to increased size of individual muscle fibers.

b) Strength changes with muscle size: muscle fiber has a contractile force roughly proportional to its cross-section area.

c) Short-term strength changes occur too rapidly to be due to muscle size, and are probably due to better nervous organization. Inhibitory impulses (designed to prevent muscle being torn away from the bone) may be allowed to weaken with learning, so that positive impulses reach the muscle sooner and produce a stronger response. Improvement in motor coordination may also help.

d) Changes in hardness are due to tighter contraction, and perhaps to muscle fiber replacing fat.

e) Development of endurance may be due to increased capillarization (see below), or, as with strength, to improved nervous organization.

f) The processes by which flexibility is increased are not yet understood. Gains in flexibility reduce the likelihood of joint injury and muscular stress.

THE HEART gains from appropriate exercise, as other muscles do. Its strength, coordination, and endurance improve. More blood is pumped per stroke, so the rate of heartbeat can be lower. In a normal adult at rest, the heart rate is perhaps 70 a minute, and 80 or 90 is not uncommon. After endurance training, 55 to 60 beats a minute is possible, increase during exertion is smaller, and return to normal more rapid. The heart may beat several thousand times fewer every day, and so suffer less from wear.

CARDIO-VASCULAR SYSTEM Regular exertion has several effects.

a) It increases the number of capillaries in active tissue, improving the blood supply so that the body cells are capable of using more oxygen and nutrients per minute. The heart especially benefits, and here the capillaries also provide alternative routes that aid recovery from heart attacks.

b) It also improves the speed of return of blood from the extremities. The action of improved muscle tone against vein walls aids flow and helps prevent thromboses and varicose veins.

c) It may also reduce some forms of high blood pressure, by relaxing the arterioles.

d) Arterial deposits are kept in check by the increased blood flow during exertion and by the effect exertion has of reducing the blood content of fats such as cholesterol* and triglyceride (perhaps because exercise metabolism uses them up). Exertion may also lower the blood's clotting tendencies. If so, thromboses are less likely.

In general, appropriate exercise can reduce the likelihood of cardio-vascular disorder and make recovery more likely if it does occur. This can be seen by comparing the rates of coronary heart disease and death in active and sedentary occupations. Exercise, in mild form, may also aid in recovery from such disorders.

RESPIRATORY SYSTEM This is strengthened and improved by exertion. Air intake increases, both in the amount that can be breathed in at one time (vital capacity), and in the amount taken in over a period (ventilation). The efficiency of gas exchange in the lung alveoli also improves, while an increase in the number of red blood cells aids blood gas transport.

BODY POSTURE Better muscle tone improves both skeletal posture and organ position. Stronger back muscles lower the likelihood of spine disorder and back pain. Stronger abdominal muscles prevent stomach sag, with widespread effects on the efficiency of the internal organs. Appetite and digestion improve, and better bowel action discourages flatulence, constipation, and piles. Also the muscle tone of abdomen and hamstrings controls the tilt of the pelvis - so here again improvement reduces the likelihood of lower back pain.

NERVOUS SYSTEM Motor responses are improved by exertion that requires quick interpretation, decision, and action. The system becomes more coordinated, and better able to judge and respond to exact requirements. In addition, there seems to be a relationship in some people between physical fitness on the one hand, and, on the other, mental and perceptual alertness, absence of nervous tension, and even prevention of emotional illness. Stress and inturned emotion may also be more specifically dissipated by exertion that is especially rhythmic, or that involves enjoyable competition.

RESISTANCE TO DISEASE The physical fitness that results from activity should make the body better able to fight off infection and to recover quickly from any illness (or injury) that does occur.

WEIGHT CONTROL For the role of exertion in weight control, see G27. In general, regular activity can use up excess Calories, stimulate the body to waste more Calories in thermogenesis, and in some cases lower the appetite. Exercise alone does not effectively reduce body fat, but it allows effective dietary measures to be - and feel - less severe.

ENERGY Someone used to physical activity usually has more energy than an inactive person.

a) His usually lower metabolic rate conserves energy resources.

b) The efficiency of his respiratory, cardio-vascular, and digestive systems makes oxygen and nutrients more quickly available during exertion, and speeds recovery afterwards.

c) He has increased oxygen debt tolerance i.e. his muscles can carry on without oxygen a little longer.

d) Any given physical demand is usually less near the limit of his acquired abilities, and so can be dealt with more efficiently. For example, he has lower oxygen needs for any specified task.

In general, a physically fit person is able to withstand fatigue for longer periods, and, after a similar work effort, he is probably more likely to have energy left for leisure activities.

WELL-BEING The physically active person is more likely to sleep well, look well, and feel the exhilaration of a healthy body.

LIFE EXPECTANCY The overall consequence of all the factors involved is that those taking regular exercise have a lower death rate for each age group than those who do not, and that, in general, the death rate is lower the more strenuous the exercise.

THE BODY AT REST
The physiological differences between active and inactive people are clear even when their bodies are at rest.

THE GAIN FROM ACTIVITY
The differences between active and inactive people are not fixed. For example, heart rate can be reduced by training, and energy efficiency increased. (Figures are averages, for a cross-section of people with different jobs.)

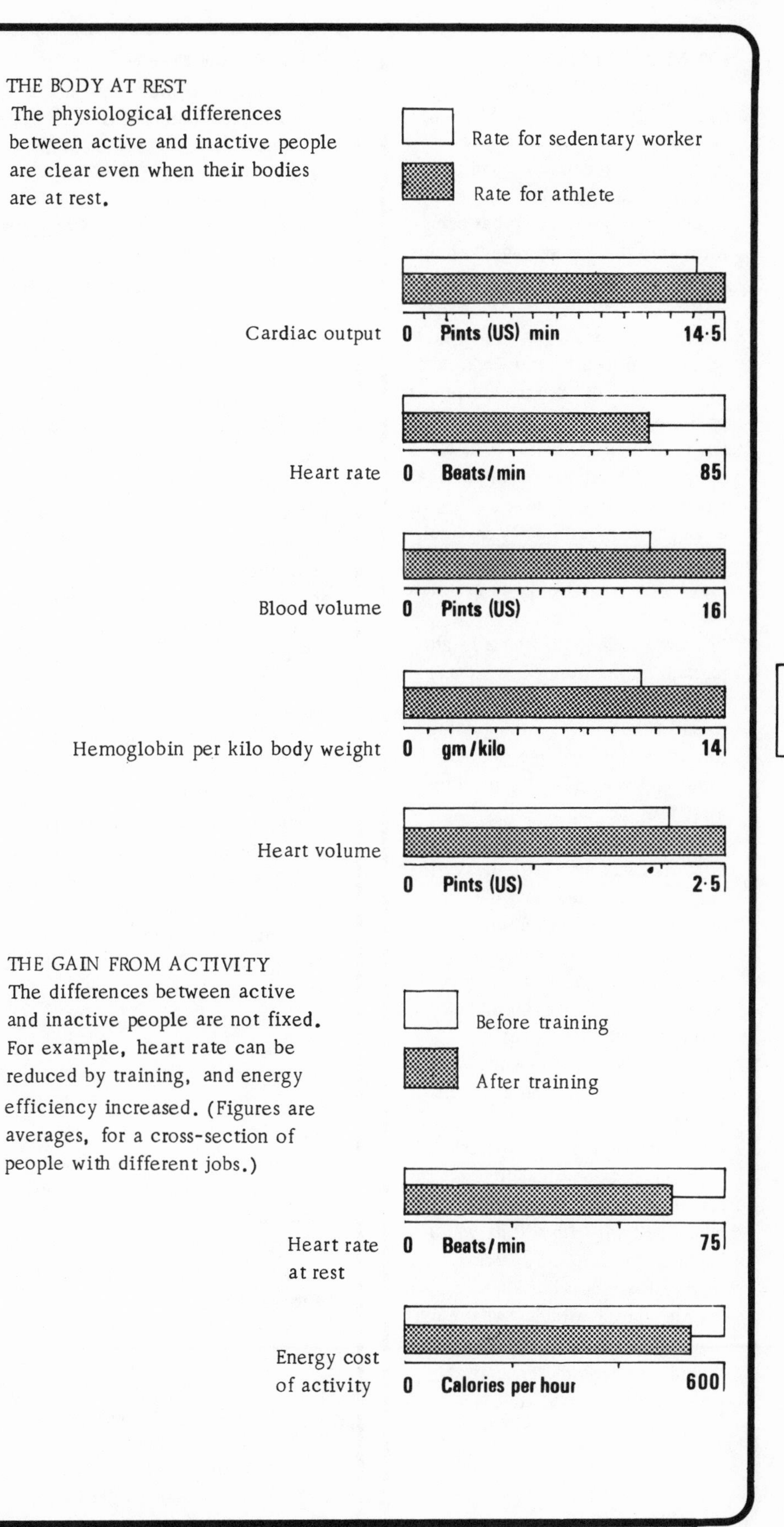

F

F09 NEED FOR EXERCISE

The natural conditions of our life no longer give us enough physical activity. Work and travel are increasingly sedentary - and leisure equally usually a matter of sitting watching something. (It has been estimated that on average 75 hours are spent by people in spectating - films, tv, sport, etc - for every 1 spent in physical participation.) So we have to plan and work, to achieve enough activity to keep us physically fit.

But if the need is there, so is the potential. A high level of physical fitness can often be reached in just a couple of months daily physical training - and maintained after that by exercising only on alternate days.

In theory, adequate fitness might perhaps be maintained every day by: walking briskly a mile or two to and from work; standing doing something for a couple of hours; using vigorous towelling movements after washing; stretching occasionally; and hurrying up a hill or stairs carrying a fairly heavy load. But in practice few have the time or taste or consistent discipline to organize even this; and most of us are well below desirable levels of fitness. So formal exercise, over and above the normal daily demands, becomes essential for the achievement of an efficient, strong, and durable body.

There are very many different approaches to physical fitness. The remaining pages of this chapter are concerned not with setting you a particular routine of exercise, but with telling you what kinds of exercise are available, what each can and cannot do, and how you should approach the general problem of keeping fit.

F10 THE MAIN TYPES

Each component of fitness has its own corresponding forms of exercise. This brief survey gives examples for lone participants. For the exercise effects of sports, see F16.

CIRCULO-RESPIRATORY EXERCISES (CR exercises) include brisk walking, jogging, running, cycling, swimming, and rope skipping and running on the spot; also cycling machines, rowing machines, etc. All are "aerobic", and therefore place demands on the circulation and respiration to supply oxygen to the muscles involved.

ISOTONIC EXERCISES consist almost entirely of weight-lifting. This gives the progressive resistance necessary to test, and increase, the maximum strength of a single joint movement.

ISOMETRIC EXERCISES are motionless. They use the force of one body muscle against another or against a fixed point such as a wall or bar. Towels or ropes provide simple accessories; more complex are machines (such as the Bullworker and Flexorciser) that provide variable resistance according to strength. Holding for 6 seconds or more produces the best strength gains, with 10 or 12 seconds recommended. Intensity of effort is more important than frequency.

MUSCULAR ENDURANCE EXERCISES consist mainly of traditional "calisthenics", with or without equipment i.e. push ups, sit ups, squat leg thrusts, pull ups to a bar, bar dips. All these are usually isotonic - as is weight lifting done with a repetitive pumping motion (used for increasing muscle size rather than strength). They are only isometric if held locked in a tense position (i.e. against gravity).

FLEXIBILITY EXERCISES usually consist of stretching and rotating movements of parts of the body.

F11 GENERAL FITNESS

The vital ingredients of a general fitness program are:

a) CR exercise;

b) endurance exercise for shoulders, arms, abdomen, back, and legs; and

c) flexibility and stretching exercises for neck and shoulders, back, and hips and hamstrings.

Not especially useful are isometric exercises and single contraction isometrics (though isometrics may be needed to make weak muscles strong enough to begin endurance movements).

For CR exercises see F17 and F18

Endurance and flexibility exercises can be obtained from gym training, keep fit classes, some sports, or from personal routines. With personal routines, the desire to persist in a movement or position is often too weak for improvement - but see F19.

Isometric exercises and single contraction isotonics (i.e. weight lifting) will not be considered in any further detail. There are many books on these subjects if required.

F13 GENERAL ADVICE

a) Take some exercise daily, if possible - especially with general fitness routines. (Some CR exercises, though, may give as good results from 2 or 3 workouts a week as from 4 or 5. Isotonic exercises should alternate work days and rest days.)

b) Whatever frequency you can manage, make it regular: don't skip allocated days.

c) Help yourself by setting aside a regular time: whether (for example) before breakfast, or in the late morning or afternoon at work, or at home in the early evening, or just before going to bed.

F12 CHOICE OF EXERCISE

The range of possibilities includes team sports, opponent sports, gym activities, keep-fit classes, companion activities (such as hiking or group jogging), lone indoor and outdoor routines, and extensions of normal activity such as walking to work or going up stairs carrying heavy shopping.
Factors in your choice of exercise will include:
a) your purpose;
b) the availability of time, money, facilities, equipment, and other people; and
c) your personal interests.
It is worth judging these things carefully before you make a decision.

PURPOSE
You may want to get generally fit, or to train for a sport, or perhaps to develop or strengthen a weak part of your body. The distinction is important because the function of different exercises is so specific. Where training for sport is the intention, the best method is to practice the sport itself. Endurance running, for example, will not help too much with endurance swimming - though some exercises may provide a near substitute.
But some sports do not raise the level of general fitness much, and so additional fitness training may bring improved performance.
Similarly, strengthening a part of the body is best done in conjunction with a general fitness program. (General fitness exercises also fulfil a useful warm-up function.)

REQUIREMENTS
Exercises vary greatly in their requirements. The same fitness may result from five minutes of daily exercise without equipment as from hours spent on (and traveling to) a specialized field with two teams and officials. Choose an activity that you know you will be able to arrange regularly.

INTERESTS
What exercise you will keep to also depends on what you enjoy. Different exercises offer varying elements of:
a) competition;
b) company;
c) being encouraged or goaded along by an instructor;
d) being pushed along by an abstract concept (such as time, or the desire to progress to the next level of fitness); and
e) associated factors, such as social life or the pleasure of being in the countryside.
You must judge which factors are most important to you. Remember that, to be enjoyable, some require success from you. Competition, or the eye of an instructor, or fighting against the clock, may not encourage you if you fail.

F

d) Also help yourself and avoid harmful effects by setting realistic targets. Start gently and progress slowly. Always underestimate your abilities. There is normally no long-term advantage in doing something "till it hurts" - and there are likely to be painfully obvious disadvantages. Something that seems all right for a day or two may result in sore muscles and the end of your resolutions. Your body is the best judge of what you can do. Take notice of it, and only adjust upwards when you are sure you are within your capabilities. Practical advice on determining your level of fitness and your safe levels of activity is given in F14 and F15.
e) Read F07, on possible harmful effects, before you start. But never feel that your health entirely rules out the possibility of exercise. Only a minimum of organic health is needed for some kind of general fitness program to be possible and desirable. Take your physician's advice.
f) Be sure to give the body a general warm up, either before a routine or as part of it (eg beginning with the less difficult exercises, and not immediately using full speed or effort).
g) Do not be discouraged if you reach a stage at which no progress is made. Ease back to a slightly lower level of effort, and progress up again from there.
h) Once the desired level of fitness is achieved, less frequency is needed to maintain it, eg general fitness routines may only require 3 workouts a week. But keeping up daily exercise may still be a good idea for relaxation, digestion, sound sleep, etc.
i) Associated factors may be as important as exercise. Get adequate sleep. Try to find ways of forgetting work worries. Eat sensibly. If you smoke, stop if you can.

F14 TESTS OF FITNESS

All components of fitness can be tested, eg isotonic strength by the weight of barbell that can be lifted, isometric strength using strain gauges and dynamometers. But only CR testing gives a good guide to general fitness. Muscular endurance tests may also be interesting for following progress.

CR FITNESS

The Tecumseh step test given here is safe for most age groups. It involves stepping up and down at a given rate between the ground and a single step, bench, or stool. Afterwards the pulse rate is taken.

General rules for any step test are:

a) face the same way all the time and always step back to the ground on the same side;

b) "one step" is one complete ascent and descent (see F18, bench stepping);

c) keep the correct step rate;

d) take the pulse at wrist or throat (but if at the throat do not press too hard, as this can alter the rate);

e) do stop before the time limit if the test is too hard (count this as putting you in the lowest fitness category); and

f) to compare performances over time, try to repeat under similar conditions (eg time of day and time and size of last meal; recent physical activity, health, and sleep; and step rate).

Do not be discouraged by apparent lack of progress: temporary factors may be involved.

MUSCULAR ENDURANCE

Isometric endurance tests judge the duration for which a certain contraction can be held (eg how long a known weight can be held at arm's length). More relevant for general fitness are isotonic endurance tests, which judge the number of times a given movement can be repeated. Typical tests (with average performances of male college students in brackets) include pull ups (8 completed), push ups (25), sit ups (40), and bar dips (9).

F15 HEART RATE AND EXERCISE

The Tecumseh step test gives you a guide to your general physical condition. You can use this to judge how high you should allow your heart rate to go during exercise.

Someone in the lowest ("very poor") category on the Tecumseh test (100 beats a minute or more) should begin exercising very gradually.

a) At the start of the first month he should exercise for 5 minutes a day at not more than 100 beats per minute. During that month he can gradually increase the time up to 10 minutes, but must keep the same heart rate limit.

b) During the second month the time allowed again increases from 5 to 10 minutes, but the heartrate limit is now 110 beats.

c) During the third month the same happens, but the limit is now 120.

d) Thereafter the person may allow his heart rate to rise to the desirable limit for his age.

Someone in the "below average" step test category should follow the same routine, but can begin at "b", and go on to "c" in the second month. Someone in the "above average" category can begin at "c".

AGE LIMIT

As the resting heart rate declines with age, the maximum possible and desirable rates also fall.

The estimated maximum possible heart rate for a healthy fit young adult is about 220 beats per minute. For a rough estimate of the maximum rate for anyone aged 30 years or older, the age should be subtracted from this figure. For example, the maximum heart rate of a man aged 40 is:

220 - 40 = 180 beats a minute.

To find the maximum heart rate that should be allowed in a fit person during exercise, the figure of 20 should be subtracted. For example, the maximum desirable rate for a man aged 40 is:

180 - 20 = 160 beats a minute.

Intensity	Heart rate	Walk/run (m.p.h.)	Cycling (m.p.h.)	Climbing (Grades)	Sports	Occupations
Maximum	200	13.0	20	12	running	digging
Very heavy	150	6.0	14	6	mountaineering	chopping wood
Heavy	140	5.5	12	5	tennis	pick and shovel
Fairly heavy	130	5.0	10	4	volleyball	gardening
Moderate	120	4.5	9	3	golf	house painting
Light	110	4.0	8	2	table tennis	auto repair
Very light	100	3.5	7	level	bowling	shopping

TECUMSEH SUBMAXIMAL TEST
For ages 10 to 69 (unless in poor health). Use 8in bench. Step at rate of 24 steps a minute for 3 minutes. Wait for exactly 1 minute after exercise. Then count heart beats for 15 seconds. Multiply that count by 4.

CATEGORIES
according to heart rate (rates for women in brackets).

Excellent	under 68	(under 76)
Good	68-79	(76-85)
Above average	80-89	(86-94)
Below average	90-99	(95-109)
Very poor	100 plus	(110 plus)

Adapted from Montoye, Willis, and Cunningham, J of Gerontology, 1968.

USING HEARTRATE GUIDES
a) Count the number of pulse beats in 15 seconds and multiply by 4. Unlike the step test, count while still exercising if possible (eg if walking).
b) With a little practice it is easy to make a rough judgement of the speed of one's heart beat at any moment, and when it is getting a bit too high. This then becomes the most practical method.
The table gives some idea of levels of heartbeat in different common activities for fit young adults.

F16 SPORT AND EXERCISE

Here we show the effect of different sports on fitness; eg, running has a high effect on CR capacity, but little on strength. The last column gives maximum recommended ages. (Note: badminton, handball, and tennis have less CR effect, and higher age limits, if played doubles.)

○ some effect
● considerable effect

	CR capacity	Muscular endurance	Strength	Power	Agility	Age
SOLO ACTIVITIES						
Archery		●	○			
Bicycling	●	○	○			
Calisthenics	●	●	○			
Canoeing	●	●	○			
Gymnastics		●	●		●	45
Hiking	●	●				
Jogging	●	●				
Skipping	●	●				40
Rowing	●	●	○			
Running	●	●				45
Skiing	●	●	○		●	45
Swimming	●	●	○	●	●	
TEAM SPORTS						
Basketball	●	●		●	●	30
Baseball	○	●		●		45
Football (US)	○	●	○	●	●	30
Hockey	●	●	○		●	30
Rowing	●	●	○			30
Soccer	●	●	○		●	45
Softball	○	○			●	50
Volleyball		○		●	●	
OPPONENT SPORTS						
Badminton	●	○			●	50
Bowling		○				
Canoeing	●	●	●			30
Golf	○			●		
Handball	●	○		●	●	45
Tennis	●	○		●	●	45
Skating	●	●	○		●	45
Skiing	●	●	○		●	45
Swimming	●	●	●			30

F17 CR EXERCISE

For improvement in the cardio-vascular and respiratory (CR) systems, considerable demand must be placed on them by:
a) the duration of exercise; and
b) its intensity (as shown by the heart rate response).
The demand needed for improvement depends on age and existing fitness; but in a fit young adult, for example, exertion at 140 to 150 beats a minute would be needed for 8 to 10 minutes several times a week. With longer duration, though, a rate as low as 120 beats gives improvement.
Intensity depends on:
a) the proportion of body muscle involved (eg jogging is more intense than sit ups); and
b) the pace of exercise (eg running is more intense than jogging).
Very low intensity exercise (eg slow walking) may not give improvement whatever the duration.
If the allowable heart rate is limited by poor fitness, this must be dealt with first; if by age, lengthy exercise of just enough intensity (eg steady walking) must be taken.
General fitness programs can give some CR fitness. But once some general fitness is achieved, the intensity of the program may not be very high and the duration insufficient. It is sensible to do additional CR exercises. An excellent source of CR programs is "The New Aerobics" by K. Cooper (Bantam).
If arranging your own CR program, start with 3 workouts a week for a fortnight, then 5 a week till desired fitness is reached. Then maintain with 3 or 4 a week.
Alternatively, follow the outlines in F18.

F

KEEPING FIT 2

F18 CR ROUTINES

Here we give simple outlines, around which CR exercise routines can be constructed. Choose an exercise, and carry it out for the required amount of time each day (included repeated occasions if specified). Also for the required number of days per week.

Start at level A. If a range of choice is given, for the number of days per week at that level, start with the lowest number and build up to the highest.
Then very gradually, and without strain or exhaustion, build up toward level B (by increasing distance and/or speed and/or duration, whichever is specified). In some cases, A1, A2, and A3 show how to start building up effort. At level B, as indicated, fitness can usually be maintained with only 3 or 4 days' exercise per week. Exercises can be alternated for variety if desired.

	Distance	Rate	Time per day	Days per week
Walking	A 1 mile	1 mile in 15 mins	15 mins	5
	B 3 miles	1 mile in 13 mins	39 mins	5
	or 4 miles	1 mile in 13 mins	52 mins	4
	or 5 miles	1 mile in 13 min	65 mins	3
Stationary running	A	70 to 80 steps a min	1 min	5
	B	80 to 90 steps a min	20 mins	3 or 4
Running	A 1) 1 mile	1 mile in 13 mins (walk)	13 mins	3 to 5
	2) 1 mile	1 mile in 11 mins (walk/run alternately)	11 mins	5
	3) 1 mile	1 mile in 9½ mins	9½ mins	5
	B 2 miles	1 mile in 8½ mins	17 mins	3
Combination	A Walking			
	1) ½ mile	120 steps per min		5
	2) 1 mile	120 steps per min		5
	B Alternate jogging and running			
	1) 1 mile	120 steps per min		5
	2) 3 miles	120 steps per min		5

	Distance	Rate	Time per day	Days per week
Swimming	A 1) 25 yds, 4 times*	25 yds in 35 secs	2½ mins	3 to 5
	2) 100 yds	100 yds in 2½ mins	2½ mins	5
	3) 100 yd increases	100 yds in 2½ mins	5 mins, 7½ mins etc	5
	B 1000 yds	100 yds in 2 mins	20 mins	3 or 4

* 4 separate occasions, with rests between

	Distance	Rate	Time per day	Days per week
Cycling	A 1 mile	12 mph	5 mins	5
	B 8 miles	20 mph	25 mins	3 or 4
Bench stepping	A 8in bench	30 steps per min	3 mins	3 to 5
	B 15-18in bench	30 steps per min	5 mins	3 or 4

"One step" is one complete ascent and descent, involving four leg movement counts: first foot up, second foot up, first foot down, second foot down. At the rate specified above this gives 120 counts per minute i.e. 2 per second.

Tennis — Also squash, badminton, basketball, handball (singles)

	Time per day	Days per week
A	10 mins	3 to 5
B	60 mins	3
or	45 mins	4

	Sequence	Times per day	Days per week
Rope skipping	A 1) ½ min skip, 1 min rest, ½ min skip	2	3 to 5
	2) ½ min skip, 1 min rest, ½ min skip, 1 min rest, ½ min rest	3	5
	etc. building gradually to:		
	3) 2 min skip, ½ min rest, 2 min skip	2	5
	4) 2 min skip, ½ min rest, 2 min skip, ½ min rest, 2 min skip	3	5
	5) 4-5 minute skip	1	3 or 4
	B 6 min skip	1	3 or 4

F

F19 5BX PLAN

With most personal exercise routines, the incentive to persist in a movement or position is too weak for endurance improvement. The following plan overcomes this by adding the pressures of time and progressive grading.

The 5BX plan for men was developed by the Royal Canadian Air Force. It gives a balanced program, requiring little space or time and no special equipment, but progressing to the fitness levels of champion athletes.

The plan consists of 6 charts, each with 12 levels of fitness. An individual starts at the bottom of the first chart, works up to the top, and then progresses to the bottom of the next one. Within each chart, the required number of repetitions increases. From one chart to the next, the exercises become more complex and testing.

An individual's rate of progress is set:

a) by whether he can do the required exercises in the time allotted;

b) by his age (on Chart One, the older he is, the more days he must spend at each level - even if he can do the exercises comfortably in the allotted time); and

c) by his own desires and responses (he can progress more slowly if he wants - and should do if he gets stiff, sore, or unduly breathless, especially if in the older age groups).

The time allotted for the basic five exercises is, on all charts, 11 minutes. The time taken over individual exercises does not matter - providing all are done within 11 minutes. But there are alternatives - walking or running - that can be substituted for the fifth exercise. If so, the first four must be done in 5 minutes, and the walking and running in whatever time is specified at that level.

The program has a built-in warming-up routine, because a stretching and loosening exercise is always first. But an individual should also begin the first exercise slowly and easily, and gradually build up speed and vigor.

The maximum levels for average individuals are indicated on the charts. For example, on the first chart, a 6 year old boy would not be expected to get beyond level B, or a 7 year old beyond level A.

Once a desired level of fitness has been reached, it can be kept up with only 3 sessions per week. After any period of inactivity, the individual should restart at any lower level that is comfortable.

The information on these pages about the 5BX has been reproduced by permission of the copyright holders: Canada Information, Penguin Books Ltd, and (for the USA) Simon and Schuster Inc. Each of these can advise about published sources from which this plan can be pursued.

SAMPLE CHART: Chart 1 (Beginners)

Exercise	1	2	3	4	5	5A	5B
	Repetitions					Minutes	
A+	20	18	22	13	400	$5\frac{1}{2}$	17
A	18	17	20	12	375	$5\frac{1}{2}$	17
A-	16	15	18	11	335	$5\frac{1}{2}$	17
B+	14	13	16	9	320	6	18
B	12	12	14	8	305	6	18
B-	10	11	12	7	280	6	18
C+	8	9	10	6	260	$6\frac{1}{2}$	19
C	7	8	9	5	235	$6\frac{1}{2}$	19
C-	6	7	8	4	205	$6\frac{1}{2}$	19
D+	4	5	6	3	175	7	20
D	3	4	5	3	145	$7\frac{1}{2}$	21
D-	2	3	4	2	100	8	21
Minutes for each exercise	2	1	1	1	6		

Alternatives to exercise 5: 5A, $\frac{1}{2}$ mile run; 5B, 1 mile walk.

Minimum number of days at each level in Chart One.

Age	Days
under 20	1
20-29	2
30-39	4
40-49	7
50-59	8
60 and over	10

Exercise 2
Each chart uses the same 5 basic exercises; but they are slightly more complex and testing each time.

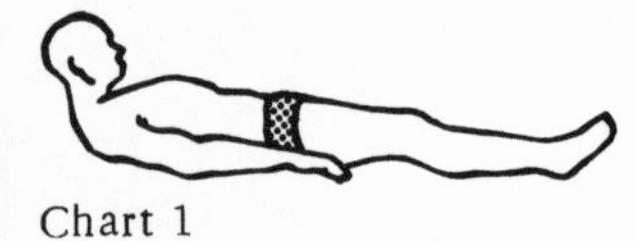

Chart 1

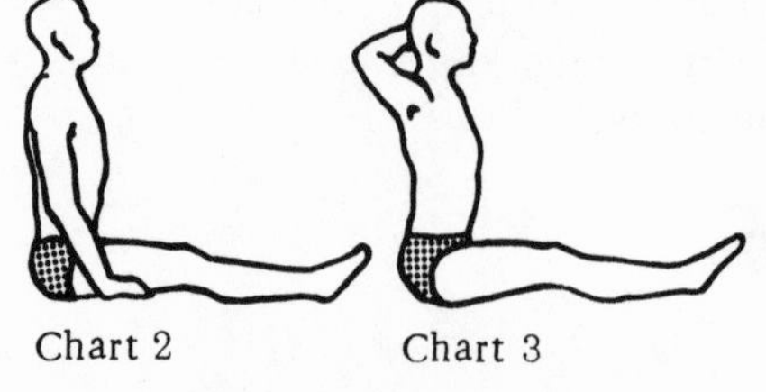

Chart 2

Chart 3

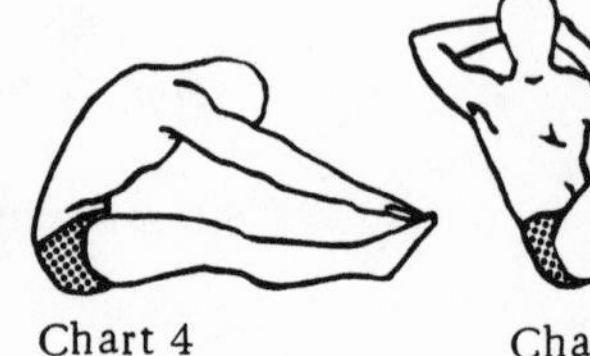

Chart 4

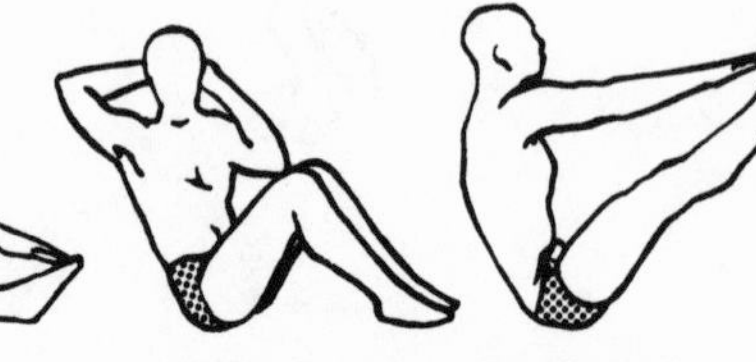

Chart 5

Chart 6

1a) feet astride, arms upward
b) forward bend to touch floor
c) return to upward stretch
d) backward bend
Do not strain to keep knees straight.

2a) back lying, feet 6in apart, arms at side
b) sit up so can just see heels
c) return to position a)
Keep legs straight. Head and shoulders must clear floor.

3a) front lying, palms beneath thighs
b) raise head and one leg
c) return to position
d) raise head and other leg
e) return to position
Above counts as one repetition. Keep legs straight at knee. Thighs must clear palms.

4a) front lying, hands under shoulders, palms flat on floor
b) fully straighten arms, lifting body, keeping knees on floor
c) bend arms and return so chest touches floor
Above counts as one repetition. Keep body straight from knees.

5 Stationary run. Lift feet about 4in from floor. Count one step every time left foot touches floor. Every 75 steps, do 10 scissor jumps. Continue till required steps completed.
Scissor jumps. Stand with right leg and left arm stretched forward, left leg and right arm back. Arm height as shown. Jump up and reverse arm and leg positions before landing. Jump and return to first position to complete one repetition.

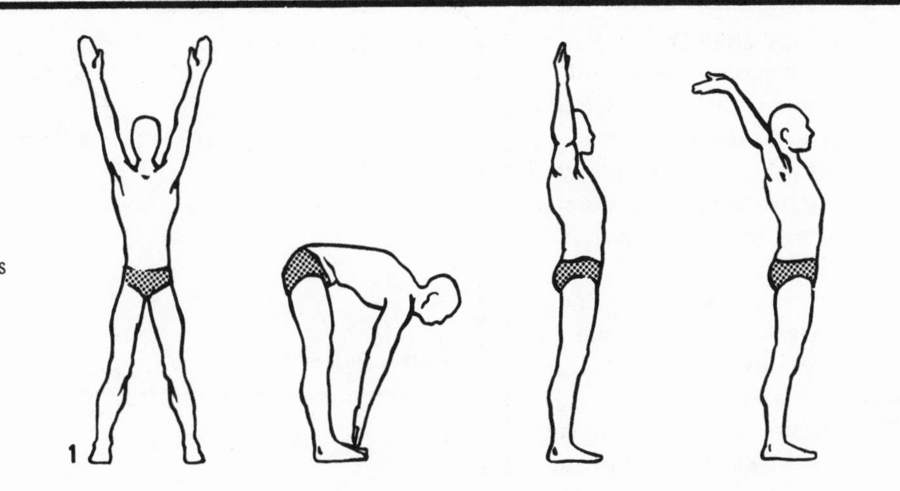

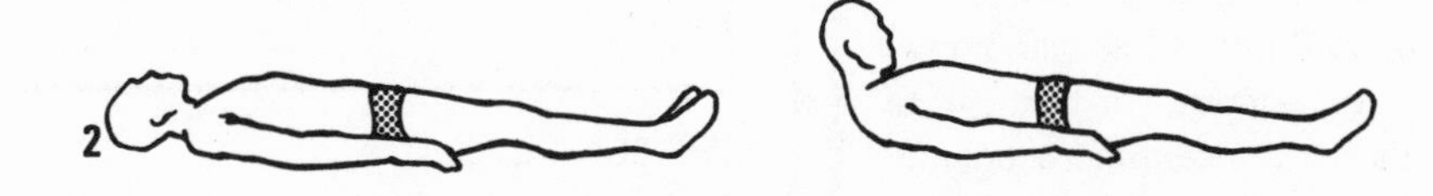

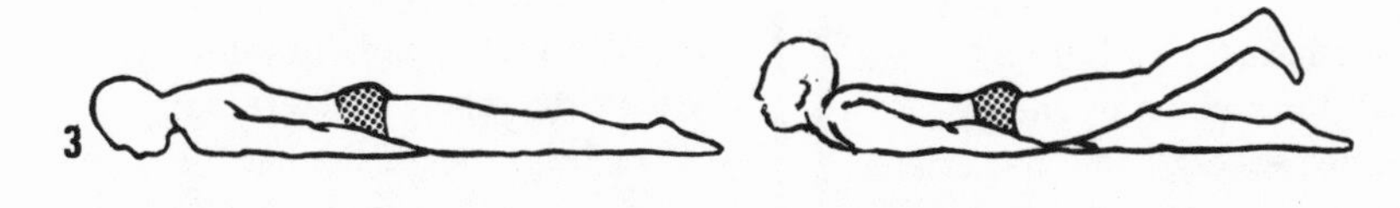

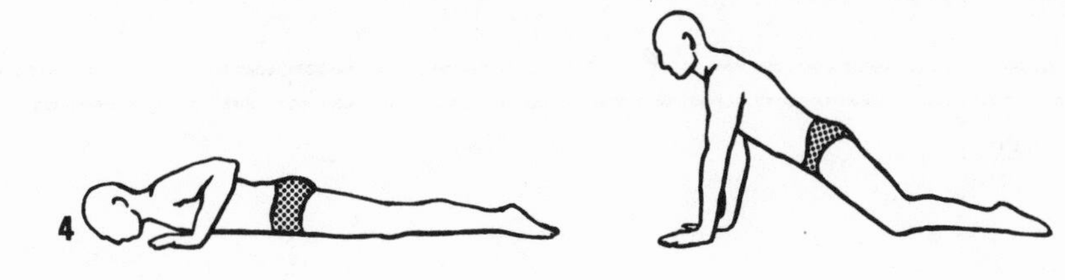

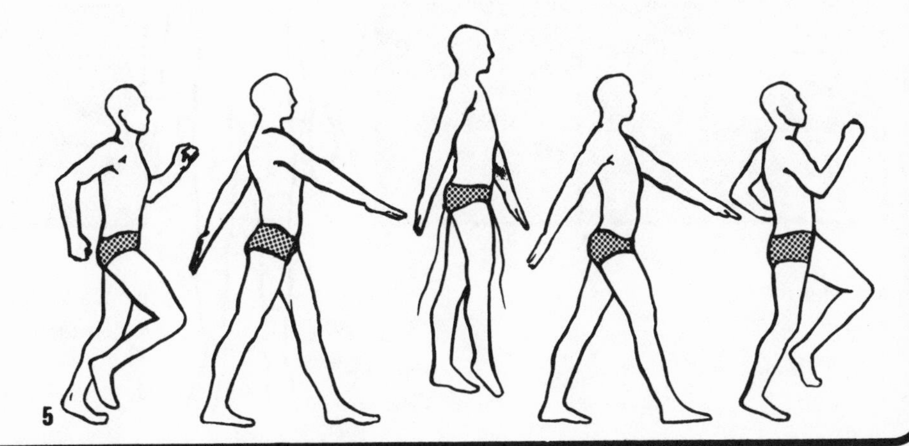

LIFE AND ENERGY

G01 LIFE AND ENERGY

All living things need sources of energy and material, because all life uses up energy and material: in movement, repair, and growth, and just in the internal processes of maintaining its own existence. Where living things find these sources is what governs their primary division into animals and plants. Most plants survive on inorganic (i.e. non-living) material - chemicals drawn from the soil and the air, and then processed within them in the presence of sunlight. They can build up complex substances out of simple ones. Animals, though, only use a few natural inorganic substances, and can only build up a few substances within their bodies. For them, food is the source of chemical energy and material. From the already complex substances in food, they break down the chemicals that they need.

So the synthesis of sunlight by plants begins a chain of energy transference: energy and matter are passed on, thereafter, because on life form consumes another as food.

G02 FOOD CHAIN

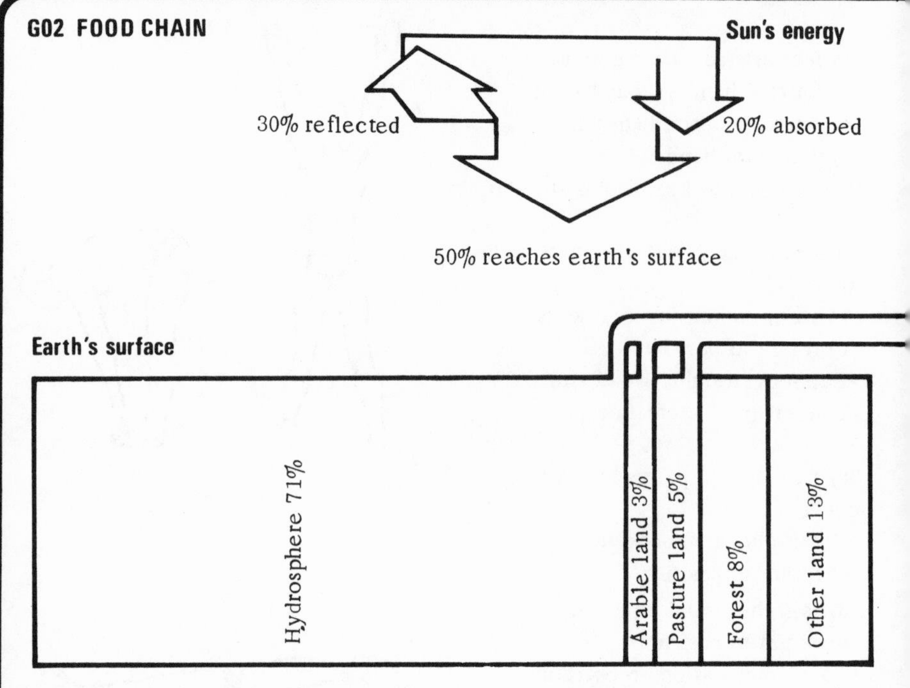

THE SUN'S ENERGY

Energy from the sun arrives at the edge of the earth's atmosphere at the rate of 2000 million million Calories per second. Of this, at least 30% is reflected and 20% absorbed by the atmosphere. The remaining 50% or less reaches the earth's surface, at the average rate of 100 Calories per square foot per day.

LAND USE

Of the energy reaching the surface, 71% irradiates areas of water, and 29% land areas. The land areas include forest and uncultivated land. Only about a third of the land surface is primarily in the food chain, as arable land or pasture.

G03 METABOLIC TURNOVER

... showing the daily input and output of a 154 lb man in a closed environment.

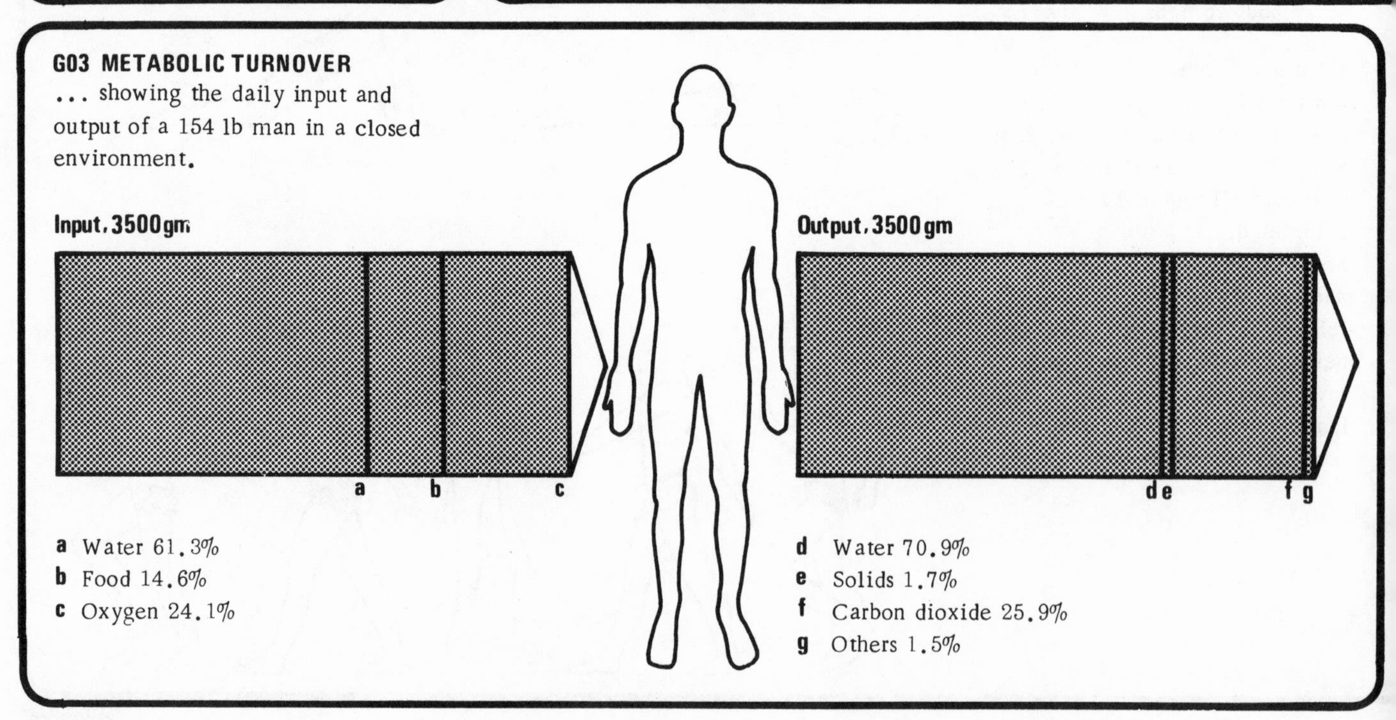

a Water 61.3%
b Food 14.6%
c Oxygen 24.1%

d Water 70.9%
e Solids 1.7%
f Carbon dioxide 25.9%
g Others 1.5%

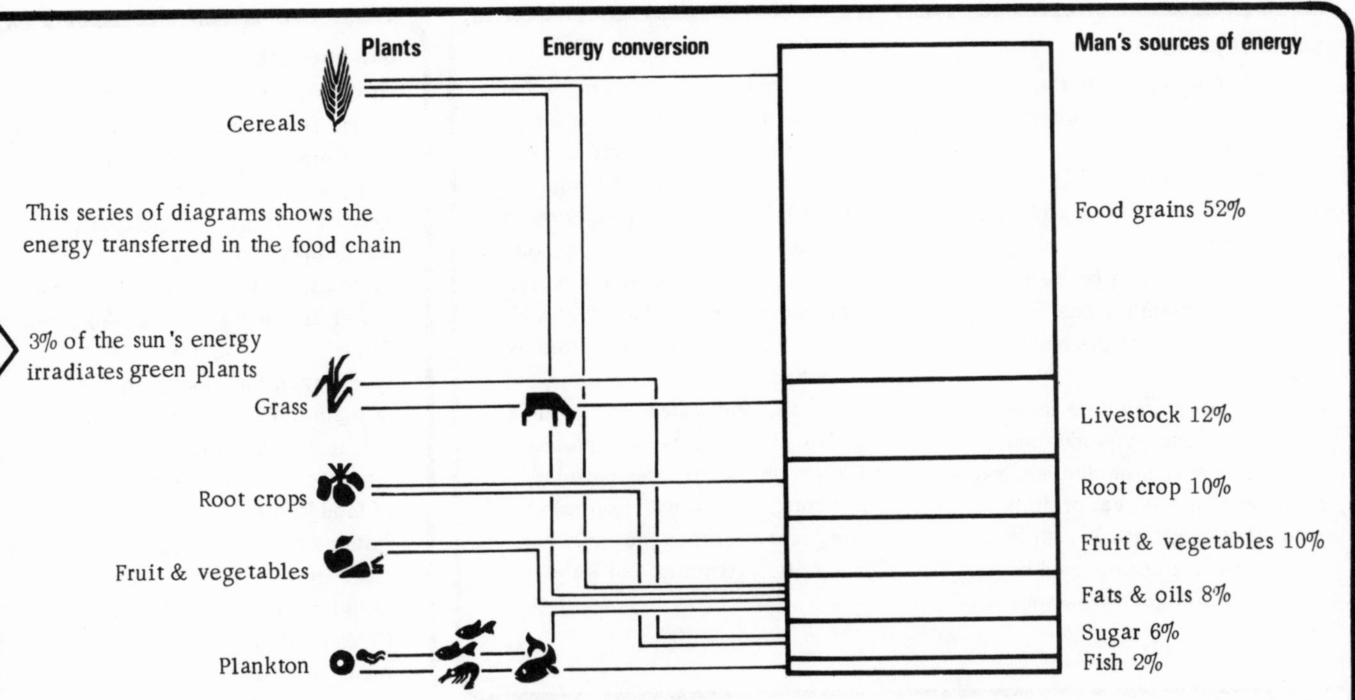

This series of diagrams shows the energy transferred in the food chain

3% of the sun's energy irradiates green plants

PLANTS
In all, only about 3% of the sunlight actually irradiates green plants on the land surface or algae in the sea. The land plants include cereals, grasses, root crops, and vegetables and fruit.

ENERGY CONVERSION
The plants convert about 1% of the energy reaching them into stored chemical energy. Some of this is stored. In the food chain, the plants are consumed, and about 10% of the plants' stored energy is stored by the animal that eats them. Similarly, when the animal is eaten, about 10% of its stored energy is stored by the eater.

MAN'S SOURCES OF ENERGY
The chain reaches man as inputs of food grains, livestock products, root crops, vegetables and fruit, fats and oils, sugar, and fish.

G04 RELATIVE EFFICIENCIES

At every step in the food chain, only 10% of the energy gets passed on. Prof. Hardin of the University of California gives an example of this: to produce 1 lb of man requires 10 lb of bass, which requires 100 lb of minnows, which requires 1000 lb of water flies, which requires 10,000 lb of algae
Meat and animal products are usually a much more concentrated source of human dietary needs than plant products. But the process of their production is far more inefficient, as there are more steps in the chain.
Here we compare energy loss in a potato crop and in beef cattle production. With potatoes, about 30% of the original sunlight energy becomes usable food energy for humans; with beef, only 4%.
In fact, an acre of land can produce, in a year, almost 9 times as much potato protein as beef protein.

POTATO
a Plant metabolic loss 37%
b Farming loss 24%
c Available for processing 39%
Available after processing 30%

CATTLE
d Plant metabolic loss 34%
e Farming and feeding loss 25%
f Animal metabolic loss 35%
g Available for processing 6%
Available after processing 4%

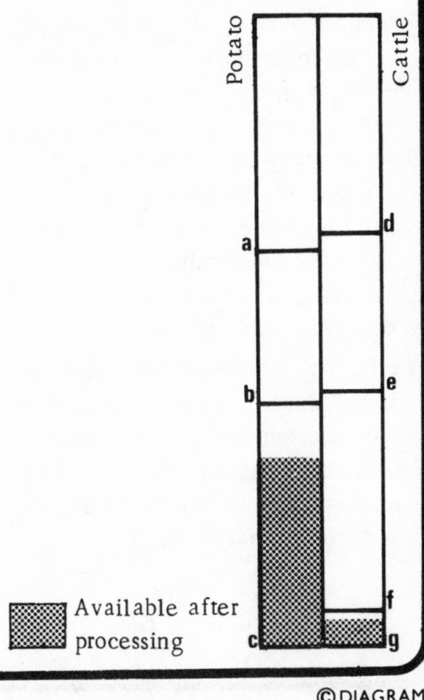

G05 WHAT FOOD IS

Food is anything that has a chemical composition which can provide the body with:
a) material from which it can produce heat, activity, and other forms of energy;
b) material that can be used in the growth, maintenance, repair, and reproduction of the body;
and/or
c) substances to regulate these processes of energy production, growth, repair, reproduction, etc.
Not everything we eat or drink is food. Flavorings such as paprika and pepper are not utilized by the body. Tea affects the nervous system and is a drug but not a food. (But alcohol, though it is a drug, also provides energy, and so falls within the definition of food.)
Bran performs a useful function as a laxative, but again is not food as it is not absorbed by the body.
The constituents of food that are of value to the body are: proteins, carbohydrates, fats, vitamins, minerals, and water. Energy uses carbohydrates, fats, and proteins. Growth and repair uses proteins, minerals, and water. Control of body processes uses proteins, minerals, vitamins, and water.

G06 CALORIES

The constituents in food that help growth and repair cannot all be measured on one scale: different constituents do different jobs, which are not interchangeable. The same applies to the constituents that control body processes. It is no good, for example, trying to add together Vitamin A units and calcium units to get so many "control units". That is like trying to add cows and washing machines. But the constituents that provide energy can be measured on a single scale, and added together. For in the end all of them can be measured in terms of the amount of heat they produce in the body.
The basic unit for measuring any energy (including heat output) is the scientist's calorie. This is defined as the amount of energy needed to raise the temperature of 1cc of water by 1°Centigrade. The measure used in talking about food and human energy needs is a thousand times larger than this: the kilocalorie, or Calorie (which should be - but is not always - written with a capital 'C').
For example, a typical number Calories for a man to use up in a day is about 3000. So this is the amount of energy his food must supply, unless he is to run down his stored reserves. Protein, fat, and carbohydrate are all sources of energy (though protein is more vital as a source of other things).
One ounce of protein produces over 113 Calories in the human body, one ounce of carbohydrate the same, and one ounce of fat 255 Calories. (An ounce of alcohol - which falls outside these three main categories - produces 180 Calories.)
Actual foods range in calorific value from, for example, 105 Calories to the pound (tomatoes) to 4200 Calories to the pound (lard).

G07 PROTEINS

Protein is the basic chemical unit of the living organism. There is no substitute for protein, for it is the only constituent of food which contains nitrogen - essential for the growth and repair of the body.
Proteins, in fact, provide the raw materials for the body's tissues and fluids. They also have certain specialized functions. They help to maintain the chemical fluid balance in the brain, spine, and intestine, and they aid the transport of food and drugs.
Proteins are very complex substances made from a number of chemicals called amino acids. About 20 different kinds of amino acid are found in protein food, and the thousands of different ways these can be linked up produce the many types of protein that exist in food.
A single protein molecule can contain as many as 500 amino acid units linked together.
The two main sources of protein are from animals, in the form of meat, fish, eggs, and dairy produce, and from plants in the form of nuts, peas and beans, grains and grain products (such as bread, especially wholemeal), and in small quantities in many tubers and vegetables.
Most animal proteins contain all the essential amino acids that humans need, and so are called complete proteins. But vegetable proteins are all, individually, more or less incomplete. They can carry out some individual jobs in the body, but cannot fulfil the vital task of cell repair and growth unless combined together, or with animal protein.
Most proteins are insoluble in water. Some are soluble - such as casein (milk), and albumen (egg white) - but become insoluble when heated or beaten.

G08 CARBOHYDRATES

Carbohydrates provide our main source of energy for immediate use. Energy is used up even during sleep, to keep body organs functioning. Carbohydrates play a vital role in the proper functioning of the internal organs and the central nervous system, and in heart and muscle contraction.

Our bodies cannot manufacture carbohydrates so we get them from plants, or from animals that feed on plants. Plants synthesize carbohydrates out of the reaction of sunlight on water and carbon dioxide. This is called photosynthesis and it occurs in the green leaves of plants.

All carbohydrates are made up from carbon, hydrogen, and oxygen. The end product of these three elements is first sugar and then starch, which is stored in plants for future use.

There are several different kinds of carbohydrates.

SUGAR

This is one kind, of which there are 5 types:

Glucose is the form in which fuel is transported in the body (though, eaten, it gives energy no more quickly than other sugars).

Fructose comes from grapes, honey, and other fruits. It can also be made out of sugar cane. Glucose converts to fructose during the process of the release of energy in the body.

Sucrose is a chemical combination of fructose and glucose and occurs naturally in sugar beet and sugar cane. It is also present in fruit and in carrots. Sucrose forms the common household sugar, which is available in various grades and in crystal sizes due to different refinement processes.

Lactose occurs naturally in human and cow's milk and is not as sweet as sucrose. It is a combination of glucose and galactose.

Maltose is derived from malt and is also produced naturally from starch when grain germinates.

STARCH

This forms the largest part of the carbohydrate in our food. It is the stored food in plant seeds, intended for use in maintaining the growing plant until it is able to feed itself by photosynthesis.

Unripe fruit contains starch which converts to sugar as the fruit ripens. Starch is composed of complex chains linked together with glucose units. Starch is indigestible unless it is cooked, when the starch granules swell and burst.

GLYCOGEN

Glycogen is similar to starch, and it serves the same purpose in animals as starch does in plants: i.e. it stores fuel - in this case in the liver and muscles. It is not found in most meat as it breaks down into glucose after the animal is killed, but horse meat and oysters do retain it.

OTHER FORMS

Fiber is a complex carbohydrate. Even though humans cannot digest fiber, it plays an essential role in helping them to move food through the body and in promoting bowel regularity.

Pectin is present in apples, other fruits, and turnips. It has no direct food value but has the property of making jam set.

Sources of useful carbohydrates include bread, potatoes, rice, wheat, sugar, honey, vegetables, fruit, jam, liver, milk, eggs, and cheese.

G09 FATS

Fat is the most concentrated source of energy. Also, when stored in the body, as a layer of fat beneath the skin and around organs, it provides insulation and protection for body structures. Finally, certain fats carry the fat-soluble vitamins (A, D, E, and K).

Fat contains the same three elements as carbohydrates - carbon, hydrogen, and oxygen, but combined in a different way. Chemically, fat is a combination of fatty acids and glycerine. At normal temperatures, fat can be solid as in animals or liquid as in vegetable and fish oil. But all fat can be made liquid on heating and solid on cooling.

Fat is not soluble in water, though it is in alcohol, ether, and chloroform. But by chemical treatment with alkalis, fat can be broken down into its separate units, and then can be mixed with water. Soap is made by this process, and it also occurs during the digestion of fat. Mineral oils such as paraffin or Vaseline cannot be saponified. They are therefore unavailable to the body and are of no value as food.

Fat in the diet falls into three categories. Sources such as butter, lard, margarine, and oils are added to recipes in a recognizable and measurable form. Other sources, such as the fat found in meat, fish, eggs, etc, are not so readily measurable, and vary with the quality of the source, the time of year, and so on. In addition, when fat is added as a cooking medium, it finds its way into the outer layer of the food, increasing its fat content.

WHAT FOOD PROVIDES 2

G10 VITAMINS

Vitamins are certain substances found in food in minute amounts. They are needed for the regulation of chemical processes inside the body, and through this have an important role in growth and development and in protection against illness and disease. The presence of vitamins in the diet is essential, as most of them cannot be made by the body.
The role of vitamins in nutrition was only discovered in the present century, but there are now known to be about 40, of which 12 or more are essential in the diet.
Because of the haphazard process of their discovery, they originally formed a jumbled list of alphabetic names (A, B_1, B_6, etc). But now their chemical structures have been identified, chemical names are often used for many of them. Identification has also meant that they can now be made artificially.
Chemically, in fact, they are proving to be an equally mixed bag - only sharing the characteristic of being complex substances needed by the body in tiny amounts. For example, a man only needs an ounce of thiamin in a lifetime - despite the vital importance of that ounce. Above an average day to day requirement, increased amounts of a vitamin do no further good, and in some cases are actually harmful.
Vitamins in the diet can be divided into two classes: those soluble in fat (vitamins A, D, E, and K), and those soluble in water (vitamins C and the B vitamin complex).
VITAMIN A is found in halibut and cod liver oil, milk, butter, and eggs. It is destroyed by cooking and sunlight.
It plays a role in the formation of bone and of the enamel and dentine in teeth. It is also responsible for the ability to see in dim light.
VITAMIN D is found in eggs, milk, butter, and fish liver oils. It is also synthesized in the skin during exposure to sunlight.
It plays a part in the digestive absorption of some minerals, such as calcium, and phosphorus. It is also necessary for retaining calcium in bones.
VITAMIN E is found in wheatgerm, oil, lettuce, spinach, watercress, etc. While the exact function of vitamin E in humans is not completely understood, it is an essential nutrient. It is an effective antioxidant and seems to preserve the integrity of red blood cells. Most Americans on a varied diet consume adequate amounts of vitamin E.
VITAMIN K is found mainly in green plants such as spinach, cabbage, and kale. But it is also synthesized in the gut by the action of bacteria.
It is a necessary factor in the blood-clotting mechanism, as it is needed for the production of prothrombin.
VITAMIN C is found in fresh fruit and vegetables, especially lemons, oranges, blackcurrants, tomatoes, and watercress. Human milk also contains Vitamin C. This vitamin is easily destroyed by cooking, especially if the food has been chopped up.
One of its most important functions in the body is to control the formation of dentine, cartilage, and bone. It also helps the formation of red blood cells, and the correct healing of wounds and broken bones.
There is no conclusive evidence that vitamin C prevents colds.
VITAMIN B is in fact a complex of fifteen different substances, but they are classed together because they occur together in the same types of food, such as yeast and wheat germ. Unlike the other vitamins, at least some vitamins of the B group are found in all living plants and animals.
The following are the most important B vitamins.
THIAMIN forms the part of the

G12 WATER

Water is not really a food, but it is an essential part of all tissues. Our bodies are composed of about ⅔ water. It acts as a form of transport: the blood, which is mainly water, carries food in its basic forms to the tissues and takes away waste products to be excreted.
Chemically, water is a simple compound of oxygen and hydrogen, but is never found pure as it contains traces of minerals, dissolved gases, and solids. The amount of these depends on what kind of soil it is from.
As well as in liquid form, water is also found in most solid food. Since it is constantly being lost in sweat, urine, and breathing out

enzyme system essential for the breakdown of carbohydrates and the nutrition of nerve cells.
RIBOFLAVIN acts with thiamin and nicotinic acid in the oxidation of carbohydrates. It is also important for the growth of the fetus, and is thought to play a part in the mechanism of vision.
PYRIDOXINE (B6) helps the breakdown of protein into amino acids and is necessary for the formation of blood cells. However, sufficient pyridoxine is produced in the intestines.
PANTOTHENIC ACID probably plays a part in the detoxification of drugs and the formation of chemicals that pass nerve impulses along the nerves.
NIACIN is needed for healthy skin and nerves, and food digestion.
FOLIC ACID is an anti-anemic factor found in green leaves and in liver and kidneys. It is especially important during pregnancy to prevent anemia.
COBALAMIN (B12) is the only vitamin containing a metal, cobalt. It is found in a high concentration in the liver and is essential for the formation of red blood cells. Unlike the other B complex vitamins, it has no vegetable source.

it must be replaced every day or dehydration of the body will occur. However, the body's need for water at any time is very accurately registered by the degree of thirst.

G11 MINERALS

Minerals, like vitamins, do not supply any heat or energy, but play a vital role in the regulation of body fluids and the balance of chemicals.

MACRONUTRIENTS

These are the minerals needed by the body in comparatively large quantities.
CALCIUM is found in milk, cheese, fish, some green vegetables, and in "hard" drinking water. It is necessary for the proper formation of bones and teeth; also for the functioning of muscles and clotting of the blood. During growth, calcium is constantly being laid down in bones and simultaneously withdrawn into the blood stream for use elsewhere. The body of an adult normally contains 2-3½lb of calcium, of which at least 99% is present in the bones.
PHOSPHORUS is found in meat, such as brains, kidneys, and liver. Dairy produce such as cheese is also rich in phosphorus.
It is important for energy transfer. Its function in the body is closely linked with that of calcium.
SODIUM AND CHLORINE occur together in the familiar form of common salt, and also in animal protein. Both are vital for life: they maintain water balance and distribution, osmotic pressure, acid-base balance, and muscular functioning. Excess sodium in the diet is believed to contribute to high blood pressure (hypertension) and stroke in some individuals.
POTASSIUM is related in function to sodium and chlorine. It is found mainly in meat, fish, vegetables, chocolate, dried fruit, oranges, and bananas.
SULFUR occurs in certain amino acids especially in animal proteins. Sulfur in the body is found especially in insulin, which regulates the level of sugar in the blood, and in the human hair.
MAGNESIUM occurs in nuts, beans, cereals, dark green vegetables, seafood, and chocolate. Its function is similar to calcium.

MICRONUTRIENTS

These are the minerals needed by the body in much smaller quantities.
IRON is found in fish, liver, eggs, "black pudding", beans, green vegetables, and oatmeal. The body of a healthy adult contains about 4gm of iron - roughly the amount of a 3in nail.
Iron is an essential part of red (hemoglobin) blood cells, which enable the blood to take up oxygen from the lungs and carry it to all cells in the body.
IODINE is important for the healthy functioning of the thyroid gland. It occurs in seafish, shellfish, iodized table salt, and vegetables grown on soil naturally containing iodine.
FLUORINE is found naturally in seafish, some "hard" drinking water, and china tea. It is also added to the water artificially in some localities.
Traces of fluorine are present in bones, teeth, skin, and thyroid gland. One known function is that it helps prevent tooth decay.
OTHER MICRONUTRIENTS are zinc, selenium, manganese, copper, molybdenum, cobalt, and chromium.

TRACE ELEMENTS

These are found in the body in tiny amounts, but their function, if any, is not yet known. They include strontium, bromine, vanadium, gold, silver, nickel, tin, aluminium, bismuth, arsenic, and boron.

DIGESTION AND ABSORPTION

G13 THE DIGESTIVE SYSTEM

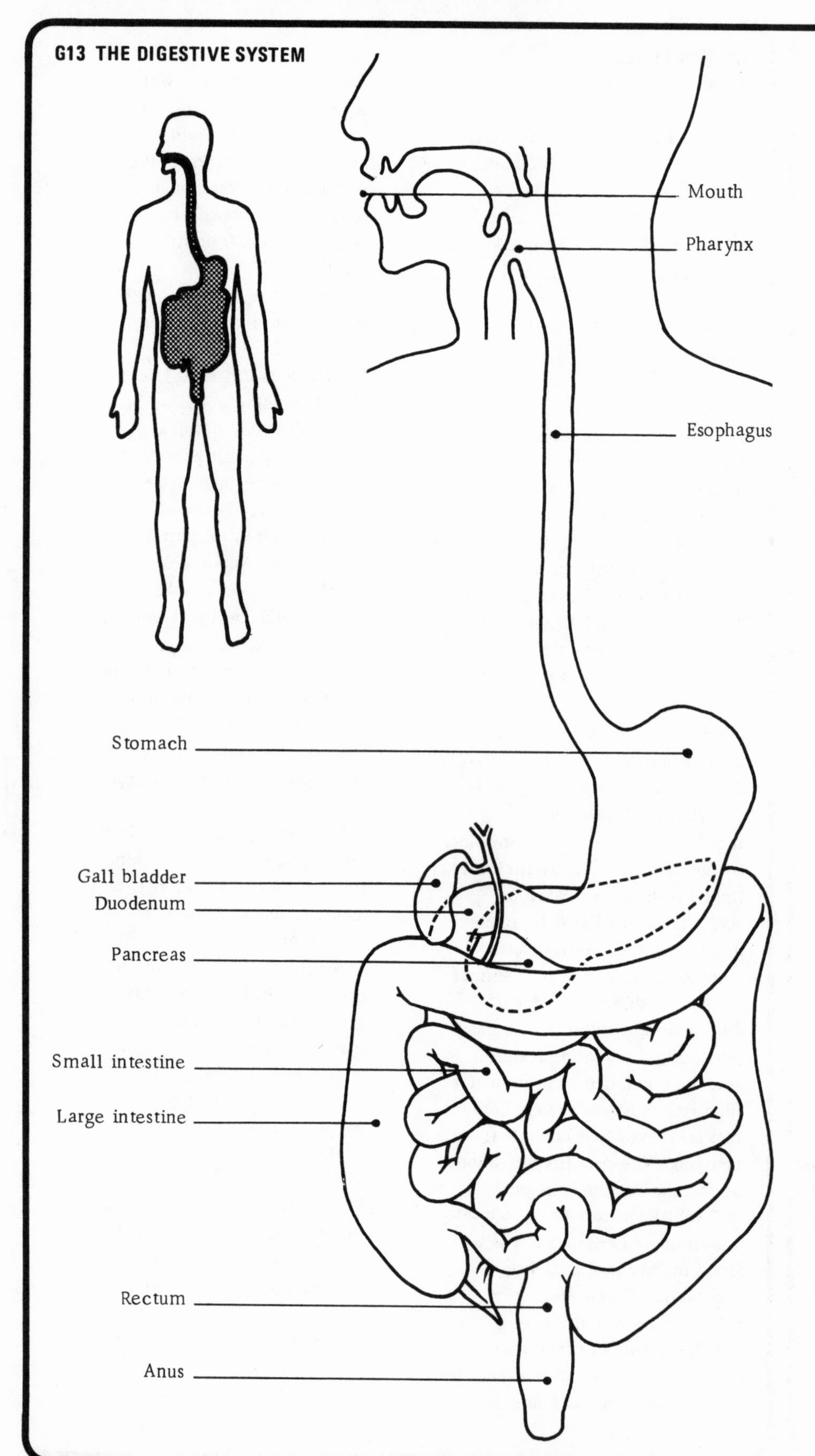

The digestive tract forms a tube over 30ft long, beginning in the mouth and ending in the anus. Between these it includes the esophagus (gullet), stomach, small intestine, and large intestine.

In the mouth, food is chewed into smaller pieces, mixed with saliva, and formed into a rounded ball ("bolus").

On swallowing, the bolus passes down the esophagus into the stomach.

The stomach varies in shape and size according to its contents. Its maximum capacity is about 2½ pints. Here food is churned into even smaller pieces, mixed with gastric juice, and disinfected with hydrochloric acid. Fat is melted by the heat.

From the stomach food passes into the small intestine. In the first 12in of this (the duodenum), the food is mixed with pancreatic and intestinal juices and with bile from the gall bladder. Then here, and in the remaining 21ft of small intestine, most of the useful elements in food are absorbed through the intestinal walls into the blood and lymph streams.

In the 6ft long large intestine, water is absorbed into the body, turning the waste product into a soft solid (feces): a mixture of indigestible remnants, unabsorbed water, and millions of bacteria. Finally, the feces pass out of the body via the anus.

Food takes from 15 hours upward to pass through the whole system. It usually stays in the stomach 3 to 5 hours, the small intestine 4½ hours, and the large intestine (where the sequence of meals may get jumbled) 5 to 25 hours or more.

G14 DIGESTION AND ABSORPTION

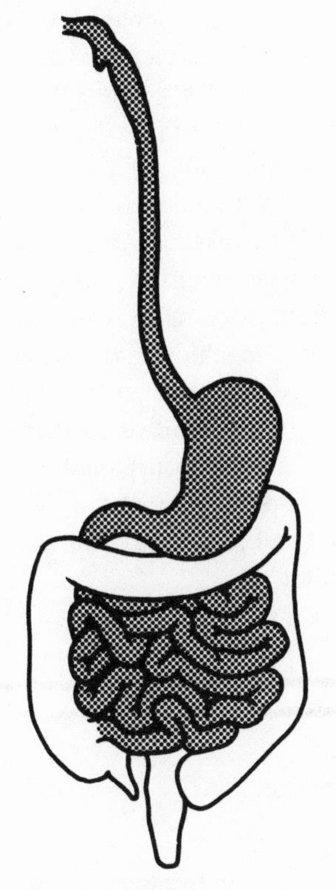

Carbohydrates

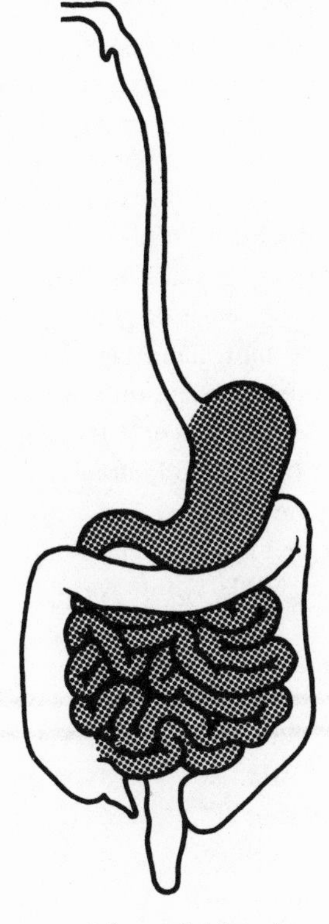

Fats and fat-soluble vitamins

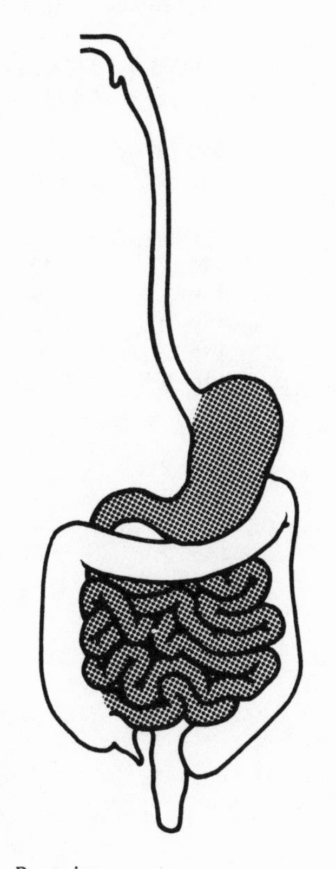

Proteins

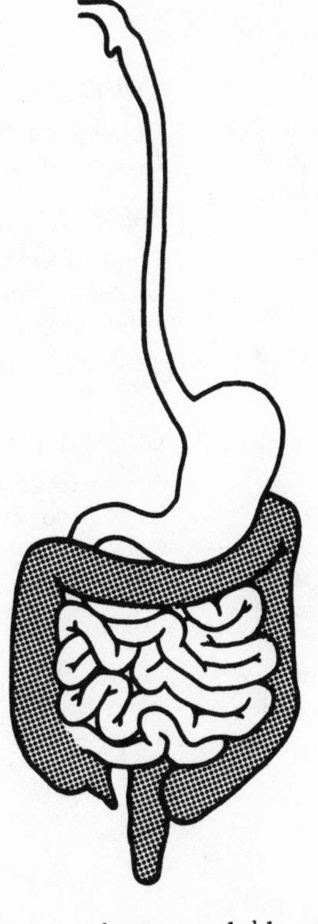

Water and water-soluble vitamins

CARBOHYDRATES Digestion of starch begins in the mouth. It continues in the stomach, but the stomach usually empties itself before this is completed. In the duodenum, pancreatic juices break the carbohydrates down into monosaccharides, which are then absorbed into the blood stream. But some forms of carbohydrate (eg cellulose) cannot be digested, while some sugars begin to be absorbed even in the mouth.

FATS Digestion begins in the stomach, where naturally emulsified fats are converted into fatty acids and glycerol. (Unconverted fat causes food to be retained longer in the stomach.) In the small intestine, bile emulsifies the unemulsified fats, and pancreatic juice converts them into fatty acids. These are absorbed into the lymph vessels (70%) or the blood stream (30%). Fat-soluble vitamins are absorbed at the same time.

PROTEINS Digestion begins in the stomach, where proteins are broken down into peptones. In the small intestine, the pancreatic and intestinal juices break the peptones down into amino acids. The amino acids are absorbed into the blood stream.

WATER is absorbed in the large intestine, into the lymph vessels and blood stream.

G15 FOOD INTAKE

What people eat varies enormously. For many people in tropical countries, a typical day's food is two small bowls of rice and a little vegetable - totaling perhaps 1600 Calories, and containing only tiny amounts of necessary proteins, vitamins, and minerals. Yet in industrial countries, the daily diet of a food lover may total over 3500 Calories, and supply in all respects about twice the body's needs.

Even taking national averages, great differences remain. In Ghana, on a diet mainly of roots, cereals, and vegetables, the average total daily intake is perhaps 2000 Calories, including 47gm of protein of which only 11 are of animal origin. In Denmark, on a diet of meat, dairy produce, cereal products, vegetables, and fruits, the average intake is perhaps 3300 Calories including 95gm of protein (62 of animal origin).

Diets also vary greatly in their variety, their range of geographical source, and their handling and processing before consumption. Perhaps 75% of the world lives on a basic diet of one food, usually a cereal (typically rice), usually grown by themselves, and usually eaten in a simple boiled form. Average individual grain intake on such a diet in a poor country totals perhaps 400lb a year. In contrast, about 1700lb of grain enters the food chain of a North American each year - but only 30% is ever eaten as cereal products. The rest goes to feed livestock for meat and dairy produce. Industrial man buys widely from restaurants, carry outs, and vending machines, as well as from an average supermarket stock of 7000 different food items that have been stored, transported (perhaps imported), usually processed and preserved, and wrapped for sale.

G16 STORING FOODS SAFELY

From the Food Safety and Quality Service, U.S. Department of Agriculture.

STORAGE TIME *Eating quality drops after time shown*	In refrigerator at 35° to 40°F. DAYS	In freezer at 0°F. MONTHS
FRESH MEATS		
Roasts (beef and lamb)	3 to 5	6 to 12
Roasts (pork and veal)	3 to 5	4 to 8
Steaks (beef)	3 to 5	6 to 12
Chops (lamb)	3 to 5	6 to 9
Chops (pork)	3 to 5	3 to 4
Ground and stew meats	1 to 2	2 to 3
Variety meats	1 to 2	3 to 4
Sausage (pork)	1 to 2	2 to 3
PROCESSED MEATS		
Bacon	7	1
Frankfurters	7	½
Ham (whole)	7	1 to 2
Ham (half)	5	1 to 2
Ham (slices)	3	1 to 2
Luncheon meats	3 to 5	Freezing not recommended
Sausage (smoked)	7	Freezing not recommended
Sausage (dry and semi-dry)	14 to 21	Freezing not recommended

	In refrigerator at 35° to 40°F. DAYS	In freezer at 0°F. MONTHS
COOKED MEATS		
Cooked meats and meat dishes	3 to 4	2 to 3
Gravy and meat broth	1 to 2	2 to 3
FRESH POULTRY		
Chicken and turkey (whole)	1 to 2	12
Chicken (pieces)	1 to 2	9
Turkey (pieces)	1 to 2	6
Duck and goose (whole)	1 to 2	6
Giblets	1 to 2	3
COOKED POULTRY		
Pieces (covered with broth)	1 to 2	6
Pieces (not covered)	1 to 2	1
Cooked poultry dishes	1 to 2	6
Fried chicken	1 to 2	4

USA
1 Green leafy vegetables
2 Citrus fruits and vegetables
3 Other fruits and vegetables
4 Milk and milk products
5 Meat
6 Eggs
7 Oil and fat
8 Sweetened products
9 Potatoes
10 Cereals

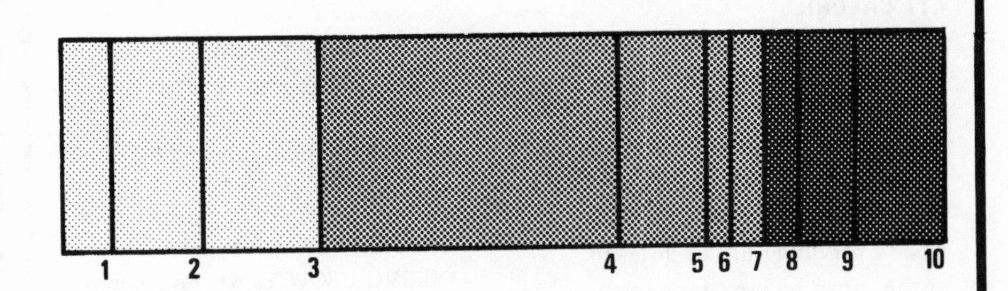

India
1 Citrus fruits
2 Vegetables
3 Legumes
4 Other fruits, sugar, meat, fish, eggs, milk, oil and fat
5 Rice

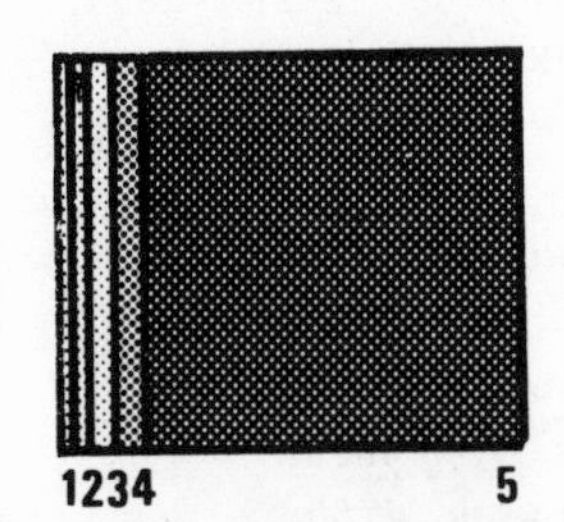

Here we show comparative Calorie consumption by food source for an average person in the USA (above) and in India (left). Calorie consumption in the USA is both far higher and far more varied in source.

RULES FOR SAFE FOOD HANDLING

From U.S. Department of Health and Human Services, Food and Drug Administration.

1. Wash hands.
2. Use clean utensils and equipment.
3. Scrub raw food products.
4. Cook food thoroughly.
5. Serve promptly.
6. Refrigerate quickly.
7. Defrost frozen food in the refrigerator before thawing at room temperature.
8. Avoid thawing and refreezing.
9. Discard questionable foods.

HELPFUL BOOKS TO ORDER

From the Superintendent of Documents, U.S. Government Printing Office, Washington, D.C. 20402. *Check with Office for current prices.*

1. "Keeping Food Safe to Eat—A Guide for Homemakers." U.S. Dept. of Agriculture Home and Gardening Bulletin No. 162. Superintendent of Documents, U.S. Government Printing Office, Washington, D.C. 20402.
2. "Hot Tips on Food Protection." PHS Pub. No. 1404. Superintendent of Documents, U.S. Government Printing Office, Washington, D.C. 20402.
3. "Cold Facts About Home Food Protection." PHS Pub. No. 1247. Superintendent of Documents, U.S. Government Printing Office, Washington, D.C. 20402.
4. "No Picnic." PHS Pub. No. 1623. Superintendent of Documents, U.S. Government Printing Office, Washington, D.C. 20402.
5. "From Hand to Mouth." PHS Pub. No. 281 48 pp. Superintendent of Documents, U.S. Government Printing Office, Washington, D.C. 20402.
6. "You Can Prevent Foodborne Illness." PHS Pub. No. 1105. Superintendent of Documents, U.S. Government Printing Office, Washington, D.C. 20402.
7. "How the Consumer Can Report to the FDA." FDA Fact Sheet No. G-3. Office of Consumer Affairs, FDA—Rockville, Maryland 20852.

G17 CALORIES

A person's need for energy from food is measured by the number of Calories* he needs. Carbohydrates and fats are the main sources of Calories for energy. Protein is only used by the body for energy when everything has been taken out that can be used for growth and repair.

The need for Calories depends on a person's daily activities.

a) An average man uses about 1650 Calories a day just for basic life processes such as heartbeat, breathing, digestion, other chemical processes, etc.

b) His work or other chosen daily activity will use up at least another 600 Calories, even in the case of a sedentary office worker, and up to 2400 (making a total of over 4000 Calories) for hard manual labor. (A highly trained person can, for a few days, do work that takes his total energy needs up to 5000 Calories.)

c) Any form of recreation or exercise adds to energy needs. Even sitting down writing - or eating - uses about 20 Calories an hour. Driving a car or playing the piano uses at least twice as much. Walking uses from 120 to 240, sawing wood over 400, and swimming 500.

However, all these figures increase with body size, for more energy is needed to operate a large body. They therefore vary between individuals according to their sex, height, weight, and (if they are still growing) their age. They also vary with climatic conditions: more food energy is needed the colder it is. And (once someone has stopped growing) they all decline with age: for not only do basic life processes slow down, but also less concentrated effort can be put into work and chosen activities. All this makes calculating Calorie needs extremely complex. It is fortunately seldom necessary. But below we give enough figures for you to have some idea of the quantities involved.

CALORIE NEEDS for men

DURING GROWTH Average needs

Age	Calories	Age	Calories
10-12	2500	14-18	3000
12-14	2700	18-27	2800

ADULT WORK

Needs at 25 years, for an average size man.

Sedentary work	2250
Light work	2750
Moderate work	3000
Heavy work	3500
Very heavy work	4250

The following are examples.

a) Light work: assembly work, light industrial, electrical, carpentry, bricklaying, plastering, painting, mechanized agricultural work, and domestic work with modern appliances.

b) Moderate work: general laboring, non-mechanical agricultural work.

c) Heavy work: coal mining.

d) Very heavy: furnace steelman.

Golf and bowling are the exercise equivalents of light work, and gardening and cycling of moderate.

WEIGHT FACTOR

The adult work figure given above needs to be adjusted to allow for a person's desirable weight*:

lb	%	lb	%
110	74	176	103
121	80	187	108
132	85	198	113
143	90	209	119
154	95	220	125
165	100	(% of work figure)	

AGEING FACTOR

This adult work-weight figure needs in turn to be adjusted with age.

Age	%	Age	%
25	100	65	84
35	95	75	79
45	92	85	72
55	89	(% of work-weight figure)	

G18 NUTRIENTS

The precise requirement for some nutrients is not yet established. For example, the minimum need for fats and carbohydrates is not certain. But people often eat these far in excess of their needs; and this also applies to most mineral and vitamin requirements that have been estimated. Only the following nutrients are worth commenting on in detail.

PROTEIN

Protein is vital to growth and cell repair - yet estimates of protein needs vary enormously. An average estimate for good nutrition is about 2½oz (65gm) a day in adulthood (with protein supplying about 7% of Calorie intake). But people have been found to adapt in a healthy way to intakes under half to over twice this amount. All this is dependent, of course, on all essential amino acids being eaten, and in good proportions. Lack of protein can be a problem in old people with little money, and in those following unusual diets.

MINERALS

Sodium intake is usually far higher than necessary, but may be insufficient for very heavy work in hot conditions.

Calcium intake depends on ordinary consumption of milk and cheese.

Iron is needed for the hemoglobin in red blood cells. It is found in meat and eggs, brewer's yeast, and wheat germ. But it is only absorbed in tiny quantities, and hardly at all if vitamin C in the body is low.

Women, with their regular menstrual blood loss, often develop a shortage of iron (anemia), with resulting fatigue and breathlessness.

Iodine shortage occurs if you eat no seafood and only vegetables grown in iodine-free soil. A lack causes thyroid deficiencies and thyroid gland enlargement. This is less common with modern food transport and availability of iodized salt.

VITAMINS

Vitamins B_1 and C can be lost by bad cooking, but both have plenty of uncooked sources.

Vitamin A may be lacking if dairy produce, margarine, or green or yellow vegetables are not eaten.

Vitamin D is only much needed in the diets of children and nursing mothers. Butter, margarine, and liver are sources. Vitamin D deficiency has been found in children in poor urban areas - especially those with pigmented skin, which impedes the vitamin's formation in the body from sunlight. It can also occur in the aged and housebound poor.

WATER

The normal requirement is about 6 or 7 glasses of fluid a day. Thirst usually provides very accurate indication of need, but in very hot conditions may not keep up with the intake needed to replace perspiration loss.

INTERACTION

Nutrients do not act totally independently of one another. The body is too complex for that. A deficiency in one can lead to a deficiency in another, because (though it may still be available in the food) it cannot perhaps be absorbed or metabolized. For example, vitamin A deficiency can lead to vitamin C deficiency; vitamin C deficiency to iron deficiency. The interactions are not just among vitamins, or between vitamins and minerals, but also between vitamins and proteins, vitamins and carbohydrates, vitamins and fats; and there are many multiple relationships.

G19 FOOD

Any survey of nutrients gives some idea of the complexity of nutrition - as a science and as a process. But to make your automobile run you only have to fill it with gasoline: not design the fuel blend or the spark plugs. The practice of nutrition is a fairly simple process - largely because nature is by far the best nutritionist.

FOOD OR NUTRIENTS?

Some people set out to eat quantities of "nutrients" and build up the "perfect diet". But you cannot buy nutrients - unless you want to live on chemicals. You have to buy food; and food is a jumble of hard-to-measure ingredients. Even drinking a glass of milk becomes a nightmare of protein, calcium, fat, carbohydrate, vitamin A, vitamin D, riboflavin, and phosphorus - together with a few other things. And if that seems too simple - what was the fat content of that hot dog? or the protein content of that lobster thermidor? Start eating for nutrients, and you will probably eat twice as much as you need to. Start buying for nutrients, and you will be trying, for example, to get your daily vitamin C out of a handful of rose hips, rather than from a morning glass of orange juice, some lunchtime potatoes, and a helping of cabbage in the evening. The search for nutrients is an excellent way of wasting time and money.

ENOUGH IS ENOUGH

Enough is enough; more is not better. You probably know that too many calories are not good for you. But other excesses are harmful, or just useless, too. It is no use eating protein above one's needs: it cannot be stored. Too much of certain minerals or vitamins can cause deficiencies in others, by upsetting their absorption or storage. For example, too much B_1 can cause deficiencies in other B vitamins. And some nutrients taken in excess are positively harmful. People have killed themselves, for example, trying to get far too much vitamin A or D. (These are not water soluble, so the excess cannot just be excreted, as excess vitamin C is.) The only nutrient that some scientists think may be useful to us in enormous doses is vitamin C - and there is far from being agreement about that.

A HEALTHY DIET

In fact, there is no one ideal diet. First, needs differ (and so does the impact of availability, cost, taste, habit, and cooking facilities and skills). But, more important, there are a million different ways of satisfying those needs, in healthy eating. It is possible to live healthily on a diet of milk, wholemeal bread, and green vegetables. It would not be very interesting, though. Variety is the spice of food.

The table on the next page shows a recommended daily food intake in our society. Only those suffering from some illnesses (such as diabetes) may need a more carefully planned diet, about which a physician should advise.

G20 DAILY FOOD GUIDE

The table gives ample intake for an average person in the course of a day.

NOTES

1) Group A uses 1 cup whole or skimmed milk as the basic measure. Alternatives are: 1 cup buttermilk; ½ cup evaporated milk; ¼ cup non-fat milk powder; 1oz cheddar cheese; 1½ cups cottage cheese.

2) If amounts in group A are doubled in the course of the day, not more than one serving of group C is needed.

3) Whole milk (not skimmed) and butter or margarine should be used in childhood, pregnancy, and lactation.

A: THE MILK - CHEESE GROUP

Age 0-9: 2-3 cups
9-12: 3 cups
13-19: 4 cups
Adult: 2 cups
Pregnancy: 3 cups
Lactation: 4 cups

B: THE FRUIT - VEGETABLES GROUP

Four basic servings daily

Serving size examples:
½ cup dark green or deep yellow vegetable (served at least every other day);
½ cup or 1 medium raw fruit or vegetable rich in vitamin C;
other, including potato (1 medium)

C: THE MEAT - POULTRY - FISH - BEANS GROUP

Two basic servings daily

Serving size examples:
2-3oz (after removal of fat, bone) cooked meat, poultry, fish;
2 eggs;
1 cup cooked dry beans, peas, lentils;
4 tablespoons of peanut butter

D: THE BREAD - CEREALS GROUP

Four basic servings daily

Serving size examples:
½ to ¾ cup cooked cereal, macaroni, spaghetti, hominy grits, kasha, rice, noodles, bulgur;
1 cup ready to eat cereal;
5 saltines or 2 Graham crackers

G21 CARBOHYDRATES

Too much carbohydrate in the diet shows itself in unhealthy weight* gain. But the type of carbohydrate is also significant. Bread and other traditional cereal products, potatoes, etc., are being increasingly replaced in our diet by highly refined and sweetened products. Pastries, cakes, chocolate, ice cream, sugar, and alcohol mostly supply little of food value, apart from their energy content. (Bread, in contrast, provides about a fifth of our daily protein.) They provide little or no roughage. And their sugar content is positively harmful. Some scientists believe:

a) that its rush into the blood stream causes the body to overreact, and withdraw too much sugar from the blood - so we are left feeling tired and irritable;

b) that eventually it can cause diabetes in people who would not otherwise contract it; and

c) that it has a role in producing heart disease.

Certainly it promotes tooth decay, and destroys the appetite for more nutritious foods.

All this applies not only to white sugar, but equally to brown sugar, raw sugar, honey, and molasses. But white sugar is the main culprit, simply because the amounts of sugar added in cooking or processing foods usually dwarf the amounts of sweetening we add at mealtime.

G22 FATS

Fats are an important part of the diet - but some fats seem to be associated with high cholesterol* levels in the blood, and so with heart disease.

Foods rich in cholesterol (which is itself a special kind of fat) include egg yolks, brains, liver, kidneys, yeast, and caviar. But the cholesterol content of food does not seem to be so important as the general type of fat we eat. There are two main types. Saturated fats harden at room temperature. Sources include most meat fat and dairy products; many solid shortening products; and also coconut oil, cocoa butter, and palm oil, which are used in many bought cookies and pastries, and in milk and cream substitutes.

Polyunsaturated fats are almost all liquid vegetable oils (eg corn, soybean, safflower). It seems that eating saturated fat raises the blood cholesterol level, while eating unsaturated fats tends to prevent this even if cholesterol foods are eaten.

G23 PROCESSING AND COOKING

It is hard to generalize, but the more processed a food is, the less desirable it is likely to be as a regular part of a healthy diet. Canned and precooked foods, mass-produced breakfast cereals, cookies, and pastries, and ready meals, all tend to be open to criticism for:

a) lower nutritional value;
b) added sugar and saturated fats;
c) added preservative chemicals and untested colorings and flavorings; and sometimes
d) unhygienic production.

In general, the "whole food" movement is a sensible one (though, incidentally, there is no agreed evidence that "organic" vegetables have higher food value than chemically fertilized ones - even though they may taste better and contain fewer pollutants).

However, nutrients can be lost in home cooking as well as in processing, and undesirable ones added. "Boiling" of vegetables should always consist of steaming in a very shallow amount of water, if vitamin C is to be preserved. (Salt should only be added at the last moment.) "Frying" should similarly use a tiny amount of unsaturated oil, not hard fat or immersion. (Grilling is better, where applicable.) Both processes are aided by use of thick-bottomed pans, especially stainless steel ones.

G24 VEGETARIANISM

REASONS FOR VEGETARIANISM

A vegetarian is a person who does not eat the meat of any animal, bird, or fish. There are two main types of vegetarian:

a) vegans, who eat nothing at all of animal origin; and
b) lacto-ovo-vegetarians, who do allow themselves animal products such as milk, cheese, eggs, and honey.

There are also people who call themselves vegetarians but do eat fish.

Reasons for vegetarianism vary from society to society and individual to individual. It has been advocated for religious, philosophical, moral, economic, and health reasons. It has also been adopted as a necessity. Many primitive peoples have lived on a diet of fruit, nuts, and berries, with meat only when it could be obtained.

Perhaps the most powerful arguments for vegetarianism in modern society are:

1) the inefficiency of the animal food production chain* in an overpopulated and underfed world;
b) the relative cheapness of the ingredients of vegetarian diet; and
c) the possible unhealthiness of eating meat that contains crop pesticides and antibiotics and hormones given to the animals, and that has been processed in many ways that are not necessarily hygienic or beneficial.

Also many people feel that the slaughter of animals is cruel and debasing, and that vegetarianism is part of a more peaceful and harmonious life.

Despite the claims of vegetarians, there is no established evidence that eating meat is unhealthy in itself. But it is certainly as possible to be a healthy, strong, and long-lived vegetarian as it is to be a meat-eater.

DIET

A person who choses to give up meat must be careful that his diet still provides enough of the right nutrients. There is no problem with:

a) healthy carbohydrates (grains, cereal products, potatoes, fruits);
b) fats (vegetable oils, dairy products, nuts, margarine); and
c) minerals and most vitamins (vegetables and fruits).

But the following need some care.

PROTEIN is readily available from eggs and dairy produce, nuts, soyabeans, raisins, grains, and pulses. But a vegetarian should be sure to get a good selection of essential amino acids at each meal. This is not difficult where eggs or dairy produce are eaten: cereal and milk, bread and milk, and bread and eggs are all good amino acid combinations. But vegans must depend on soyabeans, or on carefully planned vegetable combinations. These include: lentil soup and hard wholewheat bread; and beans and rice ($1\frac{1}{2}$ cups of beans to 4 of rice have protein value equivalent to $\frac{3}{4}$lb steak).

COBALAMIN (B_{12}) is available from dairy produce and yeast, but vegans must usually add it to their diet in synthetic form.

VITAMIN D may also need to be taken synthetically by vegans where sunlight is insufficient.

IRON AND CALCIUM These are worth mentioning, as they are sometimes deficient even in the diets of meat-eaters. But in fact there are plentiful vegetarian sources. Iron is found in raisins, wheatgerm, lentils, prunes, spinach, and other leafy vegetables, also bread, eggs, and yeast; calcium in dairy produce, dried fruit, soyabeans, sesame seeds, kale, spinach, turnip greens, etc.

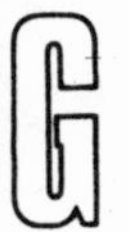

EXCESS WEIGHT

G25 EXCESS WEIGHT

ARE YOU OVERWEIGHT?

It is not easy to say what any one person should weigh. Typical weight tables show how weight varies with sex and height. But these are usually average figures, taken from people's actual weights. They are likely to be higher than "ideal", because more people in our society are overweight than underweight.

Some insurance companies have produced figures for "desirable weights", for each height and build, by noting which weights are associated with low death rates. But, though useful, the range of figures is still quite wide.

So perhaps the best way is just for a person to look at himself honestly. Fat soon shows up as: an increased skinfold thickness; a stomach bulge; or as a waist that juts beyond a straight line between hips and ribs. The waist should measure at least 2in less than the deflated chest.

Another way is to compare present weight with weight at age 20 years - when most people are near their ideal weight. The rise of weight with age, in average tables, shows what usually happens - but not what is desirable.

NUMBERS INVOLVED

Weight problems are on the increase in modern industrial society. Even by the standards of the average weight tables, perhaps 15 million people in the USA are 10% over their standard ("overweight"), and 5 million 20% over ("obese"). Some estimates put it at twice this. Obesity is more common in older people and sedentary workers. Among the poor, it is more common in women; among the well-off, in men.

EFFECTS OF OBESITY

Overweight people are not just more tired, short of breath, and physically and mentally lethargic, with aching joints and poor digestion. They are also more likely to suffer from high blood pressure, heart disease, diabetes, kidney disorders, cirrhosis of the liver, pneumonia, inflammation of the gall bladder, arthritis, hernias, and varicose veins. They have more accidents, are more likely to die during operations, and have higher rates of mortality in general (including 3 times the mortality from heart and circulatory disease). Someone who weighs 185lb when he should weight 140lb has his life expectancy shortened by by 4 years.

Some of these effects arise from mechanical causes: the burden of extra weight and its particular location as fat deposits. Others arise chemically, from the need to supply more body tissue than normal. The typical infertility of the obese is an example; the spread of hormones over increased body tissue creates problems of conception and, in women, pregnancy (including miscarriage and stillbirth).

In many cases, reduction to desirable weight removes all the symptoms of disorder, while mortality also sinks back towards normal.

G26 DESIRABLE WEIGHTS

For men 25 and over, in indoor clothing.

Height in bare feet	Small frame	Medium frame	Large frame
5ft 1in	112-120 lb	118-129 lb	126-141 lb
5ft 2in	115-123	121-133	129-144
5ft 3in	118-126	124-136	132-148
5ft 4in	121-129	127-139	135-152
5ft 5in	124-133	130-143	138-156
5ft 6in	128-137	134-147	142-161
5ft 7in	132-141	138-152	147-166
5ft 8in	136-145	142-156	151-170
5ft 9in	140-150	146-160	155-174
5ft 10in	144-154	150-165	159-179
5ft 11in	148-158	154-170	164-184
6ft 0in	152-162	158-175	168-189
6ft 1in	156-167	162-180	173-194
6ft 2in	160-171	167-185	178-199
6ft 3in	164-175	172-190	182-204

Source: Metropolitan Life Insurance Company.

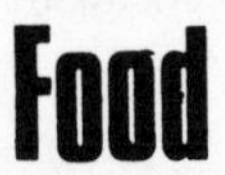

G27 THE CAUSE OF OBESITY

Overweight always - without exception - occurs because a person takes in more food energy than he uses up. The bulk of food energy is taken in the form of carbohydrate or fat. Both these supply Calories (the measure of energy); and both are converted to fat deposits, if the Calories they supply are more than the body uses. So: energy input greater than output equals fat. But several factors are involved, on each side of this equation. Energy output divides into energy needed and energy wasted. Energy input similarly divides into use and wastage - but more important is the control of total input by the appetite, and the various factors that can influence or override that.

OUTPUT

Output needs are analyzed in G17. They vary with age, sex, body size, and activity. Output wastage refers to the burning of unneeded output: "thermogenesis". It is still the subject of scientific controversy, but it does seem that some people get rid of surplus input because their bodies automatically speed up their metabolism and burn up the surplus, rathan than store it. They have not escaped the equation, input greater than output equals fat; but their bodies create another form of output. Among body types, ectomorphs have this characteristic, compared with endormorphs*. In famine conditions, the endomorphs survive better, doing more on little energy; but from the point of view of staying slim, it is the ectomorphs who are lucky.

A special category of output wastage is the rise in the body's metabolism after every meal. So two individuals may eat exactly the same, but one may waste more than the other because he eats it in several small meals rather than two or three large ones.

INPUT WASTAGE

Energy input is the Calories taken into the system in the form of food. But people's bodies vary greatly in the efficiency with which they process food. One person may eat more than another and stay slim, if his body derives fewer Calories from it.

Strictly, this does not affect the equation, energy input equals energy output plus fat. For that refers to the energy input actually finding its way into the body system. But as we have no way of measuring this, we measure food consumption - and have to accept that some people will have more input wastage than others.

INPUT CONTROL

But the main determinant of energy. input is the appetite control - sometimes dubbed the "appestat". This is usually remarkable for its precision. For example, eating an extra half slice of bread a day (30 Calories) above energy output, would bring a weight gain of 110lb over a 40 year period. Most people's people's appetites prevent them gaining weight in this way.

But the appetite control may be ignored; eg, due to:

a) social habit or custom (such as business lunches);

b) excessive love of food in general or certain foods in particular;

c) habits of overeating acquired in upbringing; and

d) eating for psychological support, whether as a general addiction or as a response to shock or stress (here food is an immediate source of pleasure, where emotional security is lacking).

APPETITE AND EXERCISE

In addition, the appetite control can be put out of action by an excessively sedentary existence.

As daily physical activity rises from moderate levels upwards, the appetite reflects well the increased needs of the body.

But when physical activity falls below moderate levels, appetite also rises, without reflecting any genuine body need. This principle is familiar from the techniques traditionally used to fatten animals, by tying down their freedom of action. In fact, studies have shown that the most sedentary people often have a food intake almost as high as the most hardworked manual laborer.

This is why exercise can be useful for combatting obesity. Exercise gets rid of some calories. But it would take 12 hours of tennis, for example, to lose 1 lb of fat; and if activity is already moderate, appetite rises to compensate. An afternoon's riding leaves us ready to eat the horse. We only get slimmer if we ignore our stomach.

But when exercise raises the general level of activity from sedentary towards moderate, energy output goes up while appetite usually decreases. The exercise puts the appestat back into action.

At the same time, the thermogenetic effect seems to work better with exercise: the body of an inactive person cannot burn much surplus energy even as waste. So sedentary living, and working, may well be the single main reason for rising obesity in the population. A sedentary person can neither reduce his appetite nor burn off the excess.

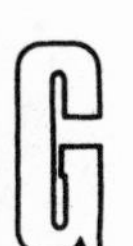

G28 LOSING WEIGHT

Excess of input over output equals fat. And you cannot do much about your energy wastage, either input or output. All you can control is what you eat and what you do: your total energy intake, and total output needs. To slim, you must eat less, and/or do more. If your activity is already moderate, it will be hard for you to do more without eating more. But, if you are overweight, your activity is probably well below moderate. Some studies of overweight people suggest that, in fact, they eat less than others - but do much less. Many overweight people would like to escape the choice of eating less or doing more. They try to blame something else outside their control: their heavy bones, their heavy family, their hormones, even their body water level. But:

a) variations in bone density cannot account for more than about 7lb weight difference;

b) though overweight does "run in families", it may be due more to acquired eating habits than genetic factors;

c) hormonal malfunctions can cause obesity, in very rare cases, but these show themselves clearly in other bodily symptoms; and

d) the body water level is very well regulated except in very hot weather and in some illnesses.

Besides - even if a person had heavy bones, an inherited tendency to heaviness, hormonal malfunction, and too much water in his body - he would still lose weight if he ate less and got more exercise. (In fact, hormonal disorders are often the product of obesity, so a sufferer who slims loses the disorder.)

G29 DIETING

Losing weight is not easy. It demands controlled eating habits, discipline, patience, and a change of attitudes. Before you start:

a) do not be tempted by any promise of easy weight loss - there are no miracles;

b) adopt a definite diet plan and stick to it;

c) if you need advice, get it from your physician.

Once weight is lost, keep a constant check, and deal with small gains as they occur.

DIET FALLACIES

Ignore any claims that you can lose weight by:

a) drinking less fluid;

b) drinking more fluid;

c) taking less salt;

d) drinking no coffee;

e) eating citrus fruits because they "convert fat into energy";

f) eating eggs because they "use up more calories than they contain";

eating heavy meals so as to "avoid nibbling in between".

h) adding lemon juice or vinegar or vegetable juice to your normal diet;

i) changing from sugar to honey or glucose; or

j) eating some kinds of fat and not others (that is, as a way of losing weight, rather than as a measure against heart disease).

Also ignore advice to take "diet pills" or Turkish baths, use weight-reducing garments or skin preparations, or have hormone injections or massage.

GENUINE DIETS

All restrict Calorie intake.

a) Low-Calorie plans set a numerical limit to daily Calorie intake; constant reference has to be made to Calorie tables.

b) Low-carbohydrate plans only limit carbohydrate. Tables are much simpler. Fat is unrestricted making the diet more palatable and socially acceptable. (Weight maintenance through excessive fat consumption does not in practice occur.)

c) No-count plans divide food into three categories: high carbohydrate food that must be avoided; high Calorie, non-carbohydrate food, that can be eaten in moderation; and unrestricted food.

POSSIBLE AIDS

Certain things may help, but are not necessarily advisable.

a) Prescribed drugs (eg amphetamines*) can reduce appetite, but are addictive.

b) Substitute meals (wafers or packaged foods) have a stated Calorie content, and often contain cellulose to give a fuller feeling in the stomach.

c) Substitute foods include saccharin (for sugar); skim milk; and some breads and crispbreads (low calorie per slice - but also less filling).

Saccharin and skim milk may be useful. Otherwise, none gives a sensible basis for future eating.

EXERCISE

Exercise uses up additional Calories as well as contributing to a sense of well-being. Alone, it will not reduce your weight significantly. Any individual about to begin a new exercise routine should check with a physician about the level of exercise that is suitable for his needs. A regular, moderate amount of exercise is usually the wisest decision.

RATE OF LOSS

It is best to aim to lose weight steadily over a long period. Constant yo-yo weight changes are as bad as overweight.

G30 WHAT'S NEW IN DIETS

The nationwide search for good health and fitness has generated a host of diet plans. Following are some of the most popular.

SCARSDALE DIET

Created by the late Herman Tarnowner, M.D. who practiced in Scarsdale, New York, this 14-day diet combines low Calories, low fats, low carbohydrates and high proteins. There is no deciding what to eat when; meals are explicitly spelled out. For example, for breakfast every day, it's black coffee or plain tea, dry protein toast, and grapefruit. Alcohol is never allowed. According to its originator, this diet causes the body to burn fat which, in turn, produces fatty acid chemicals called ketones. The ketones curb appetite and speed water loss. Maximum weight loss in the 2 weeks is 20 lb. For more details, see *The Complete Scarsdale Medical Diet* by Herman Tarnower, M.D. and Samm Sinclair Baker (Rawson, Wade Publishers, Inc.).

FAST FOOD DIET

Fast food has become an integral part of the American meal plan. According to Judith S. Stern and R. V. Denenberg, authors of *The Fast Food Diet* (Prentice-Hall, Inc.), there is no reason why you cannot lose weight while still eating Big Macs, French fries, and thick shakes as long as you stay within the 1,200-Calories-per-day regimen. The authors provide Calorie counts for fast foods so dieters know how much they can eat. For example, a McDonald's vanilla shake is 323 Calories; a chocolate shake a more fattening 364 Calories. Other rules: a variety of foods each day (vegetables, fruits, bread, milk and milk products, and foods with protein); a minimum of fats, sweets and alcohol. Exercise is crucial to weight loss in this plan. If you follow their rules, you can lose 3lb per week.

THE PARTNERSHIP DIET PROGRAM

Misery loves company or so say Kelly Brownell and Irene Copeland, authors of *The Partnership Diet Program* (Rawson, Wade Publishers, Inc.). Their theory is that by dieting with a partner, you can better stick to the diet and also enjoy it more. There are no forbidden foods, but dieters must adhere to a daily Calorie allotment - 1200 Calories for women and 1500 Calories for men. Other essentials of this diet plan: daily logs of what foods were consumed, weekly weigh-ins, eating slowly, thinking yourself thin.

THE PRITIKIN PROGRAM

Nathan Pritikin, founder and director of the Longevity Center and Longevity Research Institute in California, has received national attention in the past year for his Pritikin Program which stresses a sound diet and regular exercise. A sound diet according to him is one that is high in carbohydrates (but not highly refined carbohydrates such as sugar, honey, molasses, and syrup) and low in fats and protein. Pritikin believes that carbohydrates such as potatoes, rice, beans, vegetables, grains and fruits help a person lose weight and stay healthy, especially when they constitute 80% of a person's diet. Rules for his diet plan include eating beans or peas 1 to 3 times weekly; limiting acceptable meats and fish to 1½ lb weekly; eating only egg whites (a maximum of 7 cooked egg whites weekly and a maximum of 2 raw egg whites weekly). *The Pritikin Program for Diet and Exercise* (Grosset & Dunlap) by Nathan Pritikin and Patrick M. McGrady, Jr., explains his diet and walking regimen, and provides recipes. At his Longevity Center, patients spend 4 weeks and lose an average of 13.3 lbs.

GRAPEFRUIT DIET

Grapefruits and grapefruit juice form the cornerstone of this diet. The rules: eat half a grapefruit or drink the juice of half a grapefruit with every meal. Meats, fish and eggs are permissible, but sugars and starches are limited. Success, say its originators, is due to the grapefruit activating a burning of fat.

WEIGHT-WATCHERS

Developed by Jean Nidetch, this diet stresses reducing one's weight and then maintaining that weight. A dieter on this plan chooses from lists of legal foods, and attends weekly meetings for support (similar to Alcoholics Anonymous). There are even Weight-Watchers frozen foods available in supermarkets.

DIET AND EXERCISE

Exercise uses up additional Calories as well as contributing to a sense of well being. Any individual about to begin a new exercise routine should check with a physician about the level of exercise that is suitable for her needs. A regular, moderate amount of exercise is usually the wisest decision.

DRUGS AND DRUG ABUSE

H01 DRUGS AND DRUG ABUSE

A drug is any chemical compound which can affect the body's functioning. Drug abuse is the use of any drug for a purpose other than a medically or socially accepted one. This includes the misuse of drugs obtained in medically or socially acceptable ways.

Especially relevant here are psychoactive drugs: those having effects on the body which bring about behavioral changes - relaxation, euphoria, hallucination, etc.

H02 NERVE IMPULSES

Each nerve of the nervous system is made up of a broad chain of specialized cells, called neurons. Between every cell in the chain is a gap. When a message travels along the nerve, a chemical agent carries the nerve impulse across this gap. But some neurons try to stop the message, while others try to pass it on. Usually, how many of each are stimulated depends on the strength of the message. An impulse is only transmitted when the neurons that promote the message outnumber those that inhibit it.

H03 WHAT DRUGS DO

Some drugs have the following effects on nerve impulses:

1 They stimulate the neurons that try to stop messages.

2 They slow down or stop the production of the chemical transmitting agent.

3 They cause the agent to break down more quickly.

4 They reduce the effect of the chemical transmitter on the next neuron in the chain.

All or any of this has the effect of slowing down ("depressing") nervous activity. Fewer messages get through, and those that do get through more slowly and more weakly.

Other drugs have the opposite effect: they increase ("stimulate") nervous activity.

EFFECTS IN THE BRAIN

Different areas of the brain control different physiological and mental functions. It is because they stimulate or depress different specialized areas, that different drugs have different effects. For example, parts of the hypothalamus, when stimulated, give intense feelings of pleasure, while other areas control coordination, thought, sight and hearing, and so on.

VARIABLE FACTORS

A number of factors affect the impact of any drug. Some relate to the drug itself: the amount taken, its purity and concentration, and how it enters the body. Others concern the mental and physical state of the consumer. Mentally, drugs often heighten an existing psychic state or release a suppressed one; but the consumer's reaction to his immediate environment, and his expectations, are also important. Physically, the effects are likely to be increased by tiredness and (when the drug is swallowed) if there is little food in the stomach.

H04 REASONS FOR TAKING DRUGS

SOCIAL CONFORMITY If the use of a drug is accepted in a group to which a person belongs, or which he identifies with, he will feel a need to use the drug to show that he belongs to the group. This is true of all drugs, from nicotine and alcohol to heroin.

PLEASURE One of the main reasons drugs are taken is to induce pleasant feelings - ranging from well-being and relaxation to mystic euphoria.

ESCAPE FROM PSYCHIC STRESS

In a society which increasingly sees drugs as the answer to all physical problems, the use of drugs to escape one's psychological problems inevitably seems appropriate.

ALIENATION may underlie drug abuse. In social alienation, where the values of society are rejected, drug use may seem a valid symbol of opposition. In psychic alienation - when a person has rejected not only society but all alternatives, including himself, his hopes and his goals the resulting feelings of meaninglessness, isolation, and inadequacy will predispose him to chronic drug abuse.

AVAILABILITY relates directly to drug use. Illegal use is highest where there is a ready supply (seaports, border towns), or where the market has attracted a ready supply (large cities, university towns). Legal drug use also increases with availability, eg alcoholism is common in the liquor trade.

CURIOSITY about drugs and why people take them can often start off drug taking.

AFFLUENCE AND LEISURE can produce boredom and loss of interest in meaningful activity. Drugs can then supply an easy answer to the desire for stimulation and escape.

THEOLOGICAL REASONS account for some drug use: both the practice of certain traditional religions and the personal search for self-identity and a reason for existence. Whether abuse occurs depends on the circumstances.

H05 CLASSIFICATION

Psychoactive drugs fall into four major categories, according to their effects.

DEPRESSANTS ("downers") reduce nervous activity. They include alcohol, barbiturates, and opiates (opium, codeine, morphine, heroin). Taken in small doses, they have a sedative effect; in larger doses they bring on sleep. An overdose can kill: nervous activity is so reduced that vital functions such as respiration are impaired and may cease. Tranquilizers are a special category of depressants.

STIMULANTS include caffeine, nicotine, the amphetamines, and cocaine. They increase nervous activity, especially in the sympathetic nervous system, which mobilizes the body for action. So these drugs help prolong activity and take away the desire for sleep.

HALLUCINOGENS include mescaline, psilocybin, and LSD (lysergic acid diethylamide). They produce bizarre states of consciousness (which may resemble psychotic conditions). The interpretation of incoming sense stimuli is radically affected, and this produces hallucinations, delusions, and extraordinary reactions to normal situations and events.

MARIJUANA (cannabis) forms a separate, fourth category, although it is closely related to the hallucinogens.

Drugs can also be categorized as, eg legal or illegal, socially acceptable or unacceptable. But these really refer to drug use. A medically accepted drug may be illegal without a prescription; and social acceptability varies. One drug may be illegal but socially acceptable, another legal but unacceptable.

H06 WHAT IS ADDICTION?

TOLERANCE to a drug occurs as the body gets used to it. As tolerance increases, so does the quantity of the drug needed to produce the original results.

PHYSICAL DEPENDENCE has occurred when the cells of the body have become used to functioning in the presence of the drug. When it is withdrawn, cellular activity is disrupted and the cellular need for the drug shows itself in withdrawal symptoms. Physical dependence can only be proved, therefore, when the supply of a drug is stopped.

PSYCHOLOGICAL DEPENDENCE is the need or compulsive desire to continue using a drug - whether or not there is physical dependence. It is not necessary for the person's cellular functioning, but it is necessary for his psychological functioning.

Any drug taking - and any other activity - can create psychological dependence.

"ADDICTION" is now thought of as a general term, covering the above forms of dependence. It is usually a result of drug abuse, but it can occur through legal use (as in the case of nicotine). A drug's medical application may also give rise to addiction. Many of the first heroin addicts became addicted through the use of morphine as a pain killer in hospitals. The medical use of barbiturates has also produced many addicts.

HABITUATION refers to the repeated use of a drug when there is no form of dependence. Generalizations about habituation cannot be made for groups of drugs, because, depending on the individual, there may always be psychic dependence.

Drug		Dependence?	Tolerance?
Depressants:	Barbiturates	Yes	Yes
	Tranquilizers	Yes	Yes
	Opiates	Yes	Yes
Stimulants:	Amphetamines	Yes	No
	Cocaine	No	No
	Nicotine	Yes	?
	Caffeine	Yes	?
Hallucinogens		?	No
Marijuana		No	No
Alcohol		Yes	Yes
Wearing a hat		No	No

?: opinions differ

"Dependence" in the table refers to physical dependence.

All the above can create psychic dependence.

All those that do not create physical dependence allow habituation i.e. regular use without any dependence.

Alcohol can also be used regularly without any significant dependence. This is because its use is normally kept in check by social norms: society has, over thousands of years, gained some experience in coping with its dangers. Yet, in the numbers of individuals it destroys, alcohol remains by far the most dangerous of all drugs.

H

DEPRESSANTS

H07 BARBITURATES AND TRANQUILIZERS

Barbiturates (nicknamed "barbs", "candy" or "goof balls") are made from barbituric acid. Like all depressants, they reduce the impulses reaching the brain. Because of this they have been medically prescribed for many years to relieve anxiety and tension and induce sleep; some have also been used as anesthetics But with greater realization of their dangers, prescription is becoming less common.

TYPES Barbiturates vary in their immediacy and duration of effect, depending on the rate at which they are metabolized and eliminated; eg "Seconal" is a short acting drug, "Phenobarbital" a long lasting one.

SYMPTOMS Someone who has taken some barbiturates may well show signs of drowsiness, restlessness, irritability and belligerence, irrationality, mental confusion, and impairment of coordination and reflexes, with staggering and slurring of speech. The pupils are constricted and sweating increases. The person experiences initial euphoria, followed by depression.

When an excessive amount is taken (an "overdose"), the depressive effect upon the nervous system is such that unconsciousness occurs, followed in extreme cases by death from respiratory failure.

WITHDRAWAL SYMPTOMS The barbiturates create tolerance and physical dependence. The effects of withdrawal on a chronic user can be worse than those of alcohol or heroin. They include irritability and restlessness, anxiety, insomnia, abdominal cramp, nausea and vomiting, tremors, hallucinations, and sometimes death.

TYPES OF ABUSE Addicts are attracted by:

a) the possibility of escaping from emotional stress, through sedation;

b) the feelings of euphoria on initial ingestion, when large amounts of the drug are tolerated;

c) the ability of barbiturates to counteract the effects of stimulants. This cyclical use of "uppers" and "downers" can lead to dependence on both.

The common prescription of barbiturates to induce relaxation and sleep has resulted in the largest group of dependent people being the middle aged, especially housewives. The same ready availability also makes them a common suicide procedure, while the combination of barbiturates' depressive effects with those of alcohol has brought many accidental deaths through taking barbiturates after heavy drinking.

TRANQUILIZERS

Tranquilizers are increasingly used in place of barbiturates in medical prescription. They differ in their derivation and mode of action: they relieve anxiety and tension without any anesthetic effect. However, the majority also give rise to tolerance and physical dependence, and are subject to the same forms of abuse.

H08 BARBITURATES AND TRANQUILIZERS

Drug	Description (but this can vary, with dose and source)	Nickname
Amobarbital	Green blue	Blues, blue devils
Pentobarbital	Yellow	Yellows, nembies
Secobarbital	Red	Reds, red devils, red bird
Tuinal	Red blue	Rainbows, tooeys
Thorazine	Orange	
Miltown	White	
Librium	Green white	
Valium	White	Goofers

H09 OPIATES

The opiates are known in drug-taking circles as "the hard stuff". Opium itself and its derivative heroin are, in fact, the archetypal drugs of addiction. However, codeine and morphine, which are also derived from opium, are better known for their medical uses.

GENERAL ACTION

All depressants inhibit the activity of the central nervous system, impairing coordination and reflexes, etc, but opiates especially affect the sensory centers, reducing pain and promoting sleep. As with alcohol, this nervous action may cause initial excitement, as inhibitions are removed.

In larger doses the opiates act on the pleasure centers of the hypothalamus, producing feelings of peace, contentment, safety, and euphoria.

General symptoms of opiate use include loss of appetite, constipation, and constriction of the pupils. An overdose of an opiate is likely to cause convulsions, unconsciousness, and death.

All opiates create tolerance and physical dependence. The symptoms of withdrawal from abusive use begin with stomach cramps, followed by diarrhoea, nausea and vomiting, running eyes and nose, sweating, and trembling. These are accompanied by irritability and restlessness, insomnia, anxiety and panic, depression, confusion, and an all-consuming desire for the drug.

OPIUM

Opium is the dried juice of the unripe seed capsules of the Indian poppy. The plant is cultivated in India, Persia, China, and Turkey, and opium is then prepared in either powder or liquid form. The poppy possesses its psychoactive powers only when grown in favourable conditions of climate and soil. Poppies produced in temperate climates have only a negligible effect.

Opium is traditionally smoked, using pipes, but it can also be injected or taken orally.

CODEINE

Codeine (methyl morphine) is the least effective of the opiates. It is white and crystalline in form, and is often used with aspirin for treating headaches. Because of the inhibiting effect on nervous reflexes it shares with all opiates, it is used in many cough medicines, and sometimes in the treatment of diarrhoea, since it reduces peristalsis (the automatic rhythmic contractions of the intestine). The risk of tolerance and abusive use are very small because of the large amounts necessary to produce pleasant effects.

MORPHINE

Morphine is the basis of all opiate action - it is opium's main active constituent. It was isolated from opium in 1805, and since then has been medically important as a pain killer. It is ten times as strong as opium, and must be administered with great care to avoid tolerance and physical dependence. However, instances of abuse are not too common, as drug users prefer heroin.

HEROIN

Heroin (diamorphine) was first isolated in 1898. It is three times as strong as morphine, and has a quicker and more intense effect, though a shorter duration. Among drug takers it is often known as "H", "horse", or "smack". In the USA it is not used medically. Its production, possession, and use all connected with drug abuse. A greyish brown powder in its pure form, for retail purposes it is mixed with milk or baking powder to add bulk. This results in a white coloring. The high cost of the drug, and its necessity to those who have become dependent on it, account for the high crime rate associated with its users.

The powder may be sniffed but is usually injected - normally into a muscle when use begins, but then into a major vein ("mainlining") as tolerance develops. Mainlining gives more immediate and powerful effects. Constant injection into the same vein causes hardening and scarring of the flesh tissue and eventual collapse of the vein. Unhygienic conditions and use of unsterilized needles can also cause infection, often resulting in sores, abscesses, hepatitis, jaundice, and thrombosis.

Almost immediately upon injection intense feelings of euphoria and contentment envelop the user. The strength of these depends on the purity and strength of the heroin, and the psychological state of the user - the higher the previous tension and anxiety, the more powerful the subsequent feelings of pleasure and peace. It is the force of the initial pleasure that makes heroin more popular than morphine. In a chronic user, the ritual of injection is also important in the creation of pleasure.

Physical dependence on heroin is reached if one grain (60mg) of heroin is used in a period of up to two weeks. Withdrawal effects will then begin four to six hours after the effect of the last shot has worn off.

Chronic users become impotent.

H

H10 AMPHETAMINES

The amphetamines ("pep pills" or "uppers") generally stimulate the sympathetic nervous system, which mobilizes the body for action with the "fight or flight" syndrome*, including increase in epinephrine production, heart rate, blood sugar, and muscle tension.

EFFECTS The user experiences a sense of well being and, with strong doses, euphoria. Alertness, wakefulness, and confidence are accompanied by feelings of mental and physical power. The user becomes talkative, excited, and hyperactive. Accompanying physical symptoms including sweating, trembling, dizziness, insomnia, and reduced appetite. Mood effects are probably due to stimulation of the hypothalamus, and sudden shifts to anxiety and panic can occur.

DEPENDENCE Amphetamines create tolerance, but are not considered physically addictive. However, psychic dependence is easily produced. The extra energy is "borrowed" from the body's reserves: when the drug's action has worn off, the body has to pay for it in fatigue and depression. This creates the desire for more of the drug to counteract these effects.

MEDICAL USAGE has become rarer since realization of the dangers. But amphetamines are still used for some purposes, eg:
to prevent sleep in people who have to be alert for long periods;
to treat minor depression;
to counteract depressants;
and to suppress the appetite in a few cases of obesity.

ABUSE of amphetamines is common because of the feelings of euphoria and alertness they give. The dangers include not only psychic dependence, but also:
physical deterioration due to hyperactivity and lack of appetite;
induced psychotic conditions of paranoia and schizophrenia, resulting from prolonged overdose;
suicide due to mental depression following large doses;
and death from overdose.

H12 NICOTINE AND CAFFEINE

NICOTINE is a stimulant of the sympathetic nervous system. It is found in tobacco*.

CAFFEINE is a stimulant of the central nervous system, found in coffee, tea, cocoa, and cola drinks. Its action combats fatigue, but it is a comparatively mild drug. It is also a "diuretic" i.e. it increases the urine output of the kidneys. Medically, caffeine is often included in headache pills, to counteract the dulling effect of the pain killing ingredient. Abuse is unlikely because of the large quantities necessary, but those who drink considerable amounts of coffee probably have a mild psychic dependence, because of the feelings of tiredness experienced when the stimulation wears off.

H11 AMPHETAMINES

Drug	Description (but this can vary, with dose and source)	Nickname
Benzedrine	Red pink	Bennies
	Pink	Bennies
Dexadrine	Orange	Dexies
	Orange	Dexies
Methadrine	White	Speed, meth, crystal
Biphetamine	White	Whites
Edrial	White	
Dexamyl	Green	Christmas tree

H13 COCAINE

COCAINE (often nicknamed "coke" or "snow") is a white powder obtained from the coca plant found in South America. Synthetic derivatives are also available.
EFFECTS Cocaine stimulates the central nervous system, dispelling fatique, increasing alertness, mental activity, and reflex speed, and inducing euphoria. After an initial "rush", the effects become more steady. Accompanying physical symptoms include dilation of the pupils, tremors, loss of appetite, and insomnia.
MEDICAL USE Although it is a stimulant, local application of cocaine has anesthetic effects. It is used for minor operations on the eye, ear, nose, and throat, and can also be used to anesthetize the lower limbs by injection into the spinal canal.
DEPENDENCE Cocaine does not create physical dependence, but psychic dependence easily develops for the same reasons as with amphetamines.
ABUSE is the main use found for cocaine. As a powder it is inhaled, which eventually results in deterioration of the nasal linings and finally of the nasal septum separating the nostrils. Injection of a liquid form is an alternative, but using cocaine alone is unpopular, because of the violence of the sudden effects. So heroin and cocaine are often injected together. Cocaine is a short acting drug and must be taken repeatedly to maintain the effects.
Dangers of prolonged use include insomnia, paranoia, hallucinations in the sense of touch known as "the cocaine bugs", and loss of weight and malnutrition through lack of interest in food. An overdose causes convulsions, and a dose of 12gm or more at one time causes death by respiratory failure.

H14 EFFECTS OF PSYCHO-ACTIVE DRUGS

NARCOTICS
Possible Effects: Euphoria, drowsiness, respiratory depression, constricted pupils, nausea.
Overdose Effects: Slow and shallow breathing, clammy skin, convulsions, coma, possible death.
Emergency Treatment for Overdose: Splash victim with cold water to arouse him. Walk him around and around room to stimulate his metabolism. Give artificial resuscitation if breathing stops. Give cardiopulmonary resuscitation (if trained) if heartbeat stops. Get trained medical help quickly.
Withdrawal Syndrome: Watery eyes, runny nose, yawning, loss of appetite, irritability, tremors, panic, chills and sweating, cramps, nausea.

DEPRESSANTS
Possible Effects: Slurred speech, disorientation, drunken behavior without odor of alcohol.
Overdose Effects: Shallow respiration, cold and clammy skin, dilated pupils, weak and rapid pulse, coma, possible death.
Emergency Treatment for Overdose: Give artificial resuscitation if breathing stops. Give cardiopulmonary resuscitation (if trained) if heartbeat stops. If convulsions occur, remain calmly with person, preventing him from hurting himself. Get trained medical help quickly.
Withdrawal Syndrome: Anxiety, insomnia, tremors, delirium, convulsions, possible death.

STIMULANTS
Possible Effects: Increased alertness, excitation, euphoria, dilated pupils, increased pulse rate and blood pressure, insomnia, loss of appetite.
Overdose Effects: Agitation, increase in body temperature, hallucinations, convulsions, possible death.
Emergency Treatment for Overdose: Give artificial resuscitation if breathing stops. Remain calmly with person if he begins hallucinating. Get trained medical help quickly.
Withdrawal Syndrome: Apathy, long periods of sleep, irritability, depression, disorientation.

HALLUCINOGENS
Possible Effects: Illusions and hallucinations (with exception of MDA), poor perception of time and distance.
Overdose Effects: Longer, more intense "trip" episodes, psychosis, possible death.
Emergency Treatment for Overdose: Remain calmly with person who is on a "trip." Get trained medical help quickly.
Withdrawal Syndrome: Withdrawal syndrome not reported.

CANNABIS
Possible Effects: Euphoria, relaxed inhibitions, increased appetite, disoriented behavior.
Overdose Effects: Fatigue, paranoia, possible psychosis.
Emergency Treatment for Overdose: Restrain person if he becomes violent because of an adverse reaction to drug overdose. Get trained medical help quickly.
Withdrawal Syndrome: Insomnia, hyperactivity, and decreased appetite reported in limited number of individuals.

FOR ANY OVERDOSE OR SEVERE REACTION, CALL YOUR LOCAL POISON CENTER AND/OR PHYSICIAN FOR HELP.

Information primarily from the United States Department of Justice, Drug Enforcement Administration,

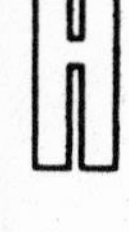

MARIJUANA AND HALLUCINOGENS

H15 MARIJUANA

MARIJUANA (cannabis) comes from the "cannabis sativa" plant. It is prepared in two alternative ways. The flowers and top leaves of the plant can simply be dried and crushed; or the resin itself - which is the active ingredient - can be extracted. The first form is called simply marijuana (nicknamed "grass") and has the appearance of a dried crumbled herb. The second form is called hashish or cannabis resin (nicknamed "hash"), and appears as a hard brown lump. A liquid "oil" of the resin is also available.

CONSUMPTION Both main forms are normally smoked, usually in cigarettes called "joints" or "reefers". The dried flowers and leaves may be used alone, or mixed with tobacco. If the resin is used, it is heated and crumbled, and then the small pieces are mixed with the tobacco as the joint is made. Alternatively, both forms may be smoked in a pipe. A water pipe is popular, as it cools the smoke before it is inhaled.

The other mode of consumption is in drinks or food. This can give longer and smoother effects; also more extreme effects, as more of the drug can be taken into the body this way. However, control over dosage is diminished, and nausea may occur.

Marijuana is not now used medically, but it has been employed in the past as a mild anesthetic in many different parts of the world.

PHYSICAL EFFECTS The neurological effects of marijuana are not yet clearly understood. It is a general sedative of the central nervous system, but some areas of the sympathetic nervous system are apparently stimulated.

Particular symptoms of use include some increase in heart rate, inflammation of the conjunctiva* of the eyes, drying of the mouth, and increase in appetite.

PSYCHOLOGICAL EFFECTS The ability to experience the marijuana

H16 HALLUCINOGENS

LSD

LSD (lysergic acid diethylamide) was originally obtained from the fungus "ergot", which is found in certain cereals. It is now produced synthetically.

Nicknamed "acid", it is the most widely used hallucinogenic drug. LSD can be injected, but is usually taken orally, either as a pill or as a drop of liquid on another substance (such as a sugar cube or a small square of blotting paper). Upon absorption it concentrates mainly in the liver, kidneys, and adrenal glands. Only about 1% is found in the brain.

ACTION The way in which LSD affects the nervous system is not completely understood. But it is known that certain chemical transmitters are interfered with and synesthesia occurs - crossconnecting of the sense responses, so one sees sounds and hears colors. Also LSD reduces the brain's ability to filter out unwanted data, so allowing more, unorganized stimuli to reach the consciousness.

PHYSICAL EFFECTS LSD causes an initial tingling in the extremities, goose pimples, and sometimes nausea, and muscle pain. The user feels cold and numb, and looks flushed. These effects soon wear off, leaving dilated pupils and increased heart rate, blood pressure, blood sugar level, and body temperature. Muscle coordination and pain perception are reduced.

THE LSD "TRIP" The psychological effects begin with the user becoming extremely emotional. This passes, but the senses are increasingly affected. Perception is enhanced and distorted: colors are more vivid, sounds more audible, inert objects seem to move. Synesthesia may occur, and orientation in time and space may be lost. Hallucinations varying in intensity and involvement are often experienced. At the same time, normal mental processes are impaired, and acquired modes of thought and behavior are disrupted. Emotional barriers are broken down, the past may be seen in a new light, and repressed experiences may be released and relived.

The emotional impact of all this on the user varies greatly. Sometimes it is utterly terrifying (a "bad trip"), sometimes euphoric. This especially depends on: whether the user is with people that he trusts, in an environment that he enjoys, and in a happy mental state beforehand; and whether the mental disruption of the drug threatens the user's sense of self-definition.

Sometimes, in presenting a completely new sense of awareness, both of himself and of the external world, LSD can be of lasting benefit to the user.

A trip lasts from 8 to 12 hours.

DANGERS In the panic of a "bad trip", the user may cause himself and others physical harm. The mental impact can also be long-lasting: the release of repressed emotions and experiences may produce psychotic conditions in a previously unstable or neurotic person. Paranoia, schizophrenia,

"high" is an acquired technique. A new user must be taught what to look for, and how to enjoy it. The ritual and special language of marijuana use are part of this process. Marijuana is a uniquely social drug.
The effects vary with the dose, from those similar to moderate amounts of alcohol, to mild hallucinogenic effects. Also, like alcohol, marijuana tends to heighten the mood prevalent at the time of consumption.
Generally there is a pleasant feeling of mild euphoria.
Inhibitions are lowered, and talking increases. Attention to the outside world is dulled, though thoughts seem rapid and involved. Sight and hearing are enhanced.
Coordination, flexibility of attention, and mental organization are impaired. Time and space are distorted and extended.
Experienced users can control their intake and maintain the pleasurable high without the depressant effects of the drug leading to sleep.
These effects last for three to five hours, reaching their peak after about 45 minutes. The user is left sleepy and hungry.
POSSIBLE DANGERS Marijuana does not create tolerance or physical dependence. However, if marijuana is mixed with tobacco, the user is also exposed to the dangers involved in tobacco smoking.
Psychologically, chronic marijuana use does seem in some cases to lead to loss of motivation and of social activity. But it does not bring the extreme mental (and physical) degeneration of alcohol.
Because marijuana is illegal and therefore part of the traffic in drugs, the user may be brought into contact with other drug abuse. If so, he may be tempted to experiment with far more dangerous drugs.

and acute depression have all been caused through use of LSD.
In addition the power of the hallucinations can produce harmful actions; eg a belief that he can fly may cause the user to leap to his death.
"Flashbacks" are spontaneous recurrences of sensory disruption at a later date. They may occur at any time up to 18 months after the drug's use. They are especially dangerous where sudden loss of orientation may cause an accident eg driving a car, or crossing the road.
It is possible that LSD can cause chromosomal damage, but this is not yet certain.
DEPENDENCE LSD does not cause physical dependence, but the desire to repeat the experience may lead to psychic dependence in some users.
MEDICAL USES LSD has been used with varying success in the treatment of some psychotic disorders, such as schizophrenia and acute depression. It is used only in certain cases, and always in very carefully controlled conditions.

MESCALINE

Mescaline is produced from the peyote cactus of Mexico and the south-western USA. It is prepared as a powder, a capsule, or a liquid, and is usually taken orally though it may be sniffed or injected. It has effects very similar to LSD, though they are longer in taking effect. 600mg can give a 12 hour trip. There tend to be side effects, such as dizziness and nausea.
Peyote itself can be eaten, but about 50 times more is needed to produce the same effect. Also the presence of other substances makes the effects slightly different.

PSILOCYBIN

This is a hallucinogenic drug produced from the mushroom "psilocybe mexicana". It has been used for centuries for religious purposes, notably by the Aztecs. It causes hallucinations and distortion of perception for up to 8 hours, followed by physical and mental depression and continued disorientation.

OTHER HALLUCINOGENS

Fly agaric is another mushroom, which causes hallucinations and visual distortion followed by heavy sleep. As with all hallucinogenic mushrooms, vomiting and diarrhoea are possible side effects.
Morning glory seeds contain six derivates of lysergic acid, and have varying effects depending on their ripeness.
DMT (dimethyltryptamine) is an extremely short acting drug, produced as a powder and usually smoked with marijuana, tobacco, or tea.
STP or DOM is typical of a group of amphetamines that can also (or instead) produce hallucinogenic effects similar to LSD. Psychotic states often result, because of hallucinogenic misinterpretation of the usual body effects that amphetamines produce.

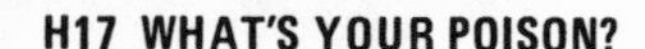

H17 WHAT'S YOUR POISON?

Bottles arranged in order of increasing percentage alcohol

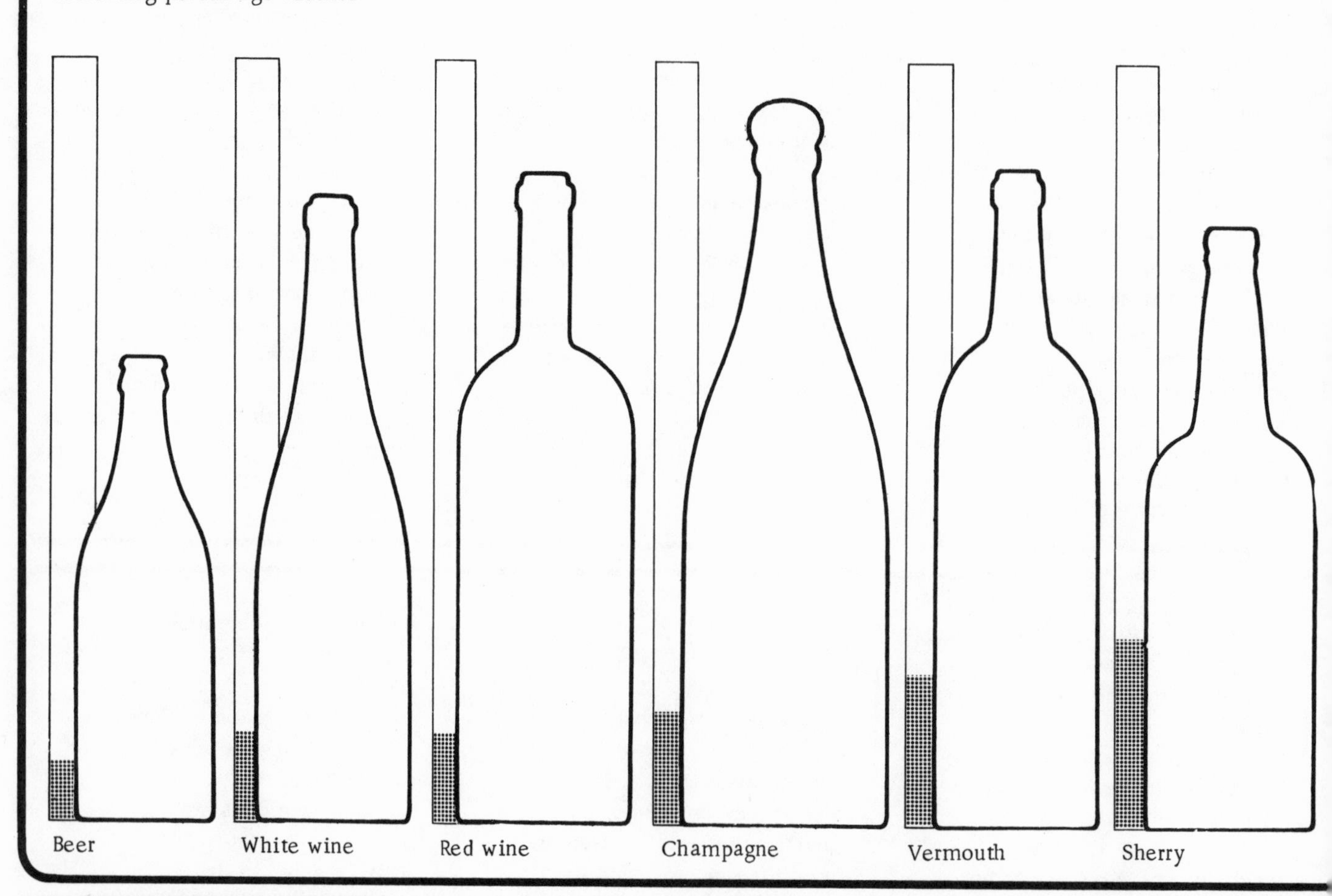

H18 THE CHEMICAL AND THE DRINK

Alcohols are volatile, colorless, pungent liquids, composed of three chemical elements: carbon, hydrogen, and oxygen. Ethyl alcohol (ethanol) is the type taken in alcoholic drinks. It may also be prescribed medically, to stimulate the appetite, or form a medicinal base in which other ingredients are dissolved.

Methyl alcohol (methanol, or "wood alcohol") is used commercially as a fuel and solvent. It is poisonous, and drinking it causes blindness and death.

ALCOHOLIC DRINKS

In the domestic and industrial production of alcoholic drinks, ethyl alcohol is produced by "fermentation": that is, the degeneration of a starch (such as maize, barley, rice, potatoes, grapes) by bacterial action. The drink that results depends on the starch used; eg malt and barley give beer, grapes give wine.

Beers and wines are produced by fermentation alone. Only about a 15% level of alcohol is possible by this method. "Spirits", with their higher alcoholic levels (whiskey, gin, vodka, liqueurs, etc) also require "distillation". That is, the alcohol is evaporated off, leaving water behind, and resulting in a higher alcoholic concentration in the eventual liquid. Distilled alcohol may also be added to wines (sherry, port, etc) and beers, to strengthen them.

ALCOHOLIC STRENGTH

Commercially, the strength of an alcoholic beverage is expressed as so many "degrees proof". This refers to the liquid's specific gravity - not to the percentage of alcohol it contains. Proof measurement regulations vary between countries. With US proof measures, the percentage of alcohol is half the figure for "degrees proof". For example, a spirit that is 100 proof (written "100°") contains 50% alcohol.

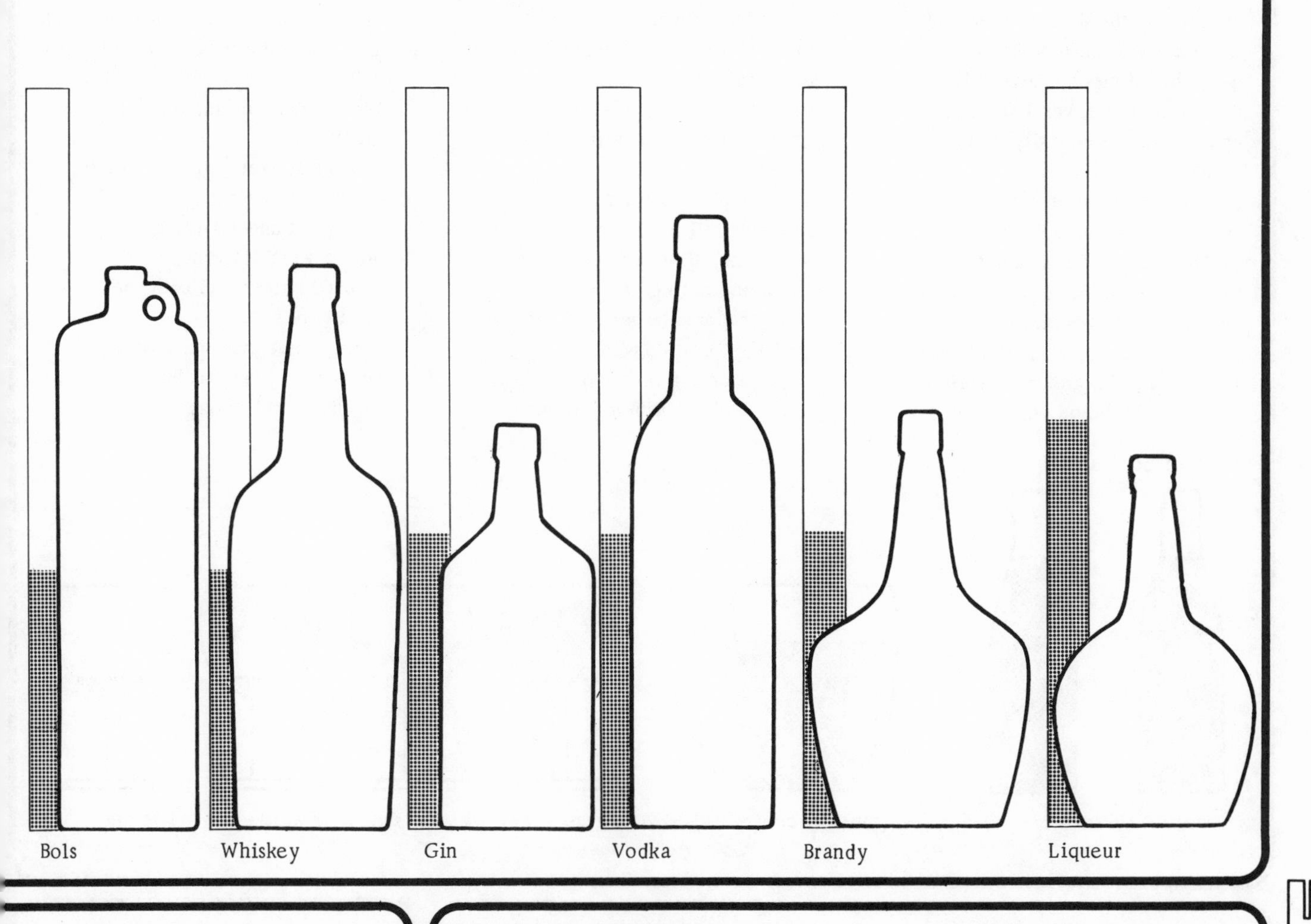

Typical alcohol contents

Lager	up to 8%
Beer	up to 8%
Cider	up to 8%
Wines	9 to 15%
Fortified wine	20%
Aperitif	25%
Spirits, liqueurs	40 to 50%

H19 ALCOHOL IN THE BODY

About 20% of any alcohol drunk is absorbed in the stomach, and 80% in the intestines. It is then carried around the body by the bloodstream. The liver breaks down (oxidizes) the alcohol at an almost constant rate: usually about 2½ bottles (1 pint) of beer or 1oz of whiskey per hour. This process eventually disposes of about 90% of the alcohol, forming carbon dioxide and water as end products. The remaining 10% is eliminated through the lungs and in the sweat. Alcohol in the body has four main effects:

a) It provides energy (alcohol has high calorific value, but contains no nutrients).
b) It acts as an anesthetic on the central nervous system, slowing it down and impairing its efficiency.
c) It stimulates urine production. With heavy alcohol intake, the body loses more water than is taken in, and the body cells become dehydrated.
d) It puts part of the liver temporarily out of action. After heavy drinking, as much as two thirds of the liver can be nonfunctioning - but it is usually fully recovered within a few days.

ALCOHOL 2

H20 BLOOD ALCOHOL LEVEL

The effect of alcohol on behavior depends on the amount reaching the brain via the bloodstream. This "blood alcohol level" is determined by several factors, apart from the quantity of alcohol drunk.

a) The size of the liver decides the rate of oxidation and elimination.

b) The size of the person decides the amount of blood in the system, because blood volume is proportionate to size. The larger the person, the greater the diluting effect of the blood on the alcohol consumed, and the more it takes to produce the same effect.

c) The speed and manner in which the alcohol is consumed is important. The longer one takes to drink a given quantity, the less effect it has.

d) Alcohol consumed on an empty stomach will have a greater and more immediate effect than that consumed during or after eating. Food acts as a buffer to absorption.

DRINK EQUIVALENTS

If we assume a person of average size (150lbs), drinking at an average rate on an empty stomach, then any one of the following would give a blood alcohol level of 0.03%:

$1\frac{1}{2}$oz (about one measure) of spirits;

$3\frac{1}{2}$oz (just over $\frac{1}{2}$ glass) of sherry or fortified wine;

$5\frac{1}{2}$oz (just under 1 glass) of ordinary (table) wine;

24oz (2 bottles) US beer; or

$\frac{3}{4}$pt UK beer.

Twice these quantities will give twice the blood alcohol level (0.06%), and so on.

Alcohol equivalents

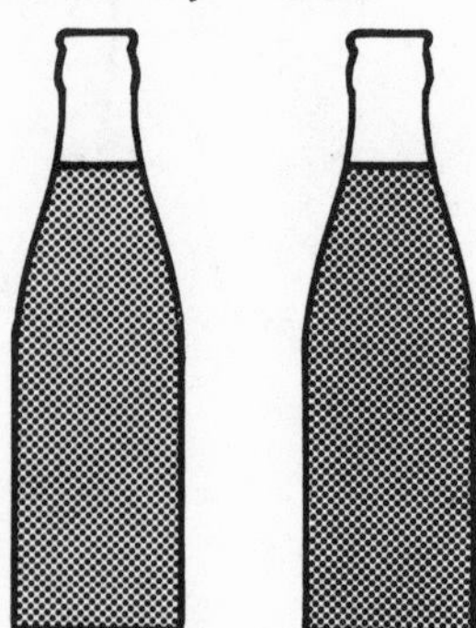

2 bottles US beer

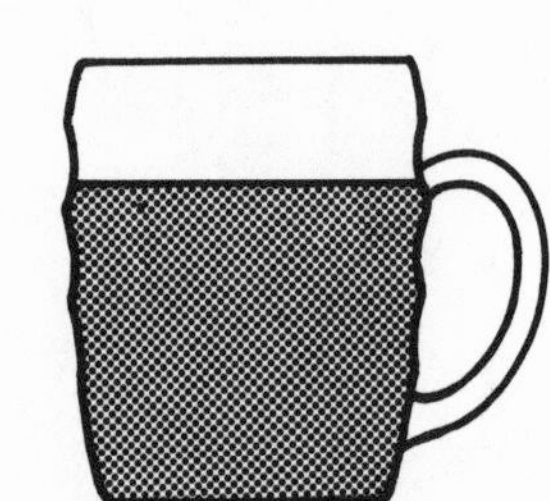

$\frac{3}{4}$ pint UK beer

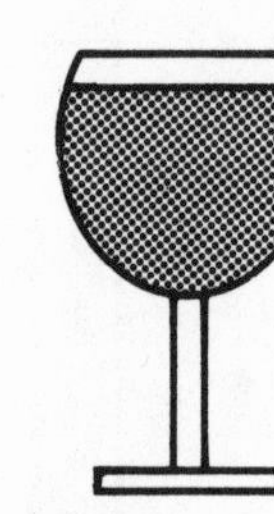

1 glass wine

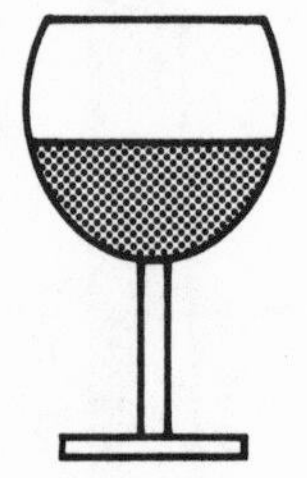

$\frac{1}{2}$ glass sherry

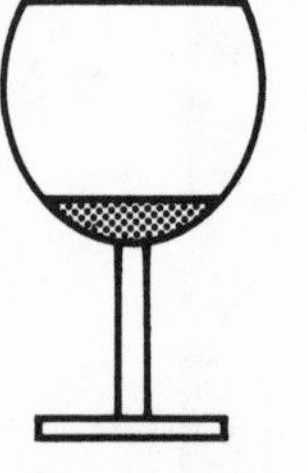

1 whiskey

1 vodka

H21 BEHAVIORAL EFFECT

As the level of alcohol in the blood rises, the drinker's brain and nervous system are increasingly affected, and changes occur in his behavior.

0.02% Sense of warmth, friendliness. Visual reaction time slows.

0.04% Driving ability at speed impaired.

0.06% Feelings of mental relaxation and general well-being. Further slight decrease in skills.

0.09% Exaggerated emotions and behavior. Tendency to be loud and talkative. Loss of inhibitory control. Sensory and motor nerves increasingly dulled.

0.12% Staggering, and fumbling with words.

0.15% Intoxication.

0.20% Incapacitation, depression, nausea, loss of sphincter control.

0.30% Drunken stupor.

0.40% Coma.

0.60% + Lethal dose. Death through heart and respiratory failure. Fortunately, lethal doses seldom occur, as unconsciousness and vomiting force the drinker to stop.

H22 DRINKING AND DRIVING

The behavioral effects of alcohol make drinking and driving very dangerous, both to the drinker and to others. Tests have shown that errors of judgement and control increase as soon as there is any alcohol in the blood stream. Therefore many countries prescribe a legal limit to the blood alcohol level of anyone in charge of a vehicle. In the USA this varies from 0.10 to 0.15%, except for Utah, where it is 0.08%. (Iowa, New Mexico, and Texas have no restrictions.) Limits elsewhere include 0.05% (Scandinavia), 0.08% (UK), and 0.15% (Australia).

H23 HOW WE GET DRUNK

Alcohol is a physiological "depressant" i.e. as consumption occurs the transmission of impulses in the nervous system becomes slowed. First to be affected are the higher levels of the brain: inhibitions, worry, and anxiety are dissolved, resulting in a sense of well-being and euphoria. As the lower levels of the brain become affected, coordination, vision, and speech are impaired.

The small blood vessels of the skin become dilated (widen). Heat is radiated and the drinker feels warm. This means that blood has been diverted from the internal body organs, where the blood vessels are already constricted by the effect of alcohol on the nervous system. So, at the same time, the temperature of internal body organs falls.

Any increase in sexual desire is due to the depression of the usual inhibitions. Alcohol is not an aphrodisiac - physical sexuality is more and more impaired as blood alcohol level rises.

Eventually, the poisoning effect of excess alcohol causes nausea and possible vomiting, and may leave the drinker with the usual symptoms of a hangover.

H25 ALCOHOL AND THE LAW

Chemically, alcohol is one of the most dangerous drugs known to man. But, over centuries of experience, society has managed to develop cultural attitudes which allow alcohol to be available without it causing too great disruption or harm.

However, legal restrictions are needed to reinforce these attitudes. Most countries have a minimum age for its purchase, restrict the number of hours of the day during which it can be sold, control the number, ownership, and location of bars and liquor stores, and keep up strict observation of their orderliness.

H24 HANGOVER

A hangover is the physical discomfort that follows the consumption of too much alcohol. Symptoms can include headache, upset stomach, thirst, dizziness, and irritability.

Three processes produce the hangover. First, the stomach lining is irritated by the excessive alcohol, and its functioning is disrupted. Second, cell dehydration occurs because the quantity of alcohol consumed exceeds the liver's ability to process it, leaving a prolonged level of alcohol in the blood. Third, the level of alcohol has a "shock" effect on the nervous system, from which it needs time to recover.

AVOIDANCE

The best way to avoid a hangover is not to drink too much. But there is less likelihood of a hangover if the alcohol is taken with meals: consumption and absorption are spread over a greater period of time, and the food acts as a barrier. Non-alcoholic drinks, taken at the same time or afterwards, dilute the alcohol; and there is usually less of an after-effect when alcohol is consumed in relaxed surroundings, and when cigarette smoking is cut to a minimum.

TREATMENT

The stomach is relieved by a fresh lining: milk, raw eggs, or simply a good breakfast! Only then should aspirin or other pain relievers be taken to help the headache. The danger of stomach irritation from pain-relieving drugs is always much worse when the stomach is empty. Fruit juice can be drunk for its vitamin C and refreshing taste, while fizzy drinks may have a soothing effect upon the stomach. Liquids of any sort help the dehydrated cells recover their fluid content.

Coffee or tea can be used to clear the head (the caffeine content stimulates the nervous system) and sugar can be taken to provide energy; but both these may leave the sufferer feeling worse when the immediate effects wear off. Similarly, for temporary relief, another alcoholic drink (in moderation) invigorates the sluggish nervous system and seems to dispel the unpleasant after effects. But this is only a postponement: the original hangover, and that of the extra alcohol, still await!

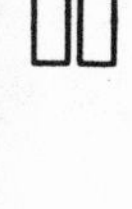

H26 THE PROBLEM

Alcoholism is the most serious drug problem in modern industrial society. In the United States in 1970 there were $5\frac{1}{2}$ million alcoholics and another 4 million pre-alcoholics. The total number of active narcotics addicts, in contrast, was 120,000 at most. In European countries there are usually not more than a few hundred narcotics addicts, but alcoholics number from 1% to 10% of the population. It is estimated that alcoholics in the USA have 7 times the normal accident rate, and $2\frac{1}{2}$ times the normal death and suicide rates, and that between 13% and 29% of the patients in general hospitals are alcoholics.

H28 SOCIAL DRINKING

Alcohol's social uses are many. The relaxing effects of alcohol reduce inhibitions and relieve anxieties, so alcohol in small quantities acts as a social lubricant, decreasing self-consciousness and increasing congeniality, confidence, and "belongingness". As a result, it has been associated with every aspect of man's nature. Sometimes casual drunkenness is encouraged and viewed with amusement; and yet alcohol has a place in much of our social and sacred ritual, even up to the celebration of religious mystery and of birth and death. The varied uses of alcohol are an accepted part of the traditions integrating the social order. As individuals, we can worship or despise the release that alcohol can bring; but a normal attitude, for our society, is that, used sensibly, alcohol is one of the earth's gifts to man - and that, taken in moderation, alcoholic drinks give pleasure at little cost to body or soul.

H27 DEFINITION

Alcoholism is hard to define, because its social manifestations vary. Some authorities define it, in effect, as any repeated drinking that is above the normal for a community. But if one looks at alcoholism as a process, what is significant is the factor of dependence. Like many other drugs, alcohol can produce psychological and, in extreme cases, physical dependence. In psychological "problem" drinking, the sufferer is constantly trying to escape his psychic difficulties into drink. In physical dependence, alcohol has become necessary for the body to function, and its removal produces extreme physical effects. The point at which drinking becomes alcoholism is not decided by the quantity drunk, or even by how far it dominates a person's social life. What distinguishes the alcoholic is that - whether he realizes it or not - his drinking is compulsive.

H29 SYMPTOMATIC DRINKING

Today the conditions of our society seem to encourage people to turn more and more often to alcohol to escape stress - whether the pressure is of work or of their own psyche. This is called "symptomatic drinking". At first, the relief the drinker seeks is easily available. But gradually he achieves it only through greater and greater quantities of drink, as tolerance to the drug increases. Eventually, his psychological dependence is supported, and finally displaced, by physical dependence - with disastrous effects upon his body, his finances, and his family and social life.

H30 WHO BECOMES AN ALCOHOLIC?

Alcoholism through symptomatic drinking is thought of by experts as an illness, relating to underlying personality disorder. It may even be linked with a metabolic defect of some sort. But also important are availability, social environment, and upbringing. Consequently, alcoholism predominates in certain social groups rather than others: senior executives and their wives, traveling salesmen, journalists, actors, and the children of alcoholics. Past cultural factors also modify society's influence: in the United States, alcoholism among Jews and Chinese is rare, that among Irish and Scandinavians much higher. And in all countries, many more men than women are alcoholics - usually in the ratio of 5 to 1. In the US, 7.3% of men are alcoholics, but only 1.3% of women. However, the proportion of women alcoholics is increasing.

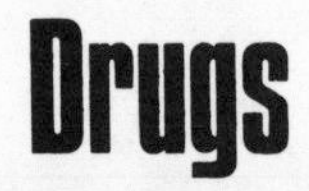

HEALTH EFFECTS

One or two average-strength drinks a day are normally no hazard to health. But sometimes any drinking is inadvisable, eg: if the person is seriously overweight; or if he has recently taken sedatives, tranquilizers or anti-histamine (anti-allergic) tablets; or if he suffers from epilepsy, liver disorders, or stomach or duodenal ulcers.

H31 INVETERATE DRINKING

There are also societies in which a very large intake of alcohol is considered normal among certain groups ("inveterate drinking"). Here intoxication and need may never be noticed: physical dependence is reached without any of the usual psychological symptoms or social and financial consequences. Yet in the inveterate drinker, alcohol may be present in the bloodstream every hour of the day and night. The physical consequences are present, too, and if the inveterate drinker is deprived of his normal intake (eg through having to go into hospital for some other reason), acute withdrawal symptoms will appear.

Inveterate drinking is most common in wine-producing countries, but it is also known in our society - among bartenders and dealers in alcohol, and in some business circles, where alcoholism may arise more through social custom and an expense account than through the pressure of psychic stress.

H32 ALCOHOLISM IN SELECTED COUNTRIES

	Percent of population	Type of alcoholic	Drinking population	Main source of alcohol
Argentina	under 0.5%	Symptomatic & inveterate	Rural	Wine
Spain		Inveterate	Urban Rural	Wine
Brazil	0.5 to 0.9%	Symptomatic	Urban•	Spirits
Netherlands		Symptomatic	Urban•	Spirits
Czechoslovakia	1.0 to 1.4%	Symptomatic	Urban	Beer Spirits
England		Symptomatic	Urban	Beer
Ireland		Symptomatic	Urban Rural	Beer
Canada	1.5 to 1.9%	Symptomatic•	Urban•	Beer Spirits
Denmark		Symptomatic	Urban•	Beer
Norway		Symptomatic	Urban•	Spirits
Peru		Symptomatic•	Urban Rural	Beer Spirits
Scotland		Symptomatic	Urban•	Spirits Beer
Uruguay		Inveterate	Urban	Wine Spirits
Australia	2.0 to 3.0%	Symptomatic	Urban	Beer
Sweden		Symptomatic	Urban	Spirits
Switzerland		Symptomatic	Urban•	Wine Spirits
South Africa		Symptomatic	Urban	
Chile	4.0 to 5.0%	Inveterate•	Urban Rural	Wine
USA		Symptomatic	Urban	Beer Spirits
France	up to 10%	Inveterate•	Urban Rural	Wine Spirits

•Substantial minority category of other type

ALCOHOLISM 2

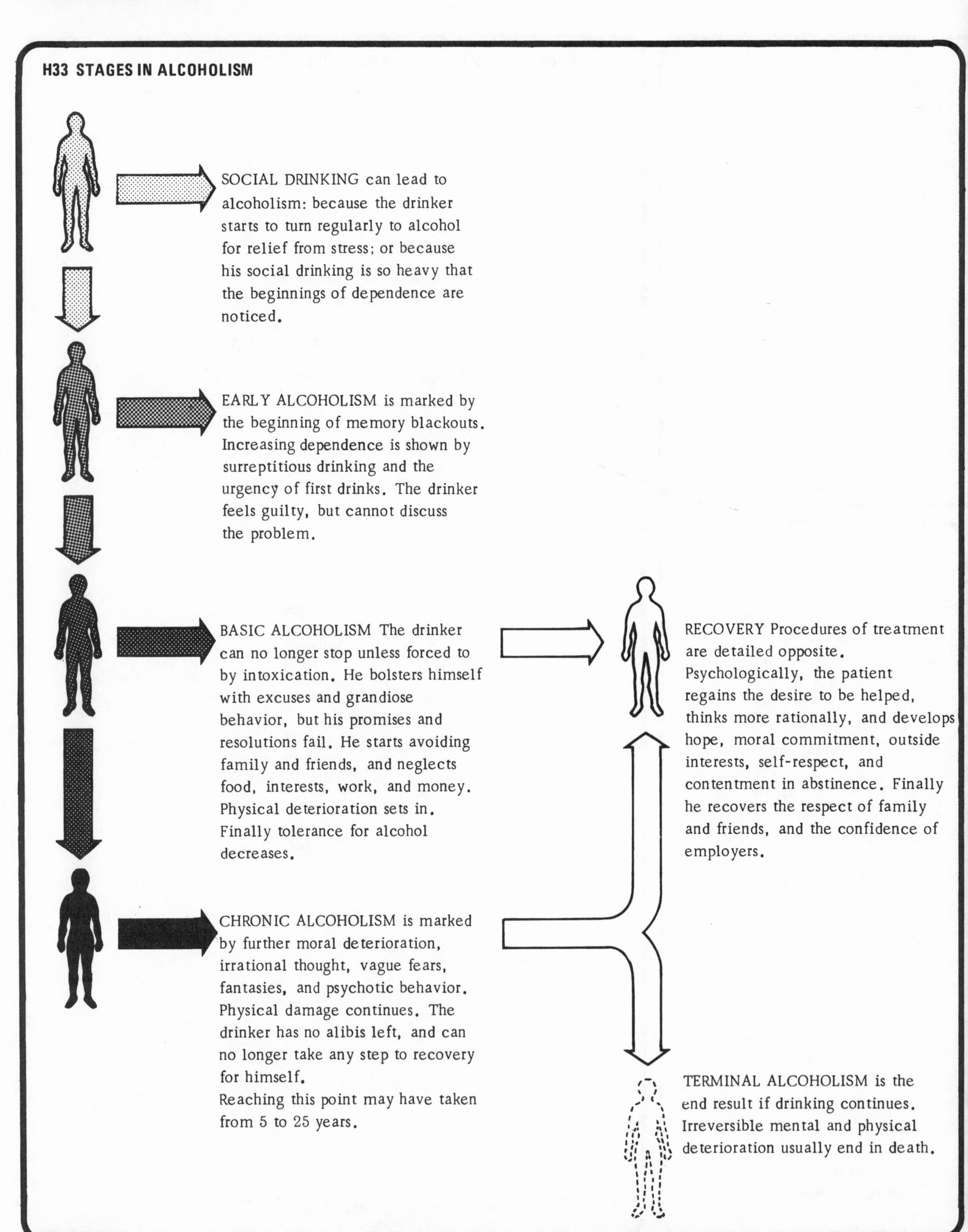

H34 PHYSIOLOGICAL EFFECTS

THE DIGESTIVE SYSTEM
The ordinary hangover shows how alcohol can irritate the stomach. In alcoholism, the stomach can be constantly inflamed (gastritis*), and eventually the intestines too (gastro-enteritis*). There are symptoms of nausea, abdominal pain, chilly sensations, and loss of appetite. The risk of ulceration and bleeding is high.

VITAMIN DEFICIENCY
The alcoholic neglects his food. Malnutrition and vitamin deficiencies result. Common manifestations include beriberi and pellagra - both due especially to B complex vitamin* deficiencies. Beriberi involves inflammation of the nerves all over the body; pellagra affects the nerves, digestion, and skin.

CIRRHOSIS OF THE LIVER
The liver soon recovers from an occasional bout of alcohol. But alcoholism often produces the condition called cirrhosis: the organ shrivels, its cells are largely replaced by fibrous tissue, and its functioning deteriorates. Ten per cent of chronic alcoholics have cirrhosis of the liver, and 75% of people with cirrhosis have an alcoholic history. The main reason is an alcoholic's self-poisoning with alcohol, in addition to his neglect of nutrition: his cirrhosis is the product of protein and vitamin B deficiencies. There are few symptoms until cirrhosis is fairly advanced. Then the victim may complain of general ill health, loss of appetite, nausea, vomiting, and digestive trouble.

ALCOHOLIC MYOPATHY is a term for muscular decay resulting from alcoholism. Causes are lack of use of muscles, poor diet, and alcoholic damage to the nervous system. The heart, as a muscular organ, may be affected.

PANCREATITIS is an inflammation of the pancreas and both a very serious and common complication of alcoholism.

NEUROLOGICAL DEGENERATION
Alcoholism destroys brain cells and causes degeneration throughout the nervous system. Poor diet upsets the brain's metabolism, through lack of B complex vitamins particularly. The sufferer experiences short term and long term memory losses; inability to think clearly; muscular convulsions in the body and limbs; and trembling, emotional disturbance, hallucinations, and fits. Eventually, the decline of nervous functioning can result in pneumonia, kidney failure, or heart failure.

DELERIUM TREMENS (The "DTs") is a state in which the sufferer experiences extreme excitement, mental confusion, and anxiety, with trembling, fever, and rapid and irregular pulse. He may have hallucinations, especially ones involving animals approaching or touching him. The onset usually occurs when a period of heavy drinking has been followed by several days' abstention, and it is often preceded by restlessness, sleeplessness, and irritability.

TERMINAL ALCOHOLISM is the stage where the physical and mental damage done to the body is irreversible. Even if the person can be kept alive, his existence becomes that of a vegetable.

H35 TREATMENT

The patient is deprived of his drug. Severe withdrawal symptoms follow: sweating, vomiting, body aches, diarrhoea, running nose and eyes, fits, convulsions, and hallucinations. Sedatives relieve these, but are terminated before they themselves become addictive. The patient's health is restored by good diet, and any physical problems due to the addiction are treated.

THERAPEUTIC TREATMENT
After detoxification, the underlying psychological causes are identified, if possible, and treated. The patient's motivation, self-confidence, and trust must be constantly strengthened.

Treatments, and their effectiveness, vary greatly. The following are the most widely accepted.

a) Aversion therapy tries to create conditioned reflexes of sickness and aversion at the presence of the drug. Techniques include electric shock therapy, and sensitizing drugs which produce severely unpleasant symptoms when the drug is taken, eg Antabuse.

b) Individual psychological therapy aims at removing the underlying psychological causes by bringing them to light and getting the patient to accept and face them for himself.

c) Group therapy aims at giving the patient objective outside views of himself, with which he must come to terms; and at the same time helps him to overcome his isolation, by giving him personal relationships, and contact with fellow sufferers.

In the case of alcoholics, Alcoholics Anonymous provides both group therapy and guidance by cured alcoholics. Their meetings also provide important support in later rehabilitation and continued abstention.

This depends above all on the patient's desire to be cured. Treatment is long-term, and its goal has to be lifetime abstention.

H36 TOBACCO CONSUMPTION

CIGARETTES account for the bulk of tobacco consumption. The tobacco they use is usually flue-cured. This gives a neutral cigarette smoke which is easily inhaled i.e. taken down into the lungs.

CIGARS are generally made of air-cured tobacco. The smoke is more pungent and seldom inhaled i.e. it only enters the mouth and perhaps the throat - but much of the nicotine content is absorbed through the linings of the mouth.

PIPE tobacco is generally air, sun, or fire-cured. It too is seldom inhaled, and there is only a small amount of nicotine absorption through the mouth.

SNUFF is a powdered tobacco that is sniffed into the nostrils. Nicotine is absorbed through the linings of the nose, and some snuff probably passes down into the lungs.

CHEWING TOBACCO is a mixture of tobacco and molasses. Nicotine is absorbed through the mouth.

With the spread of cigarette smoking after World War I, other forms of consumption declined, especially the taking of snuff and chewing tobacco. But recently, as the dangers of cigarette smoking have been recognized, there has been some slight rise in the relative proportion of cigar and pipe smokers.

Average US consumption per person, per year

	1900	1970
All tobacco•	7.5	10.5
Cigarettes	50	4000
Cigars	110	59
Pipe tobacco•	1.6	0.5
Chewing•	4	0.5
Snuff•	0.3	0.2

•weight in lbs

H37 THE PLANT AND PRODUCTION

Tobacco comes from the plant "nicotiana tabacum", and is produced in about 80 different countries, giving a world total of 8000 million lb a year. Half this is from the USA and China.

After cultivation, tobacco is "cured" (dried) in one of four ways.

Air curing takes place in a barn provided with a steady circulation of air, and takes about six weeks.

Sun-cured leaves are first exposed to the sun, and then undergo a similar process.

Fire-cured leaves are hung over wood fires, and come into direct contact with the smoke.

Flue-cured leaves are also cured by the heat of a fire, but do not come into contact with the smoke.

The method of curing affects the finished product. For example, flue-cured tobacco has a lower nicotine content than other kinds, and instead contains 15 to 20% more sugar. It also affects the leaf color. Air-cured leaves are reddish brown, sun-cured rather darker, fire-cured simply dark brown, and flue-cured light brown to yellow.

Up to 90% of tobacco is flue-cured. After curing the tobacco is left to mature, and then graded ready for manufacture. Grading is done by the size, color, and texture of the leaf. Different grades are used for different products.

H38 CONSUMPTION BY COUNTRY

... showing consumption of cigarettes and all tobacco goods per adult per year.

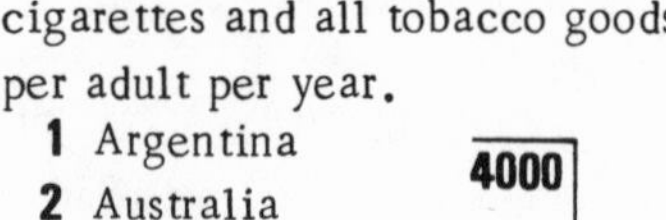

1 Argentina
2 Australia
3 Austria
4 Brazil
5 Canada
6 Finland
7 France
8 W Germany
9 Greece
10 Iceland
11 India
12 Ireland
13 Italy
14 Japan
15 Mexico
16 Netherlands
17 Norway
18 Portugal
19 South Africa
20 Spain
21 Sweden
22 Switzerland
23 Turkey
24 UK
25 US

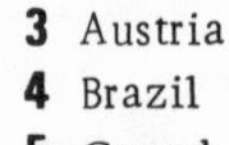

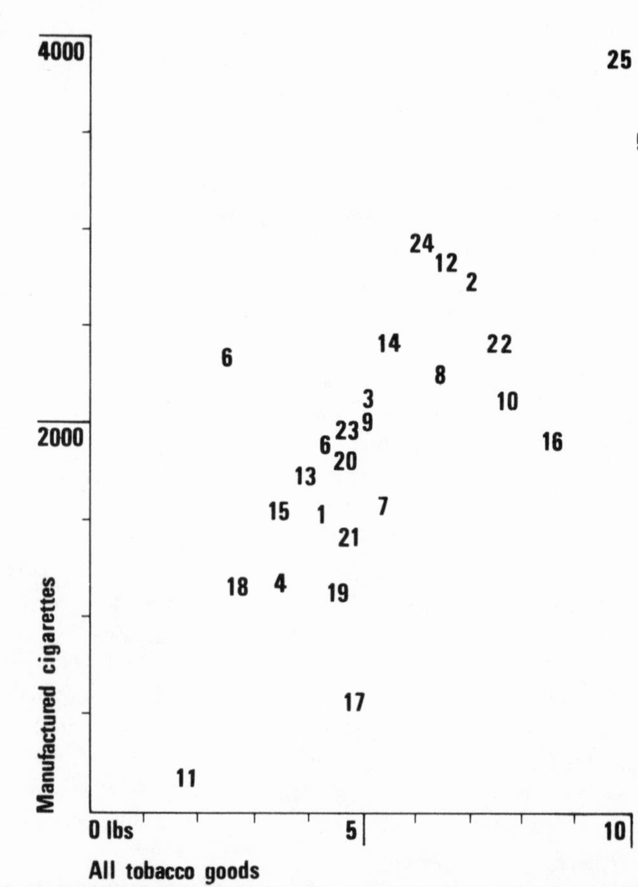

H39 TOBACCO SMOKE

Tobacco smoke contains at least 300 different chemical compounds. These enter the lungs in the form of gases or solid particles. The solid particles condense to form a thick brown tar. (The inhaled smoke of 10,000 cigarettes i.e. under 2 years' smoking, at 15 cigarettes a day, yields about 3/8 lb of this tar.) It lines the passages down which the smoke travels, and collects in the lungs. The contents of tobacco smoke fall into five main categories.

CARCINOGENIC SUBSTANCES i.e. those that induce the growth of cancer. There are at least 15 carcinogens in tobacco smoke, including certain hydrocarbons, benzpyrene, and perhaps a radioactive isotope of polonium.

CO-CARCINOGENS, or cancer promoters, do not cause cancer themselves, but accelerate its production by the carcinogens. They include phenols and fatty acids.

IRRITANT SUBSTANCES disturb the bronchial passages, increasing mucus secretion but damaging the processes for expelling this mucus from the lungs. Many are also co-carcinogens.

GASES occur at dangerous levels in tobacco smoke. They include carbon monoxide at 400 times the level considered safe in industry, and hydrogen cyanide at 160 times the safe level.

NICOTINE is a powerful poison - a 70mg injection is enough to kill. One cigarette contains 0.5 to 2.0mg, depending on how the tobacco was cured. How much of this is absorbed depends on the method of smoking. Inhalation can absorb as much as 90%, non-inhalation as little as 10%. The nicotine that is absorbed affects the nervous system, including brain activity and the control of epinephrine secretion and heart beat rate. Small amounts give the smoker a sense of stimulation, then leave him feeling more tired than before. Larger amounts sedate him. There is evidence that nicotine is the addictive constituent of tobacco i.e. nicotine gives tobacco its "kick" while the tar gives it its taste.

FILTER-TIP CIGARETTES

Seventy per cent of all cigarettes sold are now filter tipped. The filter is meant to remove the harmful substances in the smoke, but it is not necessarily successful. In fact, with any cigarette, the tobacco itself acts as a filter. But, as a result, smoking the last third of a cigarette releases as much dangerous material as the first two-thirds.

H40 WHO SMOKES CIGARETTES?

Horizontal distances measure each age group in the population. Vertical distances show the group's smoking habits. For example, there are fewer men over 65 than women, but more of them smoke - so the column is narrower, but the shaded part taller.

Non smoker

Former smoker

Present smoker

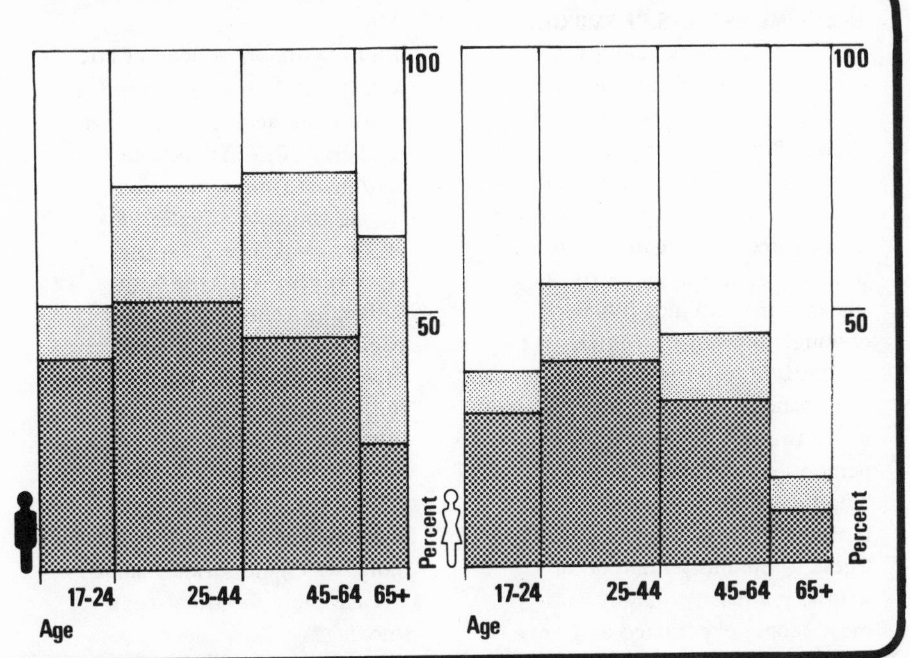

H41 REASONS FOR SMOKING

Despite the growing evidence of the dangers of smoking, old smokers go on smoking and new ones start. The reasons are many and often interdependent.

SOCIAL CONFORMITY Smoking is a socially accepted form of drug taking and for children it is an activity associated with a "grown up" way of life. Most smokers start in adolescence, copying schoolmates, friends, or workmates. Children from families in which both parents smoke are also more liable to do so themselves.

CURIOSITY Many first experiments in smoking follow from a child's natural curiosity to find out what so many adults and friends experience when they smoke.

PERSONALITY As with all drugs, the smoker's psychological make-up forms the basis of his habit and his dependence. Often those adolescents who start to smoke are those who feel unsuccessful or rebellious: smoking can give them a status symbol, a symbol of maturity. For others, of all ages, it may be used to combat or conceal nervousness, and give them confidence in company. Freudian psychology believes that smoking also provides sexual/oral gratification, acting as substitute for the loss of the mother's breast at weaning.

PLEASURE Once tolerance has developed, and smoking no longer gives unpleasant physical sensations such as dizziness, the smoker usually finds his habit comforting and pleasurable - if only because it takes away the desire experienced when he stops.

BOREDOM Smoking allows a certain amount of involvement, so it can give some release from boredom. Moreover, unlike many activities, it is socially acceptable for smoking to accompany or even interrupt work.

ESCAPE The sedative effects of smoking can provide some relief from anxiety and tension, while the physical activity of smoking can be an outlet for nervous energy, simply by giving the smoker something to do.

ADVERTISING The social acceptability of smoking means that the tobacco industry is allowed to advertise its products. Advertisements make smoking seem desirable in many ways. The constant sight of cigarettes may also result in a smoker being unable to give up.

GOVERNMENT INVOLVEMENT The high taxes imposed on tobacco products provide Governments everywhere with considerable revenue. This, and the large proportion of the population often supported by the industry, means that cigarettes will continue to be produced. As long as cigarettes are available, smoking will take place.

H42 SOME EFFECTS OF SMOKING

DEPENDENCE Smoking gives many smokers a comforting habit that helps them relax and avoid stress. For others, it is just a meaningless activity that cannot be stopped. Both cases result from the dependence that cigarettes create. Withdrawal symptoms on stopping smoking may include intense craving, depression, anxiety, instability, restlessness, sleep disturbance, difficulty in concentrating, altered time perception, sweating, drop in blood pressure and heart rate, and gastro-intestinal changes. These symptoms seldom occur with any intensity, however: most people experience only very mild discomfort or none at all.

ACCIDENTS Smokers have four times more accidents than non-smokers. This may be due to a slowing of the reflex actions, lasting about 20 minutes, that follows smoking a cigarette. (It may also be linked with differences between the kind of people who become smokers and those who do not). Smokers also run a higher risk of death or injury by fire - the most common cause being smoking in bed.

ENDURANCE The physical endurance of smokers is lower the more the cigarettes they smoke and the more the time spent smoking.

EFFECTS ON NON-SMOKERS Smoking by others also affects non-smokers, causing eye irritation, headaches, and coughing in a smoke-laden atmosphere. It exposes them to the same health risks as smokers, though in a very much reduced way.

ECONOMICS Smoking can be very expensive on a personal level, but the greatest cost is to society. Illness resulting from smoking causes 20% of the annual loss of working days in the USA. The cost of smoking to a nation also includes the impaired abilities of its members, and the extra medical expenses incurred.

H43 SMOKING AND HEALTH

Smoking is the largest single avoidable cause of ill-health and death. It can damage the cardio-vascular, respiratory, and digestive systems, and it encourages the growth of cancer in many parts of the body.

Smokers run a much higher risk than non-smokers of illness and premature death.

For example:

-Cigarette smokers are twice as likely to die before middle age as non smokers. They run the same risk of death as someone 10 years older.

-Two out of five smokers die before 65. This happens to only one out of five non-smokers.

-The average smoker aged 35 has a life expectancy $5\frac{1}{2}$ years shorter than a non-smoker.

How much damage smoking does depends on several things: the type of tobacco; the form it is smoked in; the temperature at which it is burned; the effectiveness of any filtration; whether inhalation occurs; the length of time the individual has been smoking; the amount he smokes; and the general state of his health. Smoking of all sorts is harmful, but usually cigarette smoking is the most deadly. The nicotine content of cigarette tobacco is often smaller, but the higher burning temperature and the greater tendency to inhale make up for this. Also the tendency to inhale favors lung damage and especially lung cancer, which is often not diagnosed till too late. Pipe and cigar smokers are more likely to develop the more noticeable - and so more curable - cancers of the mouth, pharynx, and larynx.

The convenience of cigarettes may also encourage more smoking than pipes or cigars.

H44 SMOKING AND DEATH

All lines below the first show mortality rates for smokers.

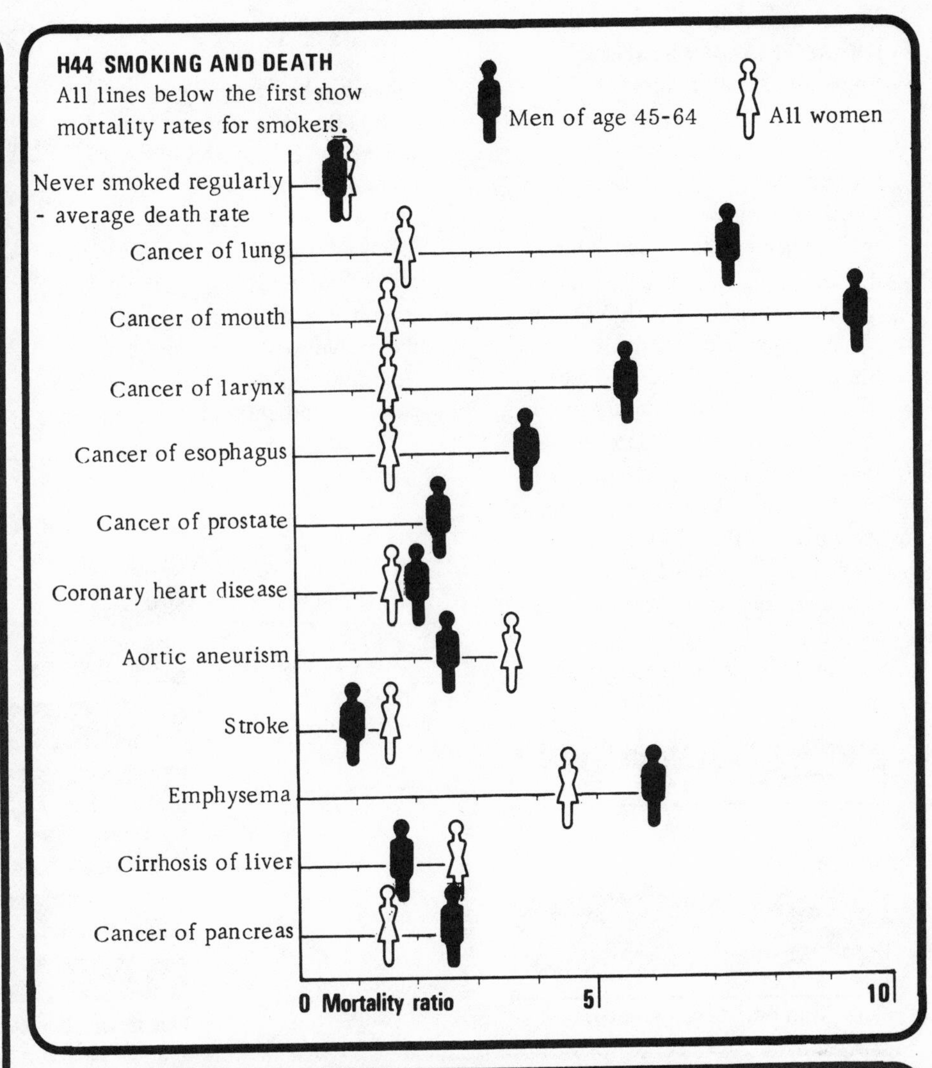

H45 YOUR ODDS OF SURVIVING

into the next age group.

Smoker A: 25 or more cigarettes per day

Smoker B: 15-24 cigarettes per day

Smoker C: 1-14 cigarettes per day

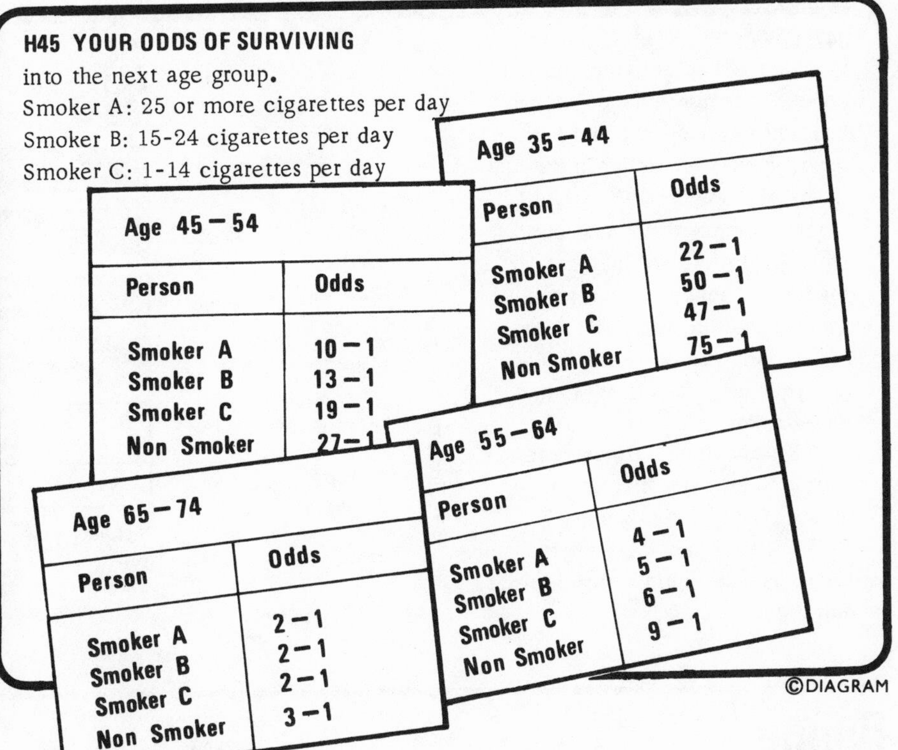

Age 35 — 44

Person	Odds
Smoker A	22 — 1
Smoker B	50 — 1
Smoker C	47 — 1
Non Smoker	75 — 1

Age 45 — 54

Person	Odds
Smoker A	10 — 1
Smoker B	13 — 1
Smoker C	19 — 1
Non Smoker	27 — 1

Age 55 — 64

Person	Odds
Smoker A	4 — 1
Smoker B	5 — 1
Smoker C	6 — 1
Non Smoker	9 — 1

Age 65 — 74

Person	Odds
Smoker A	2 — 1
Smoker B	2 — 1
Smoker C	2 — 1
Non Smoker	3 — 1

H46 RESPIRATORY SYSTEM

Smoking greatly reduces the efficiency of the lungs, especially in those who inhale.

In a normal lung, glands in the interior lining are constantly producing mucus. This captures dirt and bacteria, and the mucus and its contents are then forced out of the lungs by the action of cilia. These are small, hair-like projections that are constantly moving, pushing the mucus up into the throat, where it is swallowed. Inhaled smoke hinders the action of the cilia, whilst stimulating mucus production. As a result, mucus, tar, dirt, and bacteria collect in the lungs in festering pools, encouraging tissue degeneration and hindering gas exchange.

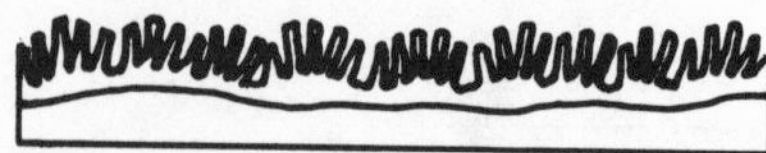
Bronchial cilia

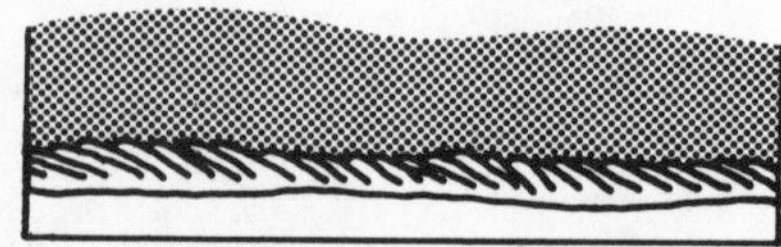
Cilia immobilized by mucus

Inhaled tobacco smoke also tends to irritate the air passages, and to reduce air flow in the bronchi and bronchioles by making them contract.

SMOKER'S COUGH The constant cough that attends regular smoking is an attempt by the lungs to rid themselves of the tar and phlegm. Healthy lungs do not collect such phlegm, and only need the normal action of the cilia.

BRONCHITIS AND EMPHYSEMA Bronchitis* is often triggered off by the irritation caused by cigarette smoke, and by the presence of bacteria in the lungs of smokers. Once established, it can progress rapidly from just a troublesome cough to a chronic condition which can kill. Emphysema* is also made more likely by the damage smoke and tar do to the lungs. Smokers, especially of cigarettes, run a much higher risk than non-smokers of contracting and dying from either of these.

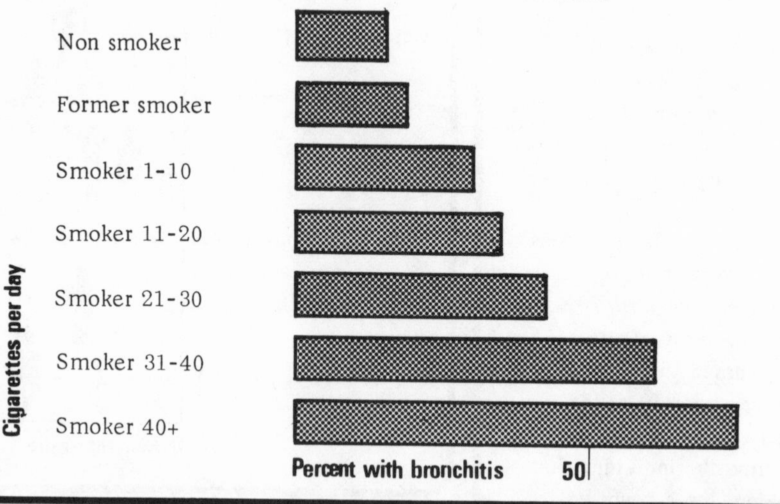

H47 CANCER

Smoking is a direct cause of much cancer, because tobacco smoke contains carcinogens, and these can set off cancer wherever in the body the smoke reaches. As a result, cigarette smokers are 70 times more likely to have lung cancer than non-smokers. Smokers in general are also more likely to suffer from cancer of the mouth and pharynx (4 times more than non-smokers), larynx (5 times more) esophagus (2 times more), stomach ($1\frac{1}{2}$ times more), and bladder ($1\frac{1}{2}$ to 3 times more). Cancer of the mouth, pharynx, and larynx are the main forms in pipe and cigar smokers.

Cigarettes per day

Non smoker
Male smoker 1-10
Male smoker 11-20
Male smoker 21-40
Male smoker 40+
Female smoker 1-20
Female smoker 20+

Mortality ratio 5 10 15

H48 CARDIOVASCULAR SYSTEM

REDUCED OXYGEN INTAKE
Carbon monoxide is the most concentrated gas in tobacco smoke. Its affinity for blood hemoglobin is greater than that of oxygen i.e. it combines with it more readily than oxygen does. The greater concentration of carbon monoxide in a smoker's lungs means that hemoglobin which should be carrying oxygen to the tissues is now carrying useless carbon monoxide. The amount of oxygen in the bloodstream can be reduced by up to 8%. At the same time, the effects of smoking on the respiratory system also reduce the efficiency of oxygen intake. All this makes heart-strain a danger, as the heart works harder and harder to keep up the body's oxygen supply.

ATHEROSCLEROSIS AND THROMBOSIS
Atherosclerosis and thrombosis are more common in smokers than in non-smokers. Smoking raises the level of fatty acids and cholesterol in the blood, and encourages blood platelets (clotting bodies) to adhere to each other and to the blood vessel walls. Carbon monoxide in the bloodstream also seems to favour atherosclerosis.

OTHER EFFECTS
The action of nicotine on the endocrine system and sympathetic nervous system constricts blood vessels, raises blood pressure and blood sugar levels, and increases the heart rate. All this makes damage to the system likely.

CORONARY HEART DISEASE
All these factors greatly predispose the smoker to coronary heart disease of all kinds. Coronary heart disease occurs, on average, up to seven years earlier in smokers than in non-smokers.

H49 THE RISK TO SMOKERS

Not only do smokers have a higher death rate than non-smokers, but the death rate is generally higher the more cigarettes smoked. These graphs show this for two age groups in two different surveys.

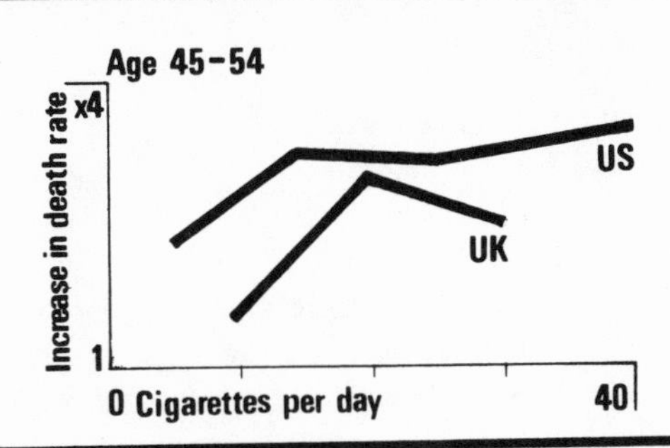

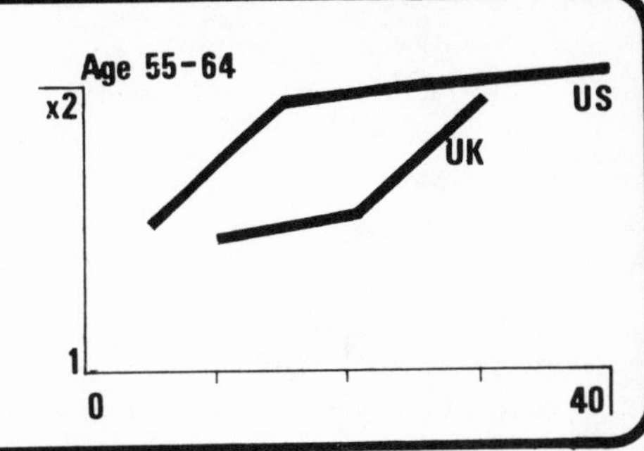

H50 OTHER FACTORS

THE UNBORN CHILD Pregnant women who smoke may retard the growth of the fetus (the babies of smokers average 6oz lighter than those of non smokers). They are also more susceptible to miscarriages, still births, and the death of the child soon after birth.

ULCERS Those who smoke are five times more likely to suffer from gastric ulcers, and twice as likely to suffer from duodenal ulcers. This may be partly due to personality differences between non-smokers and smokers, but it has also been shown that smoking hinders the healing of these ulcers.

Smoking also:
reduces the appetite (which often results in a weight gain on stopping);
stains the teeth and fingers;
increases the chances of periodontal disease*; and impairs the senses of taste and smell.

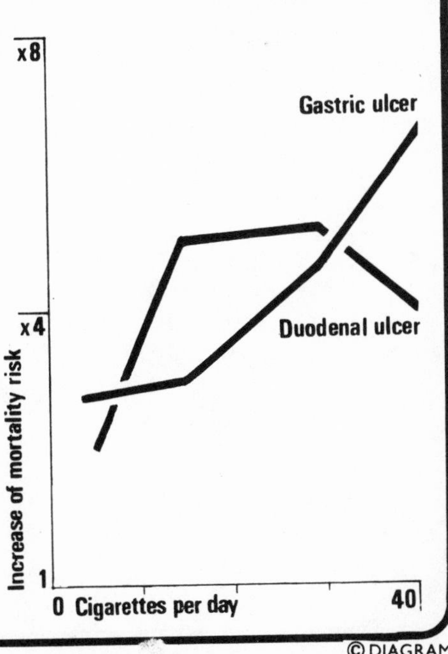

H51 CIGARETTE BRANDS

FILTER

T	N	
25	1.8	Half and Half
24	1.2	Mapleton
23	1.2	Domino
20	1.3	Tareyton
19	1.3	Camel
	1.3	Winchester
	1.3	Winston
18	1.2	Chesterfield
	1.2	L&M
	1.2	Lark
	1.1	Tramps
17	1.1	Marlboro
	1.1	Old Gold
	1.1	St Moritz
16	1.2	Kool
	1.1	Benson & Hedges k
	1.0	Raleigh
	1.0	Viceroy
15	1.0	Doral
	1.0	du Maurier
	1.0	Galaxy
	0.9	Kent
	0.9	Miyako
14	1.0	Winston Lights
	0.9	Raleigh Mild
	0.9	Viceroy Mild
	0.8	Parliament
12	0.8	B&H Multifilter
	0.8	Vantage
	0.2	Marvels
11	0.8	Tempo
	0.6	True
9	0.6	Lucky
	0.6	Pall Mall Mild
	0.5	Benson & Hedges r
8	0.3	Sano
6	0.2	Marvels
4	0.3	Carlton k
2	0.2	Carlton r

FILTER: 100mm

T	N	
23	1.4	Old Gold
20	1.4	L&M
	1.4	Pall Mall
	1.3	Chesterfield (101)
19	1.3	Lark
	1.3	Tareyton
	1.3	Winston
	1.2	Kent
17	1.2	Raleigh
	1.1	Benson & Hedges
	1.1	Marlboro
	1.1	Philip Morris
	1.1	St Moritz
	1.1	Viceroy
	1.0	Parliament
13	0.7	True
10	0.7	Lucky 10

NON-FILTER

T	N	
31	2.1	Players
30	1.2	Mapleton
29	2.2	English Ovals k
	1.8	Tareyton
	1.7	Chesterfield k
28	1.6	Fatima
27	1.7	Pall Mall
	1.6	Lucky Strike
26	1.3	Domino
	1.6	Camel
	1.5	Philip Morris k
	1.5	Piedmont
25	0.9	Marvels
24	1.4	Chesterfield r
	1.4	Raleigh
	1.2	Old Gold k
22	1.5	English Ovals r
	0.8	Sano
21	1.6	Home Run
20	1.5	Picayune
	1.2	Old Gold r
	1.1	Philip Morris r

MENTHOL

T	N	
21	1.5	Newport 100
	1.2	Spring 100
19	1.4	Montclair
	1.4	Winston (100)
	1.3	L&M (100)
	1.3	Salem k
	1.3	Salem 100
	1.2	Chesterfield
	1.2	Kool nf
18	1.5	More (120)
	1.3	Salem Extra
	1.2	Kent (100)
	1.2	Oasis
	1.2	St Moritz (100)
17	1.3	Pall Mall (100)
	1.2	Belair 100
	1.2	Kool 100
	1.2	Newport k
	1.2	Super M (100)
	1.2	Twist (100)
	1.2	Winchester
	1.1	Benson & Hedges
	1.1	Saratoga (120)
	1.0	Philip Morris (100)
16	1.2	Kool k
	0.9	Alpine 100
	0.9	Tramps
15	1.0	Belair k
13	0.9	Doral
	0.8	Alpine k
	0.8	Kool Milds
	0.8	Marlboro
	0.8	True 100
12	0.7	True k
11	0.8	Vantage
10	0.7	B&H Multifilter
9	0.6	Iceberg (100)
7	0.3	Sano
4	0.3	Carlton
	0.2	Marvels

k: king size
r: regular size
100: 100mm size
120: 120mm size
T: tar content (mg).
N: nicotine content (mg).

These tables show the tar and nicotine levels for most brands and types of US cigarettes. The higher the number the higher the content. Tar content ranges from a low of 2mg to a high of 31mg; nicotine from a low of 0.2 to a high of 2.2. Cigarettes with low tar and nicotine content make smoking less dangerous - but they do not make it safe! Use such cigarettes as a step towards giving up completely.

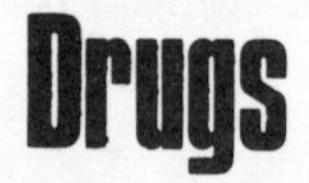

H52 GIVING UP SMOKING

JUST STOP! If you really want to you can.
But if you don't believe in yourself enough, then do make the change from cigarettes to a pipe or cigars - and stop inhaling.
If even that is impossible, at least be sure to: smoke fewer cigarettes; inhale less; take fewer puffs on each cigarette (and not longer ones); leave a longer stub at the end; avoid leaving a lit cigarette in your mouth; and change to a brand with a low concentration of tar and nicotine. Also buy, and use, a detachable filter.
Giving up is an act of self-determination, not self-denial. The benefits to your health - and your finances - far outweigh the possible discomfort of a week or two.
WAYS OF GIVING UP There are three main paths.
a) Group sessions, where the new ex-smoker gives and receives support in his attempt to stop. Some groups are organized on a voluntary basis. Others are operated by medical and health organizations. A doctor, library or local information service can advise you on these.
b) Individual medical care, in which the ex-smoker receives the personal attention and help of a physician.
c) An individual act of will and self-assertion. Probably the best way to give up smoking is to stop suddenly, either on a pre-arranged day or on the spur of the moment.
Which of these three methods would be best for you depends on your personality and on whether you smoke for support in moments of stress; out of habit; for physical gratification; to promote relaxation; or because you are truly addicted.

EFFECTS OF GIVING UP
Within ten years of giving up the life expectancy of an ex-smoker (up to 19 cigarettes a day) is the same as that of a non-smoker.
But the beneficial effects can be seen within two weeks: no more cough; better taste and smell; increased vitality; and more money to spare. At first these are often overshadowed by the initial effects of withdrawal, ranging from slight discomfort (common) to fits of anxiety, depression, and physical upset (uncommon). But however intense the symptoms, they are always temporary; and the more intense they are the greater the sense of self-esteem when they are over.
Many people turn to food for the satisfaction they previously gained from cigarettes. This, and the increase in appetite, often results in an initial weight increase.
This is usually only temporary and can be accepted as such.

PHYSICAL AIDS
There are various pills and medicines on the market that are supposed to cut down the need to smoke, or to make smoking actually unpleasant. You may find that one of these helps you - but almost all of them are unproved, and unrecognized by doctors.
There are also dummy cigarettes available, which satisfy at least the need to hold something in the mouth.
Some people change to herbal cigarettes. These contain no nicotine - but they do produce tar. They can be useful for treating a physical addiction, but they are not a safe way of smoking.

PSYCHOLOGICAL AIDS
Fix a future date on which to stop. (Then either cut down gradually before this date, or smoke as many as usual till then.)
Change from your favorite brand of cigarettes to one you don't like.
Ask yourself if you really want the cigarette you are about to light.
Delay smoking each cigarette until fifteen minutes after the initial urge.
Remind yourself continually of the harmful effects of smoking.
Become conscious of each cigarette you smoke, how much you want it, and how satisfying it actually is.
Realize, with each pleasurable sensation, the harm it is actually doing to your body. Become conscious of this each time you inhale.

ACTIVITIES
Avoid for a while friends who smoke, and put yourself in "no smoking" areas.
Change habits and activities associated with smoking.
Clear the surroundings of ashtrays and other smoking paraphernalia.
Eat fruit or sweets, or chew gum, to suppress the desire for a cigarette.
Take exercise. It will show you how unfit smoking has made you - and how rapidly you can correct this now you have stopped.
Find new interests.
The question of whether to smoke or not is up to you. Remember the damage you are doing to yourself. However well you feel, you could feel much better without cigarettes.

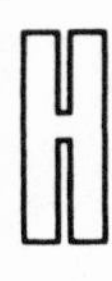

MALE SEX ORGANS

J01 LOCATION

The male sexual system is partly visible, and partly hidden inside the body.
The visible parts are the penis, and the scrotum containing the testes.
Inside the body are the prostate gland, the seminal vesicles, and the tubes that link different parts of the system.

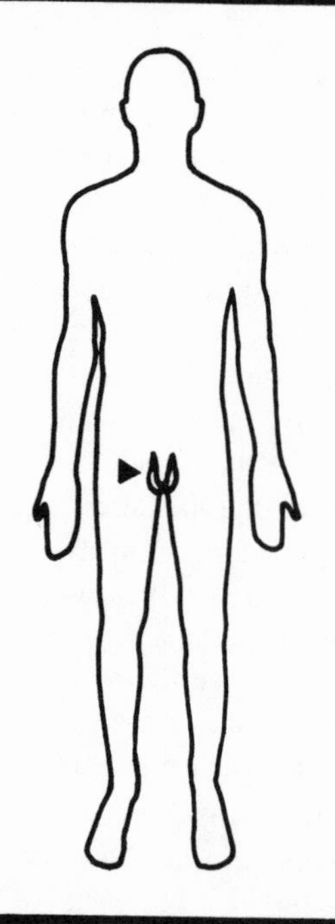

J03 ERECTION

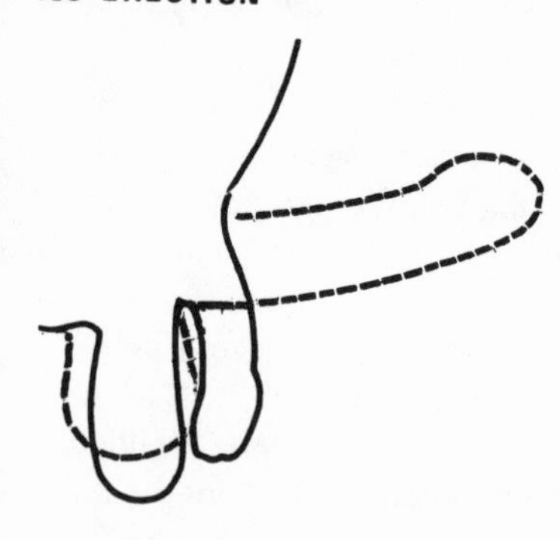

When a man is sexually aroused, the penis becomes swelled with blood. Instead of being "floppy" and hanging down, it becomes stiffer and longer, and juts out from the body. This is called "erection."

J02 MALE SEX ORGANS

THE TWO TESTES (a) are the male reproductive glands. They hang in an external pouch (the scrotum), which is below and behind the penis. Each testis is a flattened oval in shape, about $1\frac{3}{4}$ inches long and 1 inch wide.
The scrotum is divided into two separate compartments (scrotal sacs), one for each testis. (Usually the left testis hangs lower than the right, and its scrotal sac is slightly larger.)
The testes make:
a male sex hormone, testosterone; and sperm cells, which are the male reproduction cells.
The sperm cells are needed to fertilize the egg in the female body, if new life is to be produced.
THE EPIDIDYMIDES (b) are found one alongside each testis.
A number of small tubes lead to each epididymis from its testis.
In the epididymides the young sperm cells (spermatocytes) are stored and develop into mature sperm.

THE VAS DEFERENS (c) are the two tubes - one from each testis - that carry sperm from the testes to the prostate gland.
They are about 16 inches long, and wind upwards from the scrotum into the pelvic cavity.
They come together and join with the urethra tube just below the bladder.
THE PROSTATE GLAND (d) surrounds the junction of the vas deferens and urethra tubes.
Here the sperm cells are mixed with seminal fluid: the liquid in which the sperms are carried out of the body. The resulting mixture is semen: a thick whitish fluid.
THE SEMINAL VESICLES (e) make part of the seminal fluid that the prostate gland mixes with the sperm cells. More seminal fluid is made by the prostate gland itself.

THE URETHRA (f) is the tube that carries urine from the bladder to the penis. It is S-shaped and about 8 inches long.
In the prostate gland it is joined by the vas deferens - so it is also the route by which the semen reaches the penis from the prostate gland.
THE PENIS (g) is inserted into the female body during copulation.
Most of the penis is made up of spongy tissue, loosely covered with skin.
The urethra tube enters the penis from the body and runs inside it to the tip of the penis.
The external opening in the tip (the meatus) is where semen or urine leaves the body.
In its natural state, the sides of the penis near its tip are covered by a fold of skin, called the foreskin. But this is often removed - usually because of religious or social custom, shortly after birth, but sometimes for medical reasons.

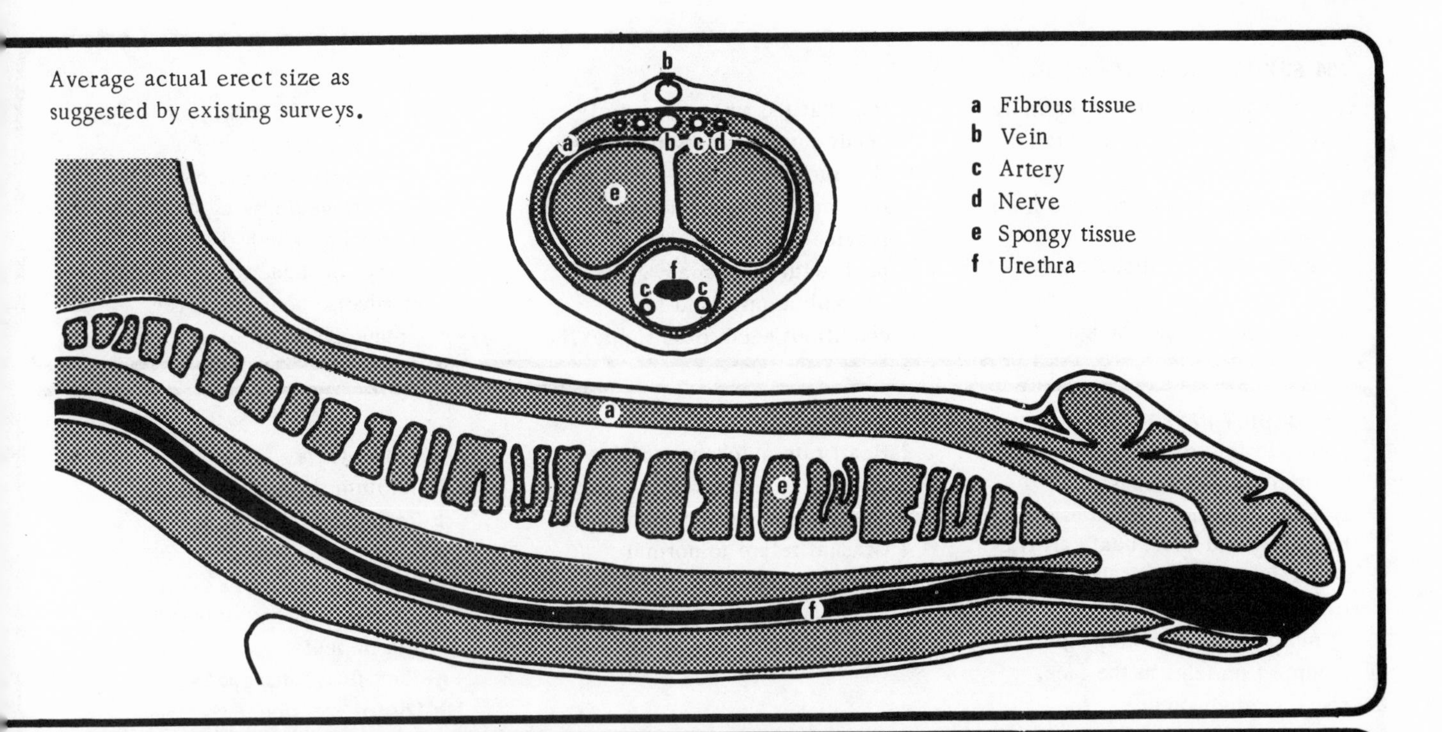

Average actual erect size as suggested by existing surveys.

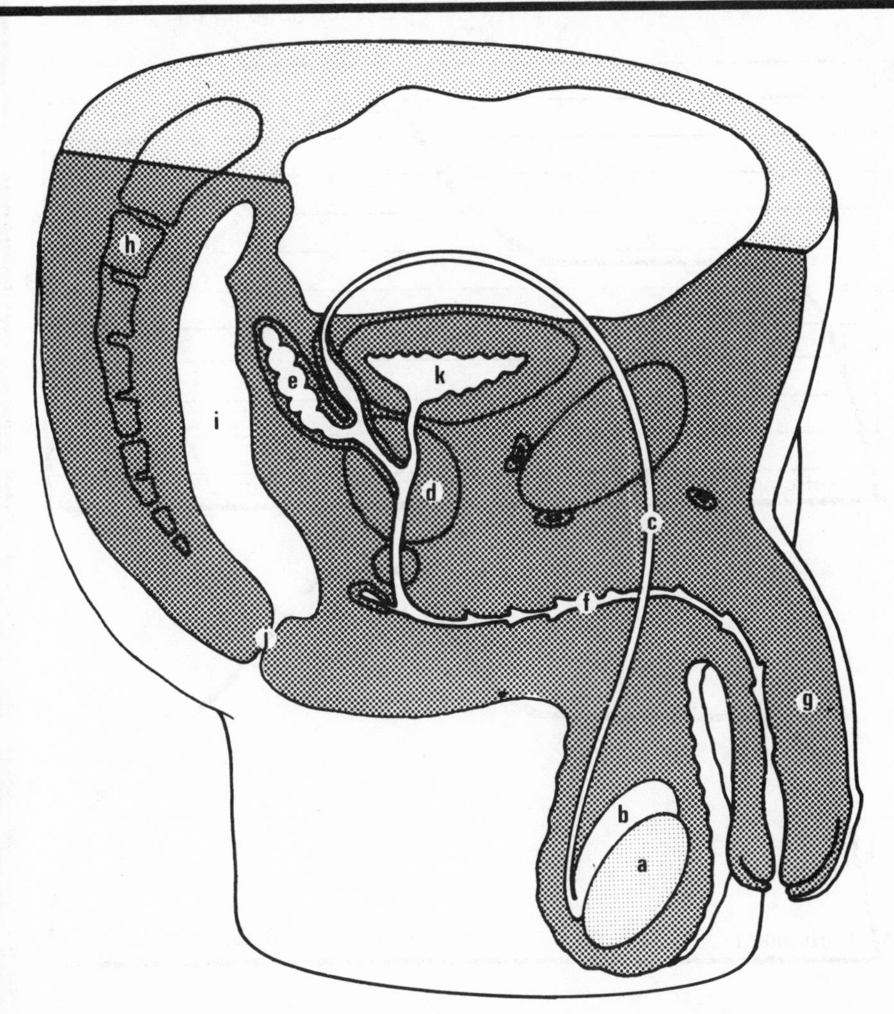

a Testes
b Epididymides
c Vas deferens
d Prostate gland
e Seminal vesicles
f Urethra
g Penis
h Pelvis
i Rectum
j Anus
k Bladder

J04 SEXUAL AROUSAL

The sexual process takes the male sexual system from its normal, inactive state, to orgasm. On orgasm, semen is discharged from the penis.
The stimulus that first arouses the system can be purely psychological - the thought of sex. But the system normally needs physical pressure on the skin surface of the penis to reach orgasm. In copulation this is provided by the contact of the penis with the female genitals.
For both arousal and for orgasm, conditions need to be right. The system can be inhibited, or the process reversed, by:
a) adverse physical conditions in the surroundings, eg cold;
b) psychological distractions (eg worry, or sudden disturbance);
c) adverse body states (eg tiredness, or too recent orgasm).

J05 BODILY RESPONSES

The following responses accompany the male sexual process:
a) blood pressure, and rates of breathing and heart beat, all rise often, on orgasm, to about 2½ times the normal level;
b) muscular spasms may affect groups of muscles in the face, chest, and abdomen;
c) contractions of the rectum occur.
In some men there is also:
d) swelling and erection of the nipples;
e) flushing of skin color around chest, neck, and forehead;
f) perspiration from soles, palms, and body, and sometimes from head, face, and neck.

ORGASM
For both men and women, the experience of orgasm can be one of very intense sexual excitement and emotional release. Yet the physical process, of irritation and spasm, can be compared with that of sneezing.
In intercourse, orgasm is usually accompanied by convulsions of the body, involuntary movements, and sounds such as sighs and groans. But orgasm can occur at various levels of sexual excitement. Evidence, in men, of a high level of excitement, are very high rates of breathing, and flushing of the skin.

1 Heart rate quickens rapidly
2 Heart rate levels off
3 Sharp rise as orgasm approaches
4 Gradual return to normal

a Penis erects
b Scrotum thickens
c Testes rise
d "Sex flush" appears
e Penis tip and testes swell
f Ejaculation, heavy breathing, and muscular spasms
g "Sex flush" disappears
h Loss of erection
i Penis returns to normal state

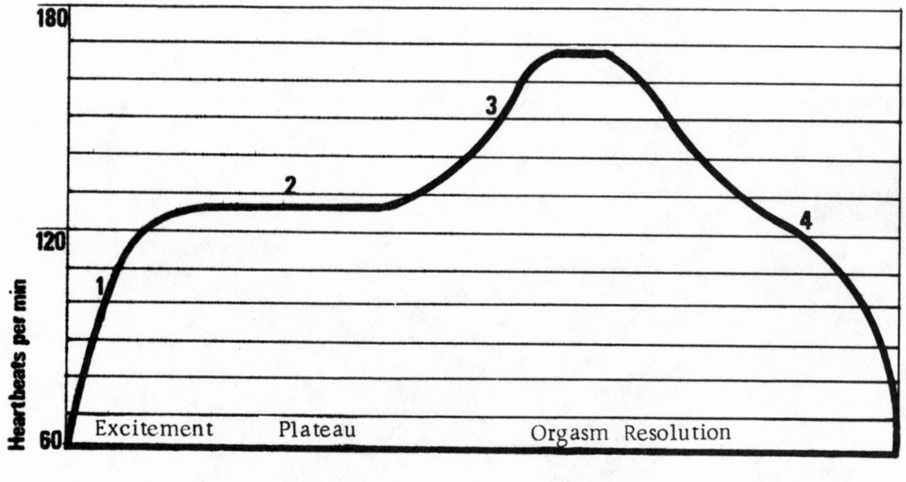

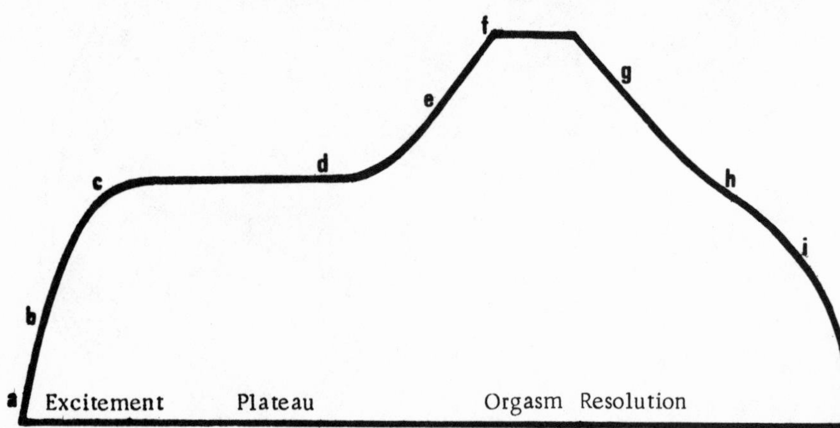

J06 BEHAVIOR OF THE PENIS

1) EXCITEMENT
The sexual stimulus triggers off an automatic reflex, which sends blood flowing into the spongy tissue of the penis.
The spongy mass swells and presses against the sheath of skin. As a result, the penis becomes stiff and sticks out at an angle from the body, usually pointing slightly upward.
Muscular contraction pulls the testes closer in to the body.
This stage can be maintained for long periods, and can be lost and regained, without orgasm, many times.

2) PLATEAU LEVEL
The testes are drawn still closer to the body. The penis increases slightly in diameter, near the tip, and the opening in the tip becomes more slit-like. The tip itself may change color, to a deeper red-purple.

3) ORGASM
The muscles around the urethra give a number of rapid involuntary contractions. This forces semen out of the penis at high pressure (ejaculation).
There are usually three or four major bursts of semen, one every 0.8 seconds, followed by weaker, more irregular, muscular contractions.

4) RESOLUTION
Often there is:
first, a very rapid reduction in penis size, to about 50% larger than its normal state;
followed by a slower reduction back to normal.
But each of these stages may be prolonged, eg if the penis remains inserted in the female genitals.
The response patterns shown here and in J05 were first described by WH Masters and VE Johnson in "Human Sexual Response" (1966).

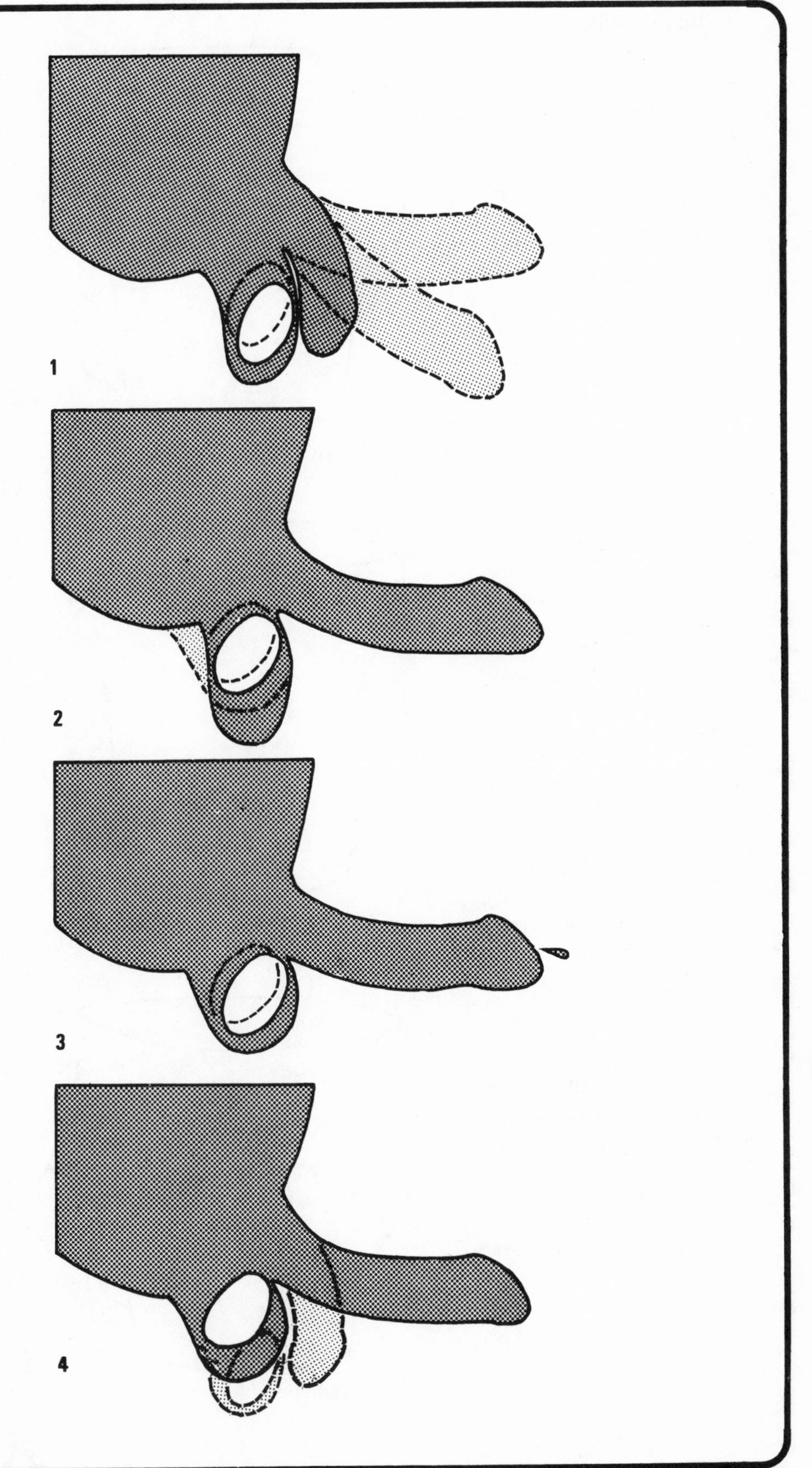

J

J07 CIRCUMCISION

In its natural state, the sides of the penis near its tip are covered by a fold of skin, called the foreskin. In primitive circumstances, this probably served as some protection to the penis at its most sensitive part. When rolled forward, the foreskin is like a hood around the penis tip but it can also be pushed back along the shaft.

In many societies, the foreskin is often removed – it is cut away, in a minor surgical procedure known as circumcision. In rare cases there are medical reasons for this: sometimes the foreskin of an adult man can become very tight and difficult to move. But usually it is a religious or social custom. Male Jews and also Moslems are circumcised as a religious requirement; and in many hospitals in the USA, and some other countries, it is routine practice to circumcise all baby boys.

The value of routine circumcision is debatable. There is no clear evidence that presence or absence of a foreskin makes much difference to sexual sensitivity, or pleasure, or time taken to reach orgasm. One practical argument for circumcision is a hygienic one When the foreskin is intact, white secretions called "smegma" can accumulate underneath it.

Unless these are regularly washed away, the foreskin can become smelly, dirty, and even inflamed. There is also a link between smegma and cancer of the penis in men; and a possible link between smegma and cervical cancer in women. However, adequate hygiene will cope with this just as well as circumcision.

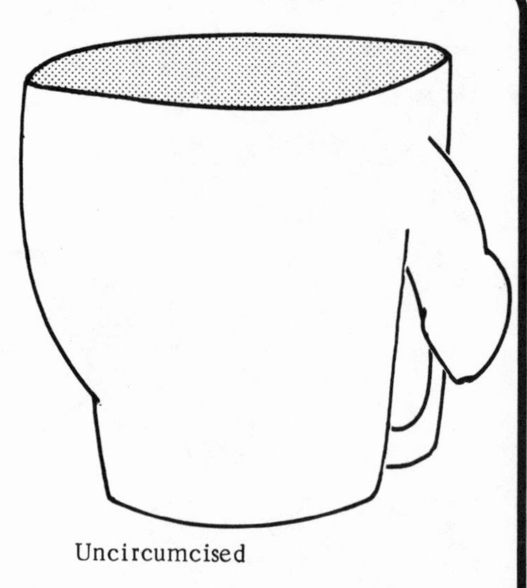

Uncircumcised

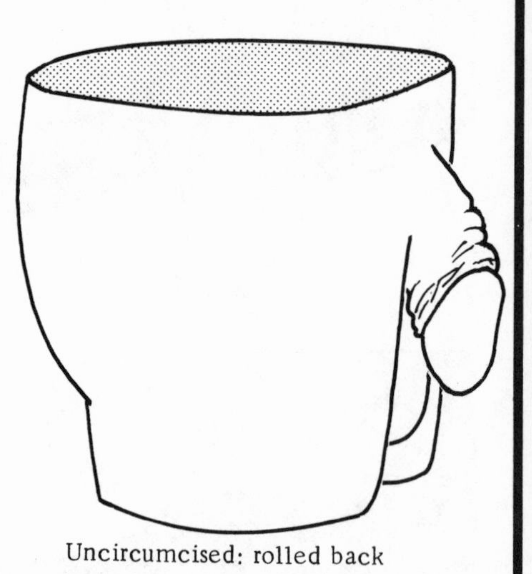

Uncircumcised: rolled back

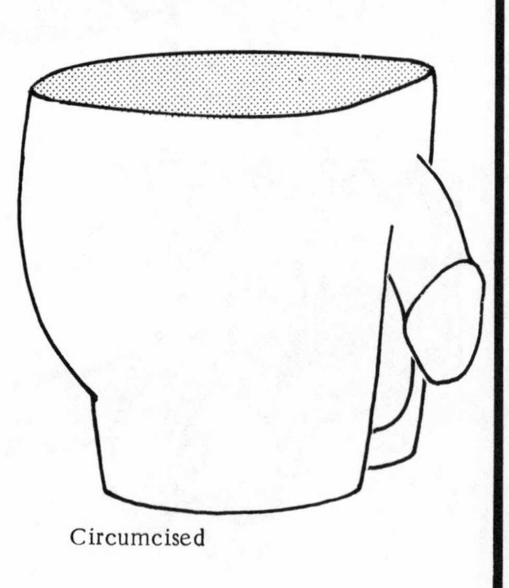

Circumcised

J08 ERECT DIMENSIONS

The longest erect penis for which there is reasonable scientific evidence measured 12in. The smallest recorded with testes and normal functioning has been under ½in in length. In other abnormal cases the penis can, of course, be totally absent.

Body size is no guide to penis size: the erect penis has a less constant relationship to body size than any other organ. Nor is flaccid size decisive: penises which hang longer when flaccid tend to gain less when erect. A short penis can gain as much as 3¾in, and a long one as little as 2in.

There is no relationship between penis size and sexual prowess or female satisfaction: the female vagina accommodates its size to that of the penis, and stimulation of the female clitoris does not depend on penis length.

J09 FLACCID DIMENSIONS

In its normal state, the penis hangs down loosely. It averages about 3¾in long, and most examples are between 3¼in and 4¼in, though a few cases will fall well outside this range.

The penis gets temporarily smaller than usual in certain circumstances, eg in cold temperatures; through immersion in cold water; in extreme exhaustion; or after a failed attempt at sexual activity. These circumstances also pull the testes and scrotal sac closer to the body.

The penis may get permanently smaller in old age, or after longish periods of impotence.

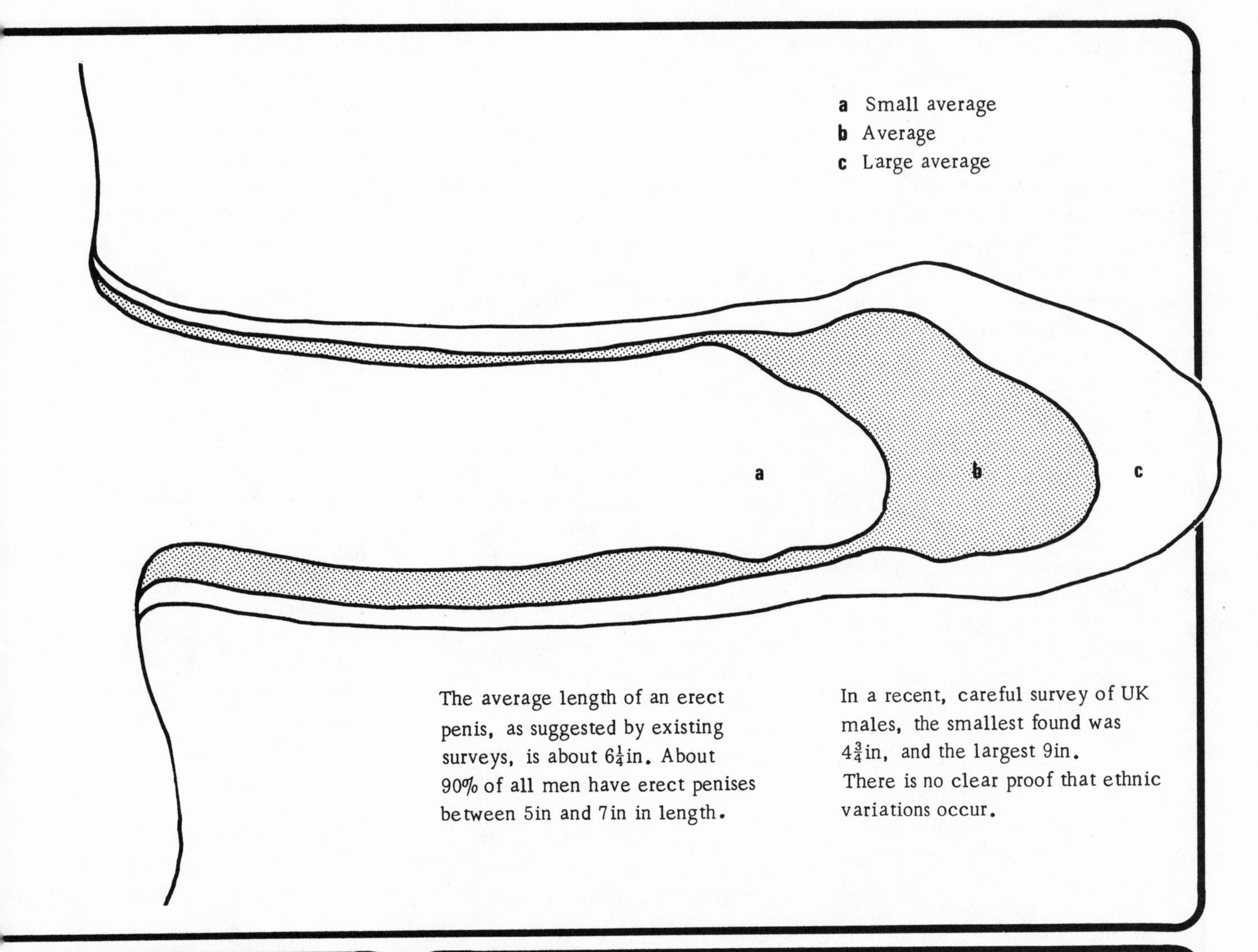

The average length of an erect penis, as suggested by existing surveys, is about $6\frac{1}{4}$in. About 90% of all men have erect penises between 5in and 7in in length.

In a recent, careful survey of UK males, the smallest found was $4\frac{3}{4}$in, and the largest 9in. There is no clear proof that ethnic variations occur.

J10 ANGLE OF ERECTION

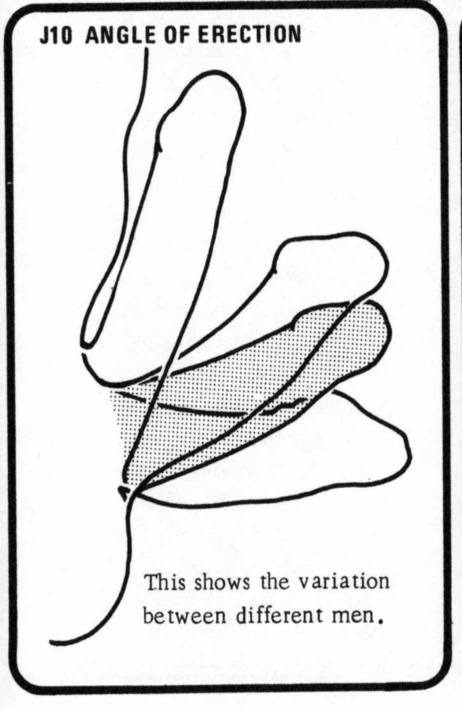

This shows the variation between different men.

J11 APPEARANCE

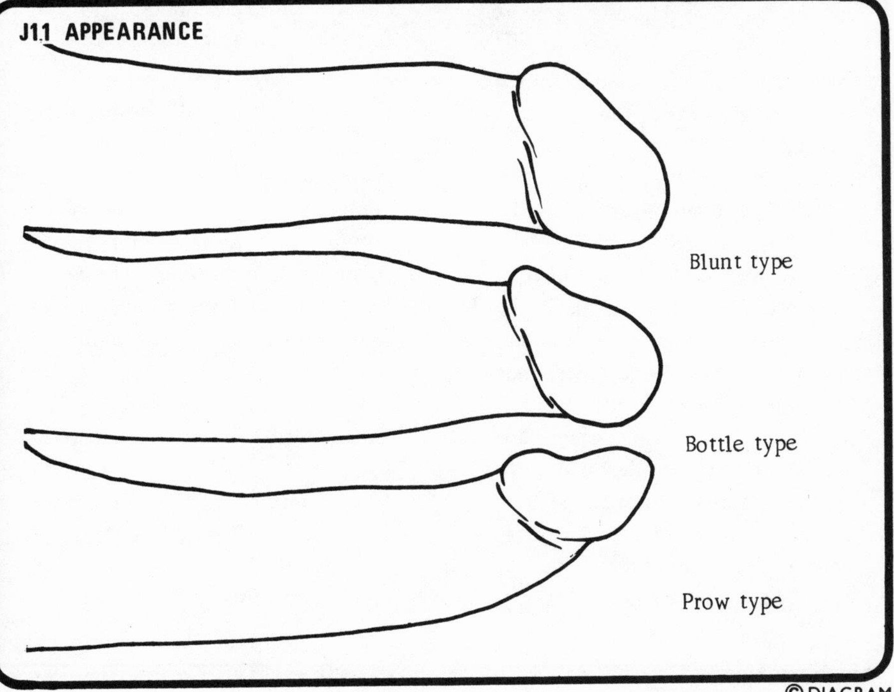

J

J12 POTENCY

The characteristics of potency are sperm production, erection, and ejaculation.

SPERM PRODUCTION

Sperm cells are formed in tiny tubes inside the testes, at the rate, in maturity, of 10 to 30 billion a month. Each is about one 500th of an inch long, and each takes about 60 to 72 days to develop. They are stored during this time in the two epididymides (tubes which would be 20ft long if uncoiled), and remain there until ejaculated from the body by sexual orgasm - or until they disintegrate, being reabsorbed into the testes.

Sperm production can only occur at a temperature 3 or 4°F below normal body temperature. That is why the testes are suspended below the body in the scrotum. High temperatures not only prevent new sperms being formed, but also kill those in storage. The effects may be temporary (infertility) or - in extreme cases - permanent (sterility). Very low temperatures also halt sperm formation, but do not kill those in storage.

Otherwise sperm production is continuous, though there is some evidence of seasonal variations (the sperm concentration in semen seems to be lower in the warmer months).

ERECTION

Erection has been recorded at all ages - from baby boys a few minutes after birth, to old men in their late 80s. But the ability usually develops with puberty, and may be lost as old age approaches. Erection can occur gradually, or in as fast a time as 3 seconds, and can also be lost rapidly or slowly. The length of time for which erection can be maintained varies considerably, and depends on circumstances, but tends to decline with age.

EJACULATION

On orgasm, a man ejaculates on average about 3.5 millileter of semen - a small teaspoonful. But the amount varies greatly, even for a given person. 3.5ml is typical after three or more days without ejaculation; but the normal variation in the same circumstances is from 0.2 to 6.6ml. Also, the volume diminishes with repeated ejaculation, while it can reach 13ml after prolonged abstinence. Whatever the volume, it is almost entirely fluid rather than sperm. Of an average volume, 60% is fluid from the seminal vesicles, and 38% fluid from the prostate (the latter gives semen its characteristic smell). The remaining 2% includes other small fluid contributions, and the sperm themselves. All this is over 90% water. Nevertheless, the sperm count in a typical ejaculation totals between 150 and 400 million. Each sperm has lived between one and 21 days since it reached maturity, and most of them 7 to 14 days.

These different elements of semen appear in a fairly set order. Ejaculation is preceded by fluid from the Cowper's gland: 1 or 2 drops of clear, colorless liquid, which neutralizes any acidity in the urethra left by urine. (This fluid can also be released after the plateau level has continued for some time, even if no orgasm occurs. It is not semen, but does contain a very large number of sperm cells. Hencc pregnancy may follow intercourse even if no semen has been ejaculated.)

This is followed, on ejaculation, by:

first, a thin milky fluid from the prostate, which usually contains few sperms;

second, the fluid containing sperms;

third, the sticky yellow fluid from the seminal vesicles.

The overall appearance of semen is milky, opalescent, and opaque. The opalescence increases with the concentration of sperms.

A forceful ejaculation, after prolonged sexual abstinence, may shoot semen, if there is nothing in the way, 3ft or more; but 7 to 10in is the average distance.

REPEATED EJACULATION

The ability to have repeated orgasms with ejaculation in a short time varies enormously, and begins to decline almost immediately once puberty is complete. Kinsey records one man who had had 4 to 5 orgasms a day, with ejaculation, for 30 years; and another man who had one ejaculation in all that period.

Within a space of one or two hours, most men can manage one ejaculation, some a second, a few three or four. Kinsey records one achievement of about 6 to 8 ejaculations in a single session; but regular multiple ejaculation is typical of only a small number of men.

IMPOTENCE

Being impotent can mean two things: being unable to get an erection, or being unable to reach orgasm even if there is an erection. They can be dealt with together because they have similar causes. Over 90% of impotence is caused psychologically: see K23. The few physical causes of long-term impotence can be categorized into: physical defects from birth; defects of physical development; and changes in the adult body state. Defects from birth concern, of course, the formation of the genitals. Defects of physical development concern the absence of puberty, due to hormonal failure. Neither of these can happen to someone who has had normal sexual functioning.

Long term impotence from physical causes can in his case only arise from changes in the adult body state, including possibly:

a) some diseases of the genitals;
b) some hormonal disorders;
c) some general disorders, such as diabetes, debilitating illnesses, and infectious damage to the spinal cord;
d) some surgery (eg for cancer of prostate or colon);
e) continual heavy drug or alcohol use; and
f) ageing.

However, none of these is certain to cause impotence.

Physical causes of short-term impotence can include almost anything that lowers the body's vitality: immediate factors like great fatigue or heavy doses of alcohol or drugs, and more mild ones like poor health, poor nutrition, and perhaps even lack of exercise.

(These things are also likely to affect sperm production. But poor sperm production does not itself cause impotence. A man can produce few sperm, but still ejaculate normally.)

There are great variations in normal potency, and almost all men experience some failure of potency at some time in their lives.

J13 SPERM DEVELOPMENT

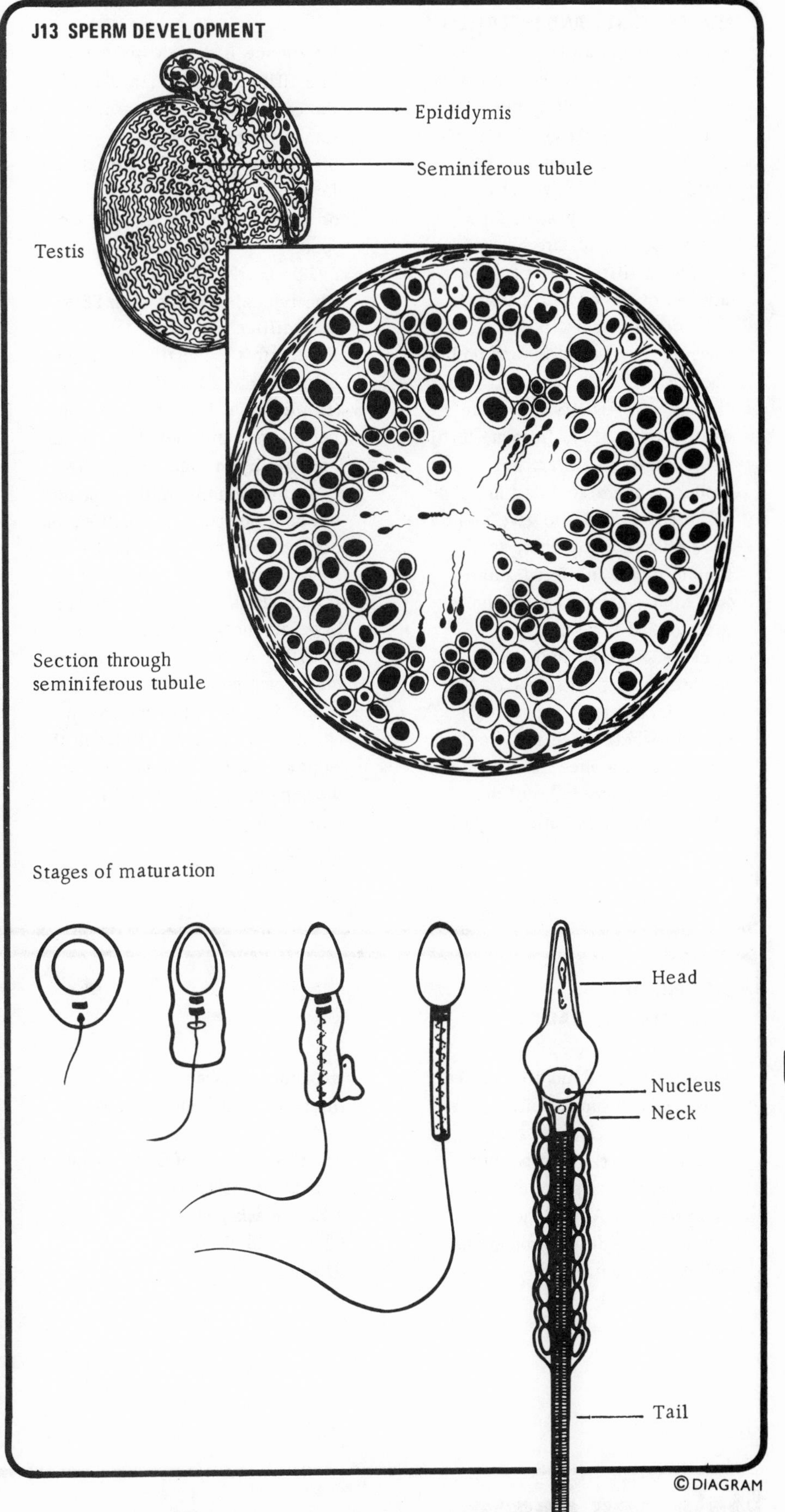

J14 FERTILITY AND INFERTILITY

Fertility is the ability to produce a child, infertility the temporary inability (and sterility the permanent inability). Out of every 100 couples, 10 cannot have children, and 15 have fewer children than they wish. So a quarter of couples are below normal fertility. The causes can involve either or both partners: the woman in 50 to 55% of cases, the man in 30 to 35%, and both in about 15%.

Causes of infertility in women are dealt with in M23. In men, fertility is lacking if sperm are not produced and ejaculated in sufficient numbers to give them a good chance of reaching the female ovum and fertilizing it (see M05). Infertility in men is therefore of two kinds:

a) cases where normal sexual performance is missing i.e. there is no ejaculation (impotence);

b) cases where there is normal sexual performance, but the nature of the ejaculate does not make conception likely (infertility of the semen).

Impotence is dealt with in J12.

Infertility of the semen is likely if the concentration of sperm in the semen is very low;

or if the sperm are abnormal in form;

or if the sperm stop moving too soon.

SPERM CONCENTRATION

The typical range is from 28 to 225 million per milliliter. The lower limit for fertility is often estimated at 60 million per ml. (However, as low as 20 million per ml may give fertility, if they are healthy in other ways.) The concentration obviously depends not only on sperm production, but also on the amount of fluid - as shown by the total amount of semen. Both very small and very large amounts are unfavorable to fertility. A small amount suggests that sperm production is also low. It also fails to buffer the sperm against the acidity of fluids in the vagina. A large amount dilutes the semen too much, and makes it more likely to spill out of the vagina.

SPERM SHAPE

Sperm appear in several forms: the normal oval shape; tapering shapes; round shapes; double headed shapes; double tailed shapes; giant headed shapes; pinhead shapes; and various other, amorphous shapes. In average semen, there are almost 90% normal sperms, but this can go as high as 99% and as low as 66%. The higher the number of abnormal forms, the less the likelihood of fertility. For example, fertility is probably impossible if the tapering shapes rise above 8 or 10%.

SPERM MOVEMENT

In newly ejaculated semen, the sperm are fairly motionless. (They may reach the uterus within 30 seconds, but that is due to the force of ejaculation and to female muscular spasm.) As time passes, most of them become mobile, travelling at about 3 millimeters a minute. In normal semen, at least 75% of the sperm show this degree of movement, while the remainder are either dead or relatively motionless.

J15 FINDING A FERTILITY SPECIALIST

After trying for 6 months to a year to conceive unsuccessfully, a couple should select a fertility specialist who can best perform the necessary tests and discover any problems. Any of the following foundations and groups will be able to provide recommendations in cities throughout the United States:

American College of Obstetricians and Gynecologists
1 East Wacker Drive
Chicago, Ill. 60601
312-222-1600

The American Fertility Foundation
1608 13th Avenue South
Suite 101
Birmingham, Ala. 35256
205-933-7222

American Medical Association
535 North Dearborn Avenue
Chicago, Ill. 60610
312-751-6000

How movement continues depends on where the sperm are. If still in the vagina, they stop moving after about an hour. In the uterus or cervix, they typically live for 24 to 48 hours.

The length of life of the sperm (as shown by their movement) is not only important because of the time they may need before encountering an egg to fertilize. For some reason not yet understood, sperm also need to stay for some time in the female reproductive tract, before they are capable of fertilizing an egg.

CAUSES OF INFERTILITY

From the concentration, shape, and mobility of sperm, it is possible to make a general estimate of the likely fertility of a man's sperm production. Causes of poor sperm production can include:

a) heat around the testicles, due, for example, to tight underclothing, obesity, or working conditions;
b) factors of general vitality, such as poor health, inadequate nutrition, lack of exercise, excessive smoking and drinking, etc;
c) emotional stress; and
d) too prolonged abstinence (this can increase the number of abnormal sperm).

More specialized factors (some of which can cause sterility) include:

a) some birth defects;
b) failure of the testes to descend before puberty;
c) some childhood illnesses, and some other illnesses (eg mumps if it occurs in adulthood;
d) some hazards such as exposure to X rays, radioactivity, some chemicals and metals, gasoline fumes, and carbon monoxide; and
e) some genital disorders*, such as varicocele and blocked ducts, and tuberculous infection of prostate.

Antibody reactions can cause infertility. A woman can have an antibody reaction to a man's sperm, or the man can have an adverse reaction to his own sperm. In one of the tests for such allergies, called the Kibrick Test, recently ejaculated semen is mixed with blood samples from the man and woman. If the sperm clump together, there is proof of an immunological problem. Sometimes the test is performed more than once.

AIDS TO FERTILITY?

Many of the causes of infertility are treatable. But, more generally, we do not yet know of any substances that will improve fertility. Severe lack of vitamins will impair fertility; but no special vitamin intake seems to raise the fertility level of a well-fed person. As for hormones, the pituitary hormones have only limited effect, while testosterone actually hinders sperm production - it is only useful where infertility is due to genital underdevelopment or impotence. However there are techniques to aid fertility. One is the medical technique of artificial insemination. Another is a practical sexual technique. It seems that the second half of a man's ejaculation - the fluid from the seminal vesicles - is actually likely to harm the sperm, while that of the prostate, in the first half, protects it. So a couple can increase their chances of parenthood if the man withdraws from the vagina halfway through his ejaculation.

Barren Foundation
6 East Monroe Street
Chicago, Ill. 60603
312-346-4038

New York Fertility Research Foundation, Inc.
1430 Second Avenue
New York, N.Y. 10021
212-744-5500

Planned Parenthood
810 Seventh Avenue
New York, N.Y. 10019
212-541-7800

Resolve
P.O. Box 474
Belmont, Mass. 02178
617-484-2424

J

J16 DEFECTS AT BIRTH

DISPLACED OUTLET

The outlet of the urethra should be at the tip of the penis. Epispadias is the condition in which the urethra comes out on the upper surface of the penis, instead of at the tip. Hypospadias is the condition in which it comes out on the under surface. Both cause difficulties. During urination, the man may have to sit, or tilt his penis. During intercourse, he may be effectively infertile, because too little semen finds its way to the uterus. Both conditions can be dealt with by surgery. If the foreskin is still present, it can be used to form a new passage for the urethra; if not, skin grafts are needed.

UNDESCENDED TESTES

The testes normally move down from the fetus' abdominal cavity to his scrotum during the eighth month of pregnancy. If they are still in the abdominal cavity at birth, the condition is called cryptorchidism. It can be corrected surgically. If this is not done before puberty, sterility results.

INTERSEX

Otherwise normal people can be born with genitals that are intermediate between those of the two sexes: for example, an unusually short penis, perhaps surrounded with folds of skin, and a half or fully formed vagina. In such cases, the dominant hormonal activity that begins at puberty may well be different from that of the sex they have been brought up as.

BLOCKED DUCTS

These can be birth defects, but are usually due to infection: see J19.

J18 DEFECTS OF DEVELOPMENT

GENETIC ABNORMALITIES

Some people, from the moment of their conception, do not have the normal sex chromosomes of either a male (XY) or a female (XX). This occurs because of errors in cell division or fertilization, and the consequences generally appear at puberty. Among such people, those that appear to be male fall into two groups. The first group have an extra Y chromosome (XYY): they have normal male functioning, though they often have other, non-sexual difficulties. The second group have one or more extra X chromosomes, sometimes with extra Y ones as well: XXY, XXXY, XXXXY, XXYY, XXXYY. All these are male, but usually their genitals fail to develop at puberty, and they may also show some female secondary sexual characteristics. The first three types listed (with the single Y chromosome) are always sterile. The fertility of XXYY and XXXYY cases is not yet clear.

HORMONAL ABNORMALITIES

People with normal sex chromosomes can nevertheless have hormonal defects. At puberty, normal sexual growth and functioning may be late or never develop, even though the genitals in childhood were the normal shape and size. Hormone treatment may be needed, with occasional pauses to see if the body hormones have started up yet.

J19 SCROTUM

VARICOCELE

This is a condition in which there is a collection of varicose veins around the scrotum. The blood carried in the dilated veins makes the testes warmer than they should be, and infertility can result. Regular bathing of the testes in cold water may be enough to counteract the temperature change. Also weight reduction will help prevent the veins getting worse, if obesity has been one cause of the condition. If the problem continues, surgical removal or tying of the swollen veins may be needed. This does not interfere with the general blood supply to the testes.

SCROTAL FLUID

Hydrocele is accumulation of fluid in the layers of cells around the testes. It can cause overheating

J17 SITES OF DISORDERS

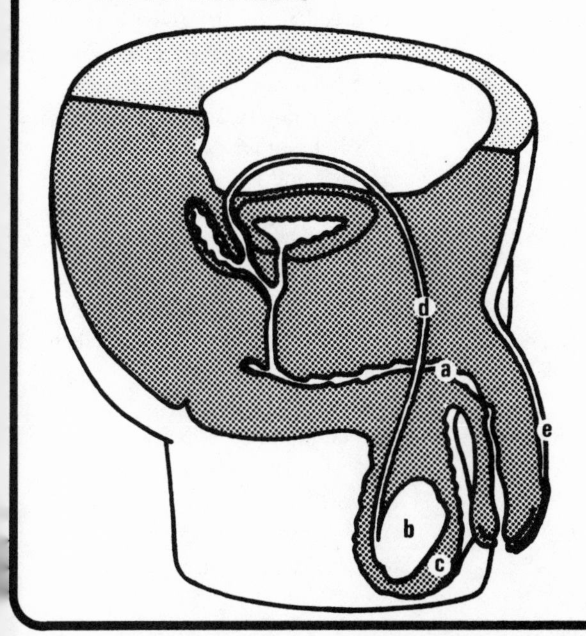

a Urethra
b Testes
c Scrotum
d Vas deferens
e Penis

and infertility, and may require surgical drainage. Hematocele is a similar condition resulting from injury; blood is mixed in the fluid. Spermatocele is accumulation of seminal fluid.

SCROTAL SWELLINGS

These can be caused not only by fluid accumulation, but also by cysts, tumors, inflammations, and hernias in the area, or by an attack of mumps.

BLOCKED DUCTS

Blockage can occur in the vas deferens tubes, that carry sperm from testes to urethra. Infertility results. Infection, such as venereal disease, is the usual cause. Corrective surgery bypasses the blockage, joining the unaffected part of the tube directly to the end of the urethra.

J20 PENIS

PAINS

Pains in the penis can be caused by trouble either there or elsewhere, due to inflammations, stones, or growths.

SKIN DISORDERS

Growths on the penis surface can include warts, ulcers, sores connected with sexual infections, and cold sores. None are especially hard to treat.

Cancer of the penis may appear as irritation and discharge from beneath the foreskin, or simply as a pimple on the penis surface that does not heal. In most western countries it accounts for only 2% of all male cancers, and usually responds well to radium treatment.

PRIAPISM

This is non-sexual erection of the penis; it may be painful also. It is commonest in the elderly, when causes can include prostate enlargement, inflammation, piles, etc. In children, it may be due to penis inflammation, circumcision, over-tight foreskin, or worms; in adults, to drug abuse, gonorrhea, epilepsy, leukemia, back injury, or just convalescence from an acute illness.

Continual priapism can be due to severe spinal injury, or to a clot in the prostatic veins.

CROOKED ERECTION

This can be due to short term inflammation of the urethra, especially from gonorrhea. Otherwise, usually in older men, it is linked with the spontaneous formation of scar tissue along one side of the penis. In this case, it gradually stops being painful, and the condition itself may eventually disappear without treatment.

SEXUAL INTERCOURSE 1

K01 ACTIONS BEFORE INTERCOURSE

The following types of activity can occur.

a) Kissing of the partner's mouth progresses from gentle kissing of the lips to a probing action of the tongue deep into the partner's mouth. The teeth may also be used in nibbling or biting actions on the partner's lips and tongue.

b) Touching/stroking/fondling/grasping of parts of the partner's body. Often this occurs in a sequence that begins with parts of the body that are not specifically sexual, and ends with those that are: eg, first hair, then body, arms, breasts, abdomen and buttocks, legs, and lastly genitals.

c) Kissing/biting/tongue exploration of any or all of these parts of the partner's body. Especially notable here is male mouth contact with the female breasts, and with the nipples in particular.

d) Specific manipulation of the partner's genitals. This includes the following male actions:
caressing of the labia*, which are the lips at the entrance to the female vagina*;
separation of the labia to expose the clitoris, which is very sensitive and plays an important part in the sexual arousal and enjoyment of the female;
insertion of one or more fingers into the vagina itself;
movement of the fingers in and out of the vagina, in the manner of the penis in intercourse.
Apart from giving pleasure, and sexually exciting the female, these actions help prepare the female genitals for intercourse.

e) Pressing and rubbing of the genital areas against the partner's genitals and against other parts of the partner's body.

f) Mouth contact with the partner's genitals, using tongue and lips (see "Oral sexuality", K25).

The order of the list given here also forms a typical sequence of events. But almost any pattern is possible: real situations are in any case often complicated by clothing, and its removal!

The early stages of love-making may take place in standing, sitting, or half-reclining positions. But by the later stages the couple will usually have taken up the position in which intercourse is to occur.

All techniques used can vary in application from very gentle to very forceful. Hasty intercourse may omit any or all of these preliminary activities.

K02 READINESS FOR INTERCOURSE

Sexual intercourse begins when the male penis is inserted into the vagina of the female.

This requires: a stiff (erect) penis; and a vagina that is sufficiently moist and relaxed to allow the penis to enter.

THE PENIS

Usually the penis becomes erect early in love-making, or before love-making begins. But some bodily states - such as general fatigue, or too recent orgasm - will interfere with t is. Erection may then develop only slowly, or not at all.

Where there is only partial stiffness, it may be possible to give the penis enough support by hand to allow entry.

THE VAGINA

The female genitals are described in M01 to M02.

A woman's desire for sex and the excitement of love-making cause her vagina to prepare itself for intercourse.

Quantities of moisture appear on the interior surfaces of the vagina, having "sweated" through the skin. This moisture runs down toward the vaginal entrance.

(It used to be thought that glands in the labia produced much genital moisture, but it is now known that this is not so.)

At the same time the muscles controlling the vagina automatically relax. This will allow it to expand when the penis is inserted.

During love-making, caressing of the female genitals by hand takes these processes further. It normally raises the level of excitement, but also:
the action of the fingers helps spread the moisture over the labia;
and the insertion of one or more fingers into the vagina stimulates the vagina to relax further.

Sometimes a couple will use an artificial lubricant. This gives the vagina additional moisture, if the natural moisture is lacking for some reason.

K03 ENTRANCE

The couple take up one of the positions that allow sexual intercourse to take place. The penis tip points at the entrance to the vagina.
Then the man may only need to push forward from his hips: his penis slides immediately into the woman's vagina. (Alternatively, in some positions, the woman lowers her vagina onto the man's penis.)
But very often the following techniques are used:
a) either partner holds the penis, to help direct it into the vaginal entrance;
b) either partner holds the woman's labia apart to help the penis slide between them;
c) the penis is inserted only very gradually, beginning with the tip and progressing at first with several small forward movements and half retreats. This spreads the vaginal lubrication over the penis surface, and helps the vagina to accommodate itself gradually to the penis's size. (Also it is used as a tantalizing technique, to heighten the sensation of entrance.)
DELAYING ENTRANCE
Once physiological readiness has been reached, the penis can be inserted into the vagina. But a couple may choose to delay this for many minutes. During this time they continue love-making without intercourse. In fact, during love-making, the highest levels of sexual excitement before intercourse are usually not reached until the body has been physiologically ready for some time. This is true of men and (especially) women.

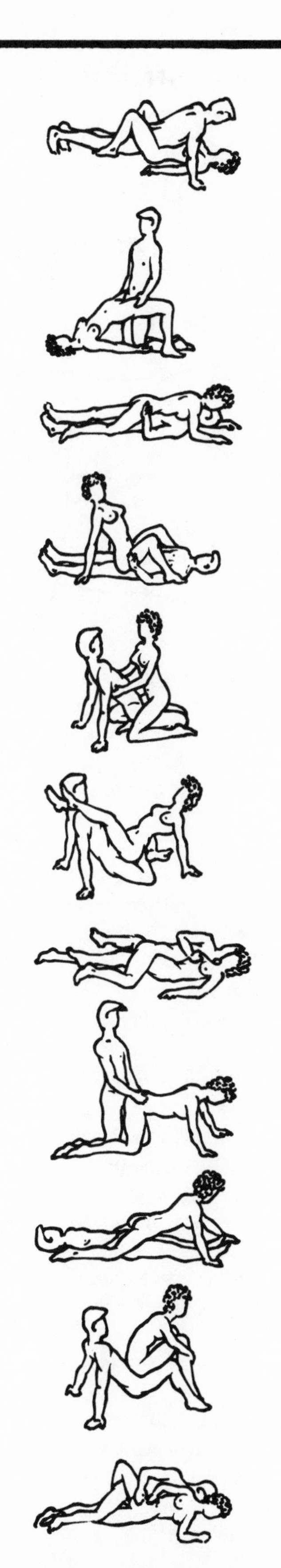

K04 DIFFICULTY OF INSERTION

This depends on:
a) the relative sizes of penis and vagina;
b) the stiffness of the penis and the degree of relaxation and lubrication of the vagina.
The second set of factors is much more important. A vagina, however small, can normally accommodate a penis of any size providing that the vagina has become sufficiently relaxed.
So problems of insertion usually arise because sexual arousal in the woman has not gone far enough.
THE HYMEN
A woman who has not had intercourse before will usually have a hymen*: an unbroken ring of flesh tissue just inside the vaginal opening. This may need to be stretched or broken, to allow entrance. If so, it is encountered by the penis as an obstruction, beyond the labia.
Hymens vary greatly in strength and and stretchability. If a hymen has to be broken, a more forceful pressure of the penis may be needed (or the fingers can be used). (In extreme cases, a minor surgical operation may be necessary.)
But, today, hymens have often been stretched by physical exercise, use of tampons, and the "petting" of boyfriends i.e. insertion of fingers into the vagina. Often, in this case, a woman's first experience of intercourse will just take further the slow process of stretching and breaking down the tissue of the hymen. The normal techniques of insertion are all that is needed.
This is especially true if entrance is not attempted until the woman is highly aroused and her vagina fully relaxed.

SEXUAL INTERCOURSE 2

K05 DURING INTERCOURSE

In sexual intercourse, the man's penis moves repeatedly into the woman's vagina and out again. This is done by rhythmic hip movements: so the genital areas move apart and then together again. Both of the partners may move their hips, or one of them may move while the other stays still. (This partly depends on what position they are in.)
Sometimes the range of movement is small, so the penis stays within the vagina; sometimes large, so the penis leaves the vagina completely, and then is thrust back deep inside it. In a single intercourse, a couple may use many kinds of movement: large and small, gentle and forceful, fast and slow. Either or both partners may take the initiative, and changes of movement may be gradual or unexpected. The couple may also choose to stop and then begin again several times.
At the same time, they usually continue many of the actions of love-making that preceded intercourse: kissing, fondling, etc.
How a man's genitals react to intercourse - or to any other stimulation - is described in J06.
How a woman's genitals react is described in M03.
Intercourse may be very brief or very protracted: a matter of seconds or hours. This depends partly on circumstances and the couple's wishes - but also on how the man's genitals react. Some men usually (and many men sometimes) reach orgasm almost immediately, and then are too tired, or satisfied, or uninterested, to continue. In other cases, a man may hold off his orgasm indefinitely; or regain enough energy and erection to continue after it; or (in some cases) to be able to reach a second and even subsequent orgasms.

K06 POSITION OF INTERCOURSE

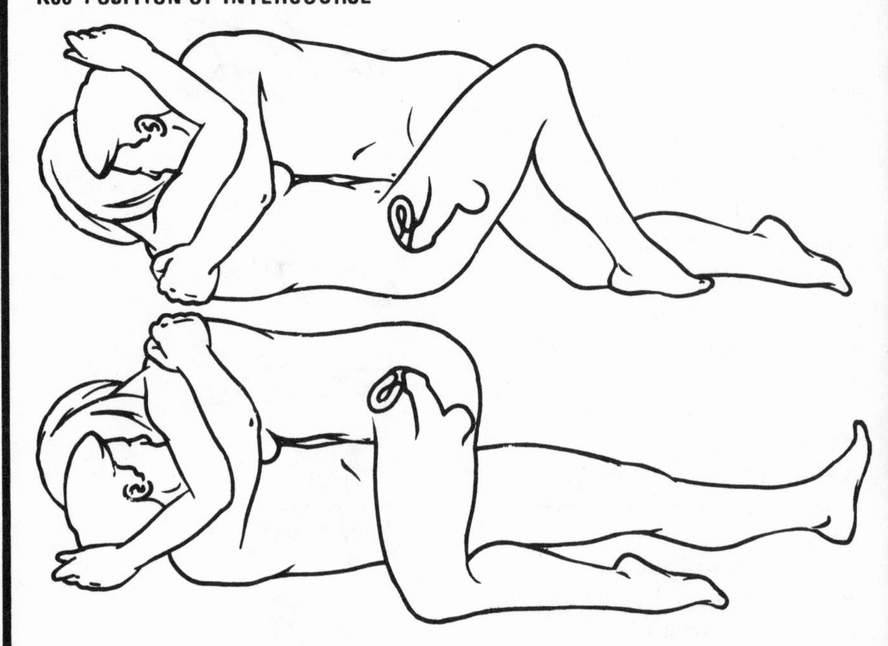

By far the most common position in our society is that in the top drawing above. This contrasts with ancient civilizations, where the woman was normally on top of the man.
Some of the range of possibilities is shown in K08. Variety is mainly of psychological significance, but there are practical differences, including whether:
a) each partner can move;
b) one has to bear the other's weight;
c) the hands have free access to the partner's body;
d) the partner's body can be seen;
e) deep penetration is possible; and
f) satisfactory genital stimulation occurs.
Also positions fall into groups, with easy movement between those in the same group.
Distribution of movement and weight are significant if one partner is weak or tired, or intercourse is prolonged. Also one partner may find it hard to reach orgasm unless in control of movements. (In particular, a woman may find orgasm easier in a woman-above position.)
Penetration can usually be deeper the greater the angle between the woman's body and her legs. In side positions, it is deepest where the angle between the partner's bodies is greatest i.e. they form a cross shape. In rear entry, deep penetration is difficult if either partner is overweight.
Stimulation does not necessarily relate to depth of penetration. There may be more pressure (between penis or pubic bone and clitoris) where penetration is more angled but less deep. However, direct contact between penis and clitoris usually decreases the woman's pleasure (see M04). Full penetration in a frontal position does give suitable indirect stimulation, because of pressure between the partners' pubic bones.

K07 PATTERNS OF INTERCOURSE

MUTUAL ORGASM (a) Both partners reach orgasm, perhaps simultaneously. Awareness of the partner's impending orgasm may trigger off one's own. However, simultaneous orgasm is not common, and concentration on it as a goal can reduce both partners' pleasure.

BRIEF INTERCOURSE (b) The man begins after few preliminaries, and reaches orgasm very quickly, usually leaving the woman dissatisfied (see M04). Unfortunately, ability for very rapid orgasm is typical of male mammals. Kinsey found that $\frac{3}{4}$ of all men can reach orgasm within 2 minutes after intercourse begins, and some within 10 to 20 seconds.

WITHDRAWAL (c) The man withdraws just before ejaculation (usually for contraceptive* reasons). The woman may already have reached orgasm, or may find that withdrawal leaves her dissatisfied.

PROLONGED INTERCOURSE (d) The woman has one or more orgasms before the man does. This usually results from conscious control by the man. In particular, he may lie still for a while, just after entrance, when his excitement is at a peak. Some couples find it better if their orgasms do not coincide. Most women like pelvic movement to go on during their orgasms, while most men want to stop or slow down during theirs.

REPEATED MALE ORGASM (e) With some men the "refractory period" after orgasm may be so brief that erection occurs again, and intercourse continues, without the penis leaving the vagina. Alternatively, manual or oral contact by the woman may help. However, the number of men who can have two orgasms within a short time is not very high (see J12).

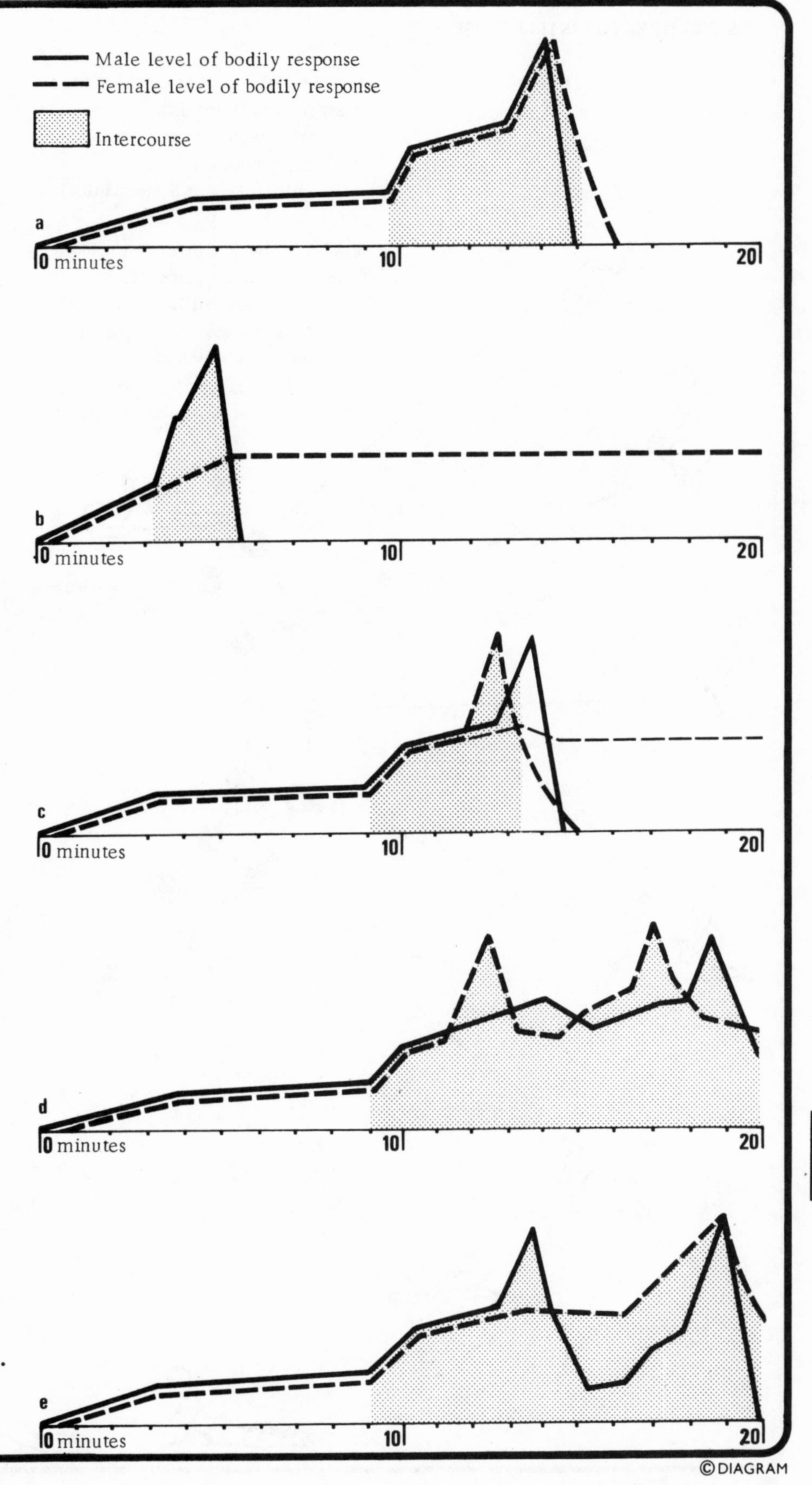

K

POSITIONS FOR INTERCOURSE 1

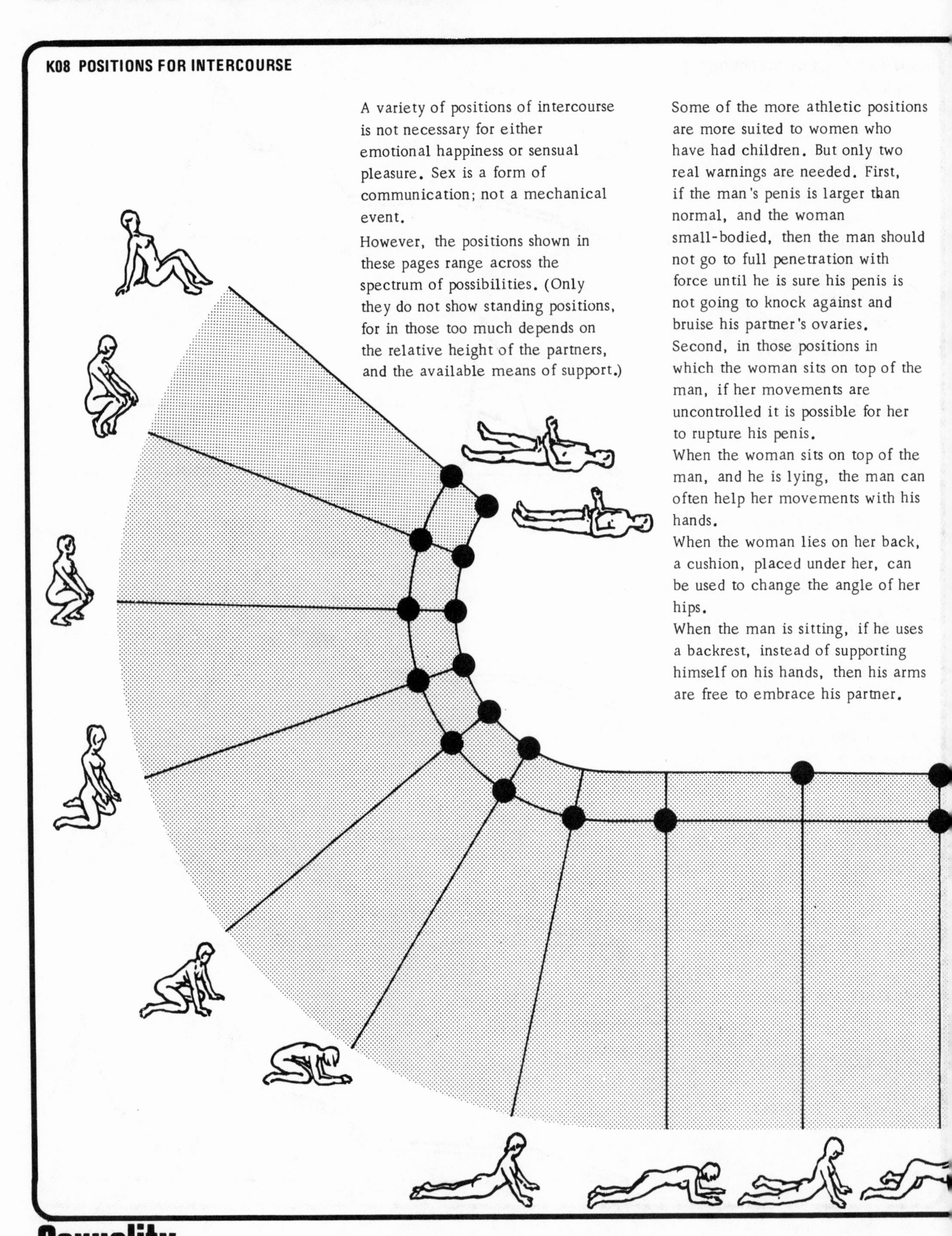

A variety of positions of intercourse is not necessary for either emotional happiness or sensual pleasure. Sex is a form of communication; not a mechanical event.

However, the positions shown in these pages range across the spectrum of possibilities. (Only they do not show standing positions, for in those too much depends on the relative height of the partners, and the available means of support.)

Some of the more athletic positions are more suited to women who have had children. But only two real warnings are needed. First, if the man's penis is larger than normal, and the woman small-bodied, then the man should not go to full penetration with force until he is sure his penis is not going to knock against and bruise his partner's ovaries. Second, in those positions in which the woman sits on top of the man, if her movements are uncontrolled it is possible for her to rupture his penis.

When the woman sits on top of the man, and he is lying, the man can often help her movements with his hands.

When the woman lies on her back, a cushion, placed under her, can be used to change the angle of her hips.

When the man is sitting, if he uses a backrest, instead of supporting himself on his hands, then his arms are free to embrace his partner.

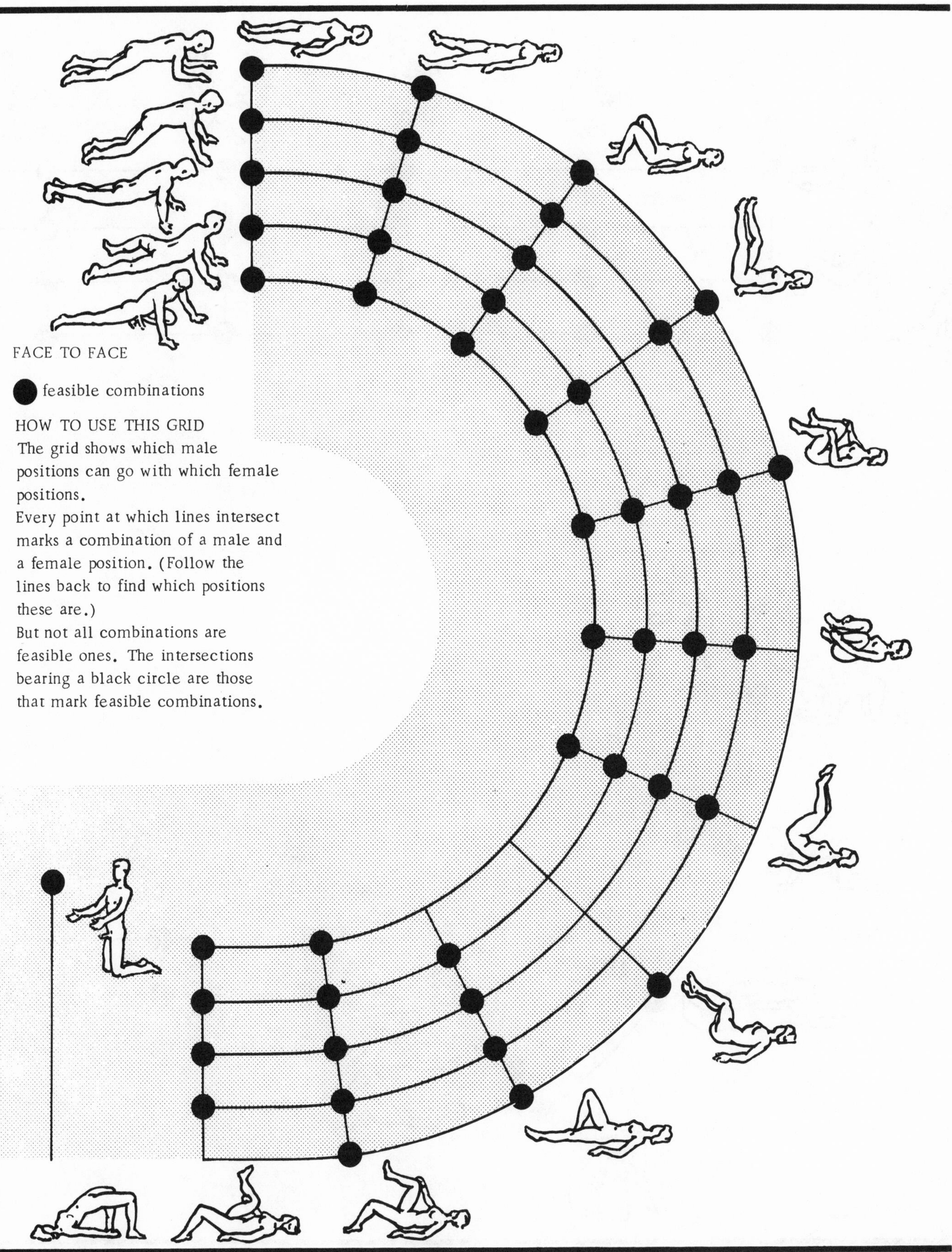

FACE TO FACE

● feasible combinations

HOW TO USE THIS GRID
The grid shows which male positions can go with which female positions.
Every point at which lines intersect marks a combination of a male and a female position. (Follow the lines back to find which positions these are.)
But not all combinations are feasible ones. The intersections bearing a black circle are those that mark feasible combinations.

POSITIONS FOR INTERCOURSE 2

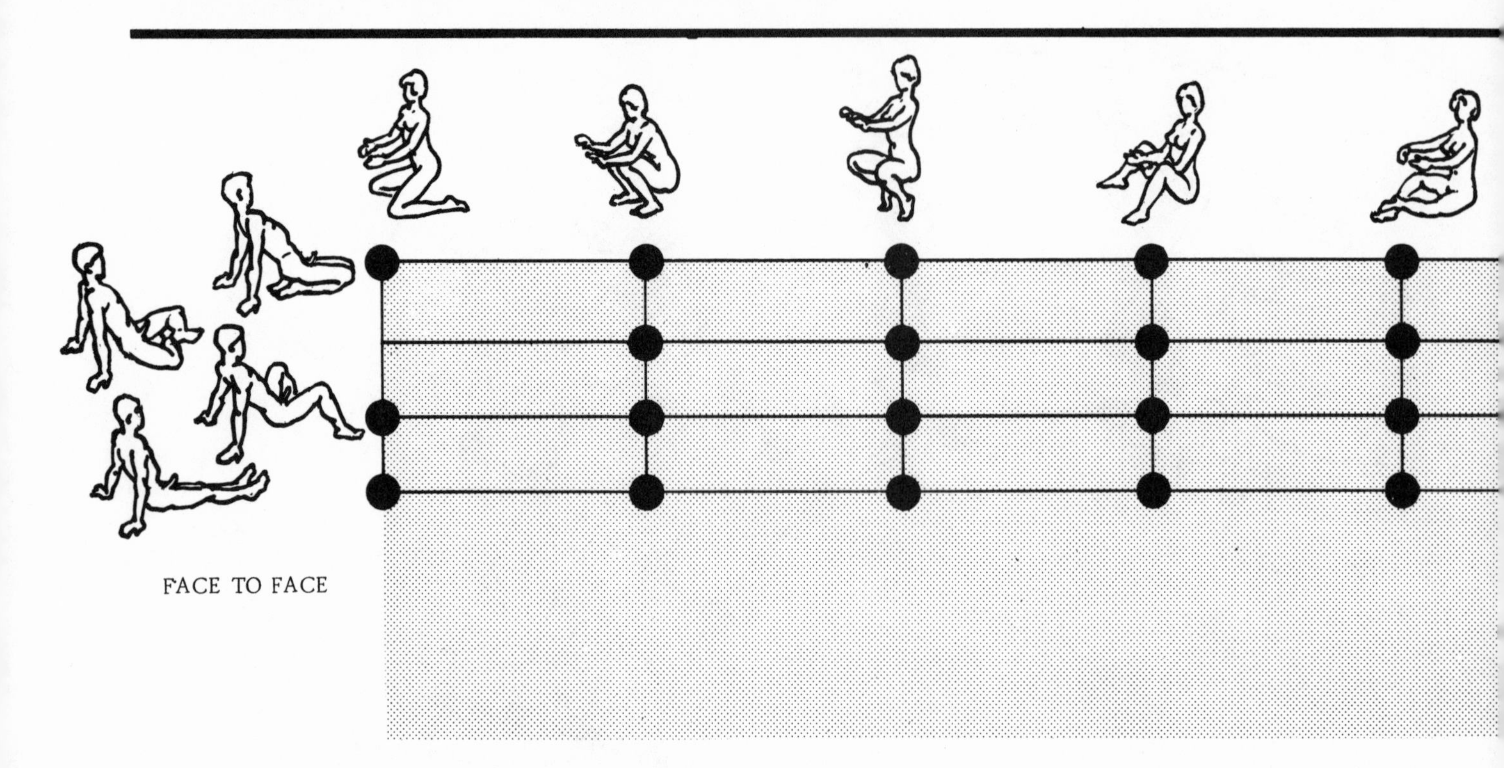

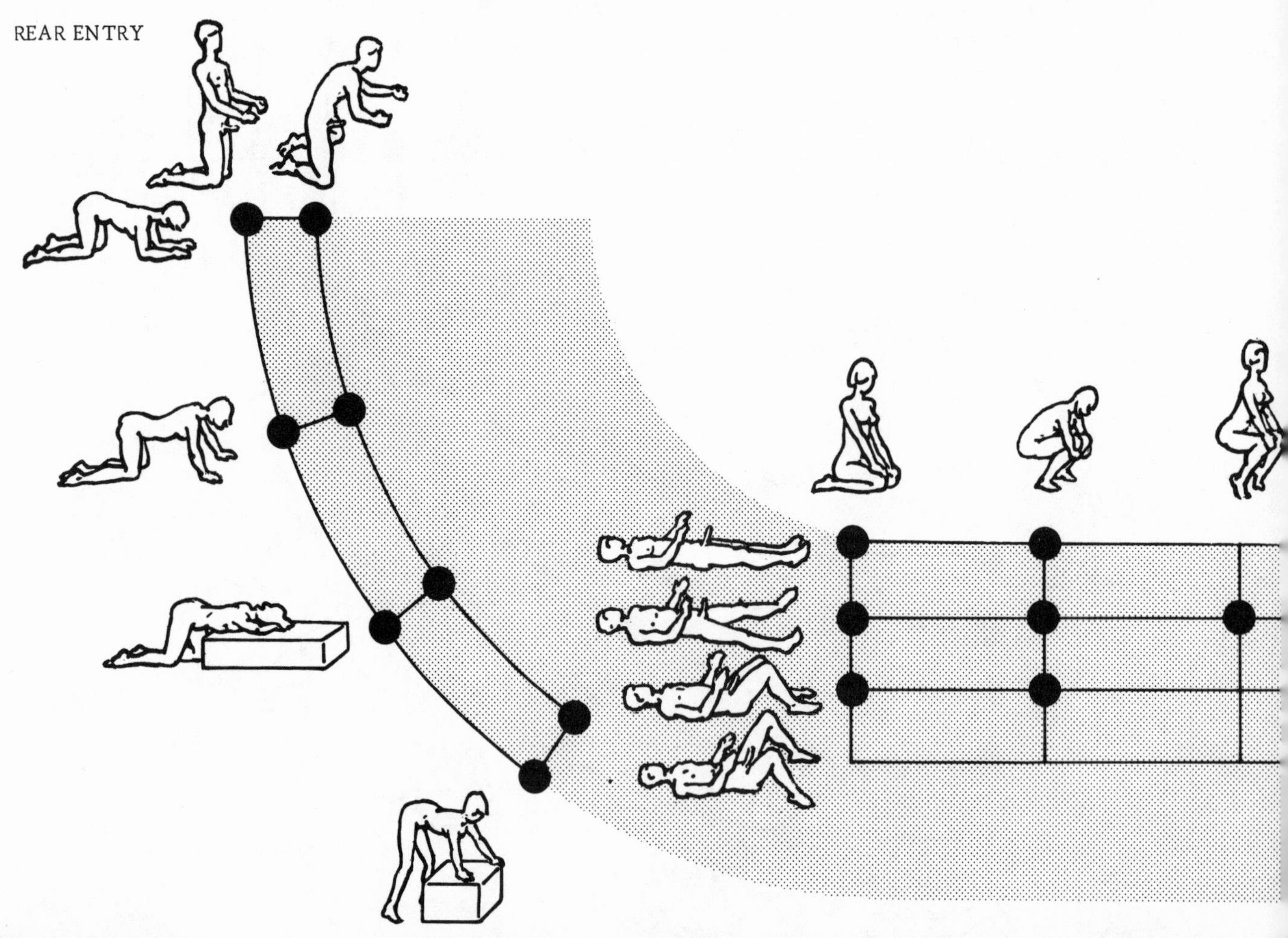

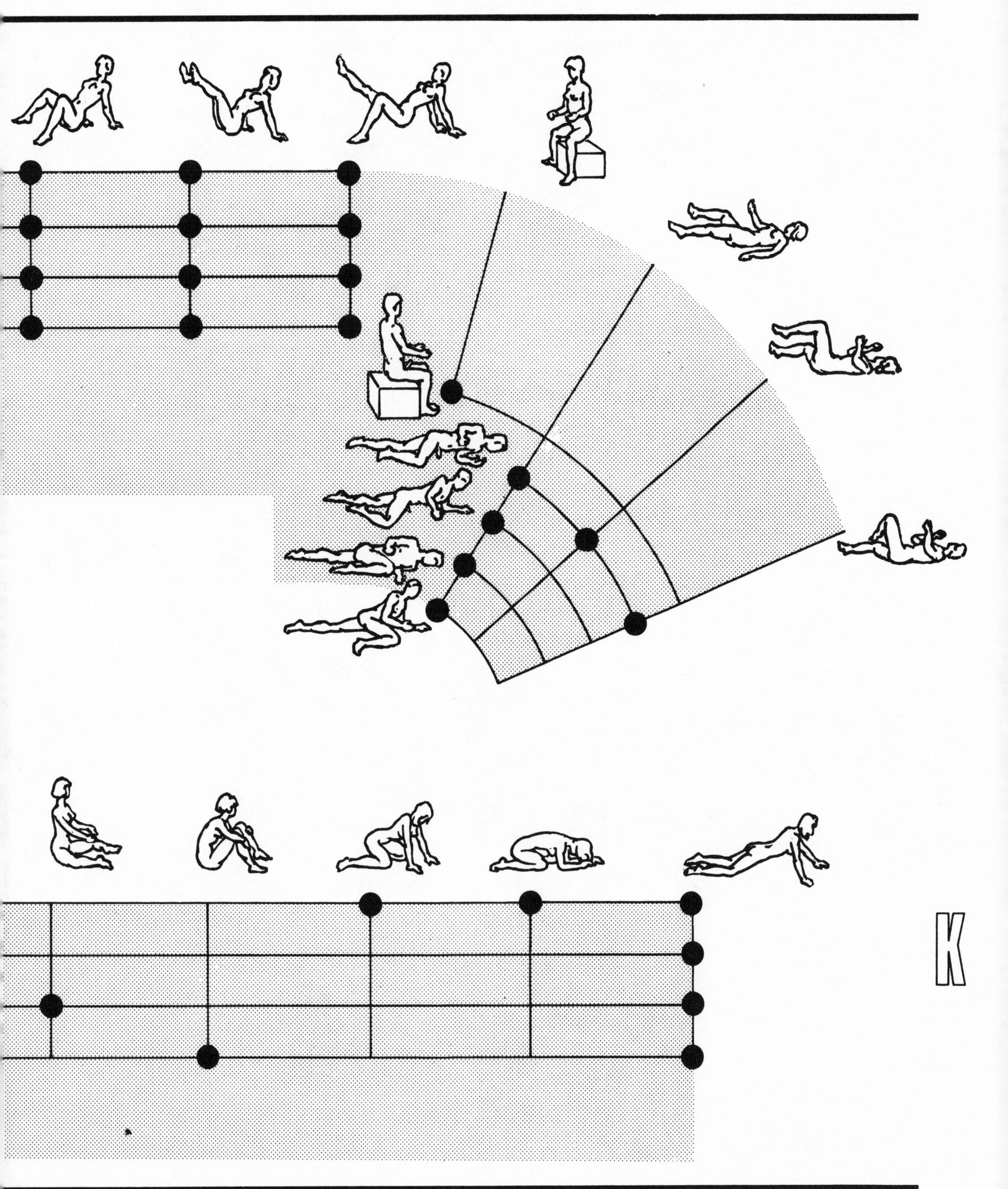

POSITIONS FOR INTERCOURSE 3

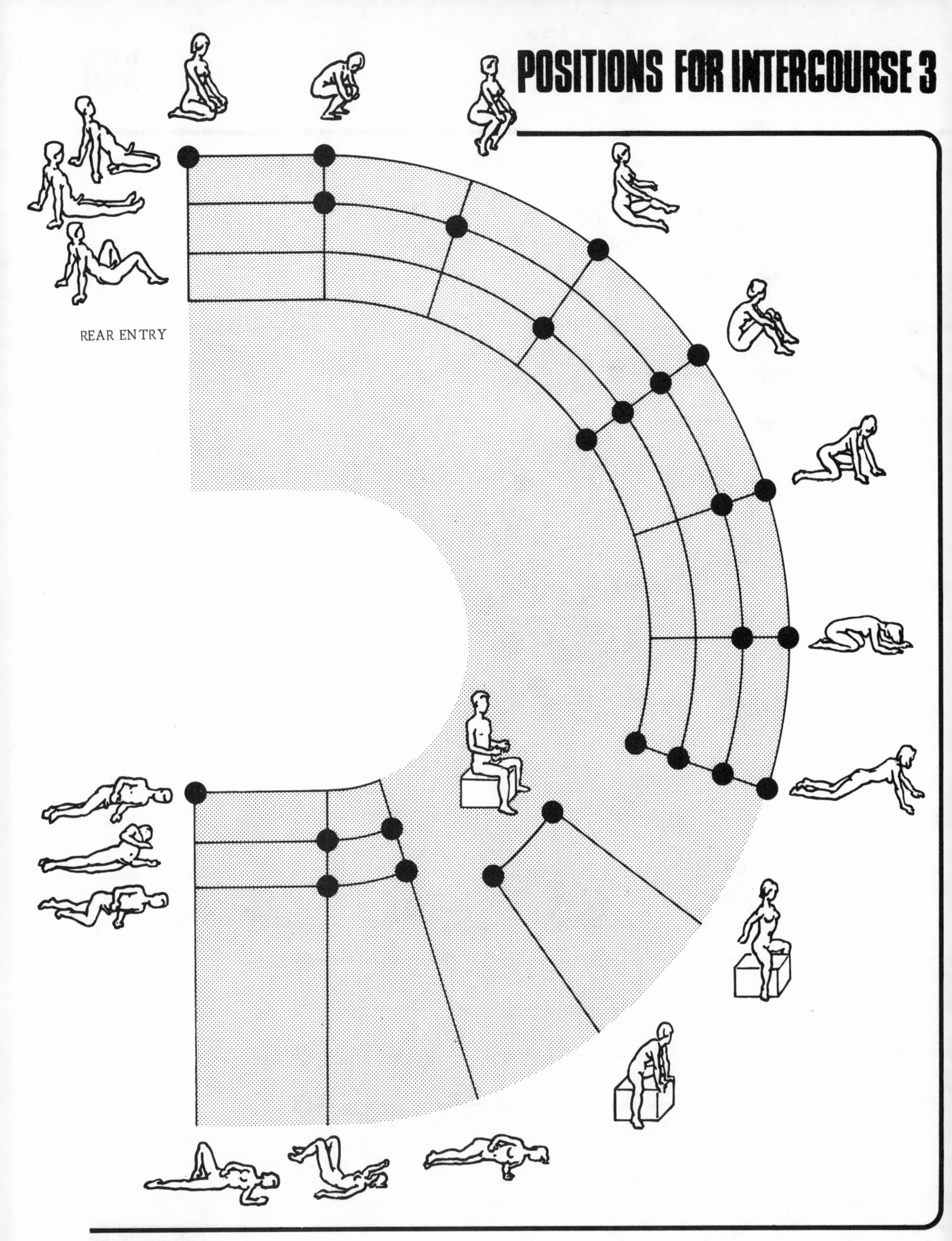

K09 EJACULATION AND CONCEPTION

Here we show the genital coupling, and the route of the semen. Ejaculation occurs in two stages. Rhythmic muscular contractions begin in testes and epididymides (a), and continue along the vas deferens (b), also involving seminal vessicles and prostate (c). Sperm and seminal fluid collect in the urethra inside the prostate. Then a sphincter relaxes, letting this semen pass down toward the penis. Contractions along the length of the urethra (d) cause ejaculation. Inside the woman's body semen passes from vagina into uterus and fallopian tubes. For conception, sperm must find their way into a fallopian tube containing a ripe ovum (see M05).

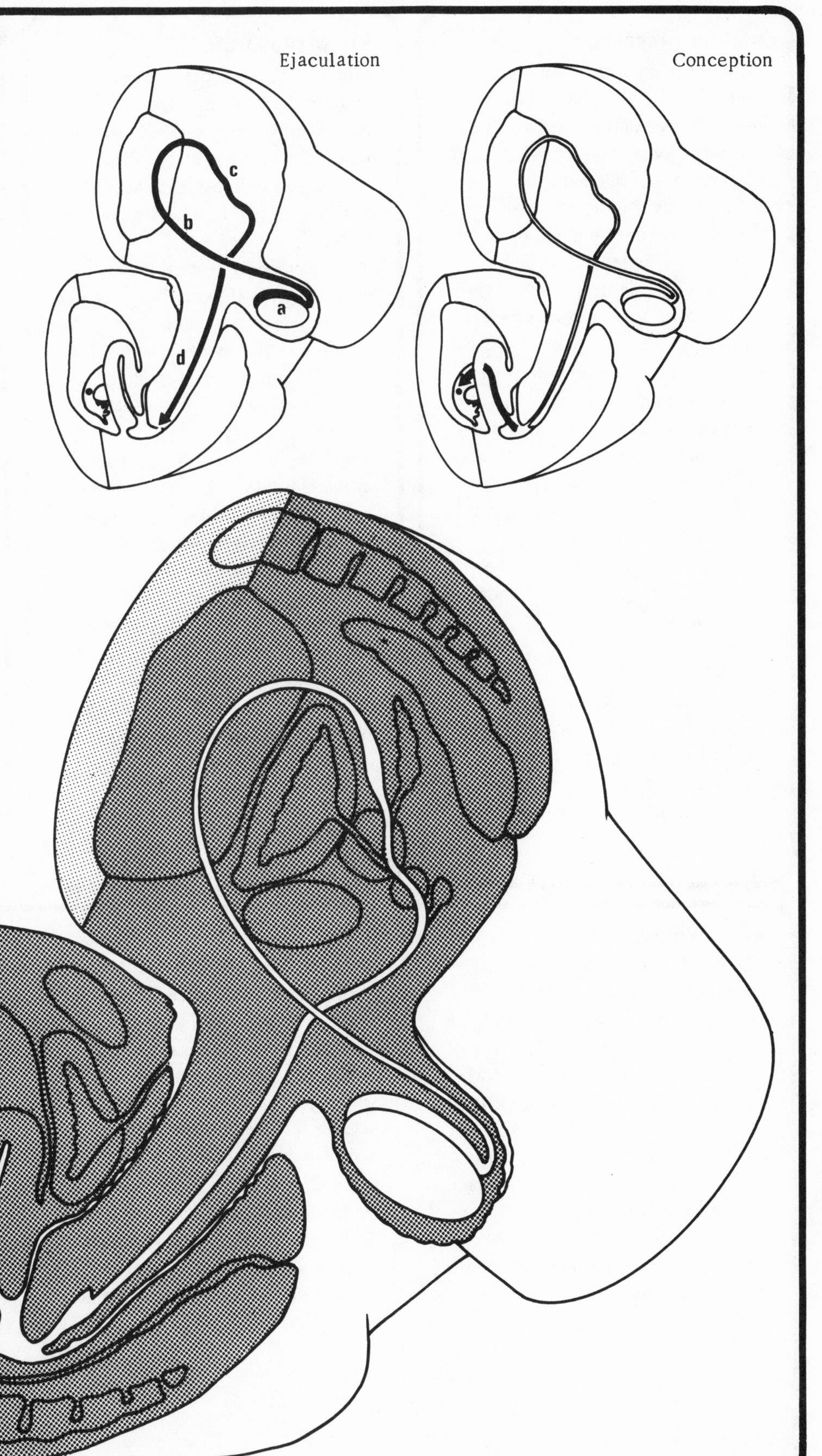

CONTRACEPTION 1

K10 CONTRACEPTION

Contraception tries to ensure that heterosexual intercourse does not result in pregnancy. Contraceptive techniques vary greatly in effectiveness. But there is no one method that is best, for choice also depends on the needs of a particular couple.

For a child to be conceived from intercourse, several things have to happen:

a) semen from the man must enter the woman's vagina;

b) the semen must contain healthy male sperms;

c) the sperms must find conditions in the vagina in which they can live;

d) the living sperms must make their way into the woman's uterus and fallopian tubes;

e) they must find an egg there that is ready for fertilization; and

f) the egg, once fertilized, must be able to make its way into the uterus and implant itself there.

By preventing any one of these, contraception is achieved.

K11 WITHDRAWAL

Withdrawal (or "coitus interruptus") is the oldest and simplest of contraceptive techniques. The man takes his penis out of the woman's vagina just before his orgasm. His semen is ejaculated outside her body.

This only works as certain contraception if every bit of semen is kept out of the vagina (and, in practice, even away from the lips of the vagina). For even the smallest amount of semen can cause pregnancy.

There are two main difficulties:

a) some fluid containing live sperm may "weep" from the penis before orgasm, especially when sexual need is intense or sexual excitement prolonged; and

b) in the pleasure of orgasm a man may not be able to bring himself to withdraw properly - especially since some couples find prolonged use of the withdrawal technique frustrating.

K12 SPERMICIDES

These are chemical products which are inserted in the woman's vagina before sexual intercourse. They work as contraceptives in two ways: they kill the sperm; and they coat the entry to the uterus with foam or fluid through which the sperm cannot pass. There are five types: creams, jellies, aerosol foams, suppositories, and tablets.

The foams, creams, and jellies are sold with a special applicator with which the spermicide can be deposited high in the upper part of the vagina. They are used up to an hour before each intercourse the nearer to intercourse, the better.

Suppositories and tablets are in solid form, and must be inserted deep into the vagina by hand. Suppositories are cone-shaped, and melt at body temperature to release their spermicide, while tablets dissolve and foam in the vagina's moisture. They are also used up to an hour before each intercourse - but not less than a few minutes before, since they

K14 CONDOMS

The condom works by preventing semen entering the woman's vagina. It is a sheath or tube about 7 or 8 inches long, usually made of of thin rubber or similar material, open at one end and closed at the other. It stretches to fit closely over the man's erect penis, and when the man ejaculates his semen is trapped in the sealed end of the sheath. Most condoms are used once only, but some are designed to be washed and reused.

The condom is the most widely used male contraceptive. Choices range from plain rubber to lubricated animal-skin sheaths. It can be bought easily and without prescription, and its effectiveness can be increased by using a spermicide as well (see above). Used consistently, from the beginning of each intercourse, it works very well - providing that it does not tear or (more likely) slip off after orgasm, releasing semen into the vagina. The other difficulty is psychological: both man and woman may find that use of the condom lowers their sense of pleasure. They may be tempted to "take the risk" sometimes. Incidentally, the condom was invented as a protection against venereal disease, not as a contraceptive, and it is still one of the few ways of reducing the risk of such infection.

need time to melt or dissolve.
The main difficulty with all these methods is that the chemical may not form a complete barrier to sperms. In particular, the thrust of the penis may drive a path through. So they are best used together with another contraceptive technique. They greatly increase the effectiveness of diaphragm or condom (or, for that matter, withdrawal.) Used alone, only the aerosol foams can be rated as even reasonably effective.
Apart from this, their main disadvantage is that a couple may find it hard to remember, or to bother, to turn to chemicals before intercourse. Also some women, and occasionally some men, may find that the chemicals irritate their genitals.
The spermicide action of all these products is, of course, only temporary. It cannot cause sterility. Incidentally, the foams, jellies, and creams also act as some additional lubrication during intercourse.

K13 DIAPHRAGM

Various devices can be placed in the vagina to cover the entrance to the uterus, and so prevent sperms passing. Examples include sponges that can hold spermicide, and small plastic caps that fit tightly over the cervix. But by far the most common is the large rubber cap called the "diaphragm".
A diaphragm is folded for insertion into the vagina, and placed in position by hand (or with a plastic inserter), so that its bottom edge rests against the rear of the vagina, and its upper edge against the vaginal wall behind the bladder.
When released, the diaphragm regains its circular shape, under the tension of a circle of flexible metal concealed in its rim. The vagina stretches to accommodate it, and so the diaphragm is held in place, covering the cervix.
Diaphragms are available in various sizes. The size number represents the diameter, in millimeters. The size needed must be decided by a physician's examination. He will also supply instructions for its use.
Re-examination for size is needed every two years, and after each pregnancy. A gain or loss of more than 15 lb. may necessitate a new diaphragm. A diaphragm should be checked periodically for holes.
A diaphragm is not felt, when in place. It can be put in position several hours before intercourse, and left in position for up to 24 hours or more. It should be left in at least 6 hours after each intercourse. When removed, it is washed, dried, and placed in a case until needed again.
The effectiveness of a diaphragm is quite high, providing it is used with a spemicide. Spermicide cream or jelly is placed in the cup and on the rim before insertion. In the vagina, the spermicide spreads itself over the cervix.
Tubes of spermicide cream or jelly can be purchased at a pharmacy for under $10.00.

Diaphragm in position

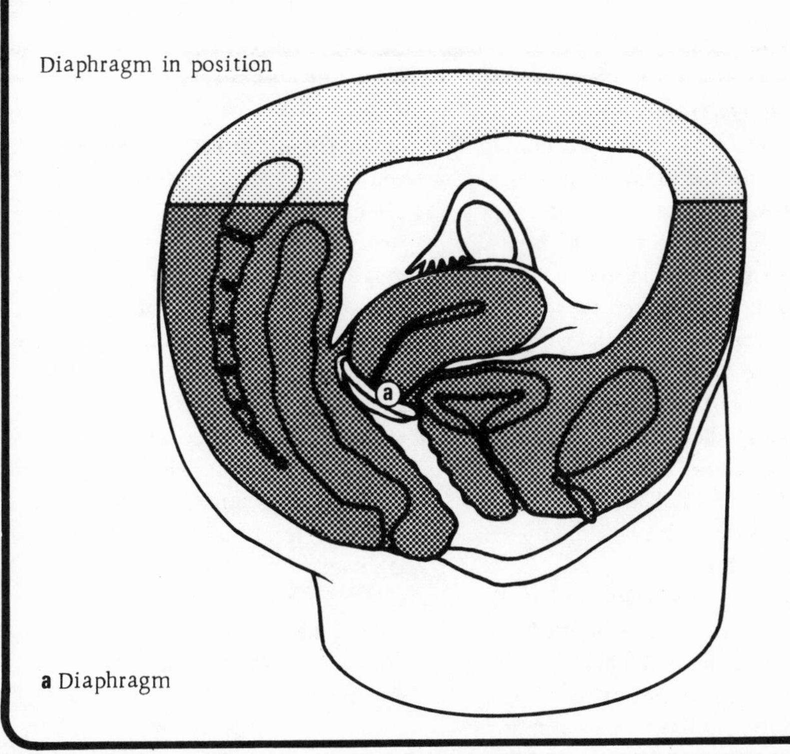

a Diaphragm

K15 VAGINAL DOUCHE

This method is so ineffective that it does not really count as contraception. A rubber bulb or syringe is used to spray large amounts of water into the vagina, immediately after intercourse.
The intention is to wash out the pool of semen, and sometimes a spermicide or other substance is added to the water. But, whatever is used, douching cannot wash out the uterus - and many sperms may be safe inside the uterus within 30 seconds of ejaculation.

K

K16 INTRAUTERINE DEVICE (IUD)

This is a small plastic or metal object, placed in the uterus on a long-term basis. So long as it stays there it prevents pregnancy, and intercourse can occur without any restriction. Fertility returns 1 month to 1 year after the device is removed.

It is not known for certain why an IUD works as a contraceptive. Possibilities include:

a) it makes the egg pass down the fallopian tube very rapidly, so that the egg cannot be fertilized or else arrives in the uterus too early for implantation;

b) it prevents the normal cyclical growth of the uterus lining, and so implantation cannot occur;

c) it does not affect transport, fertilization, or uterus lining, but interferes directly with the implantation process.

But, despite uncertainty about the process involved, several shapes and types of device have been tested and proved effective.

The most common are known as "loops" and "coils". They all need a trained person (usually a physician) to put them in place. For this, loops and coils are usually placed inside a thin tube. The end of the tube is then inserted into the uterus through the cervix. The IUD is pushed out of the end of the tube, into the uterus, and springs back into its normal shape. Other shapes may need to be put in place under anesthetic. All IUDs can be removed by a physician at any time.

A woman with an IUD should have a follow-up visit and annual checkups. Some IUDs, such as the hormone-releasing and copper types, need to be replaced periodically.

Any IUD is intended to stay in the uterus for years without damage or discomfort, and not to fall out or be expelled by normal muscular contractions. Most have nylon threads or stem projections, that are designed to hang down into the vagina so a woman can feel with a finger whether the IUD is still in place (they also indicate its type, to a trained person unfamiliar with the case). Otherwise, a woman should be unable to detect its presence.

However, an IUD may cause pain, bleeding, or nausea, and/or uterine contractions to expel it (though any significant damage to the uterus from an IUD is rare). In other cases, it may simply fall out. All these may be cured by use of a different design. But only 80% of those fitted with IUDs can use them in the long run.

Moreover, women who have not had children are usually not fitted: their cervix is too narrow and their uterus usually less tolerant to an IUD. (But some new IUD designs are meant for such women.)

When in place, an IUD is highly effective, only the pill being more so. It is also cheap, and requires no effort of memory or of preparation before intercourse.

The IUD is better removed if pregnancy does occur, as it increases the risk of miscarriage.

Potential users should know that the FDA issued a warning in 1974: "... limited data suggest that certain serious hazards to IUD use may exist." Some IUDs have subsequently been recalled.

K17 STERILIZATION

Vasectomy is a surgical operation that sterilizes the man, so the semen he ejaculates no longer contains sperm. The vas deferens* tubes are cut and tied, where they pass through the scrotal sac. After that sperms can no longer get from the testes to the urethra. (The man is not sterile immediately, because of sperm that are already in the seminal vesicles*. It takes about six weeks before he can be sure he cannot father a child.)

The vasectomy operation is short and simple: it can be performed in a few minutes under local anesthetic. It does not affect a man's ability to have an orgasm or ejaculate just as before; and as a contraceptive is it virtually 100% effective.

However, vasectomy is still usually irreversible - so sterilization must be thought of as permanent. Even if the tubes are successfully joined up again, there is no guarantee that fertility will be regained. Also, even where a couple are sure that no further children are wanted, they may feel psychologically that sterilization is somehow too drastic, or that it will impair sexual pleasure - even though they would usually find afterwards that their fears were groundless.

FEMALE STERILIZATION

This involves cutting or tying the fallopian tubes, or removing all or part of them. The effect is immediate: sperms can no longer reach the eggs, and the eggs can no longer reach the uterus.

The operation involves general anesthetic and a few days in a hospital, followed by a few weeks of limited activity. It usually leaves a small scar 2 to 3 inches long just above the pubic hair (another, quicker technique leaves only two tiny scars).

As contraception, this only fails in rare cases where the tubes later rejoin naturally. Also it does not interfere with the menstrual cycle,

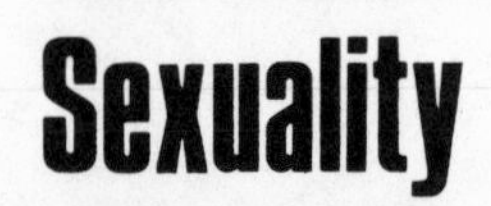

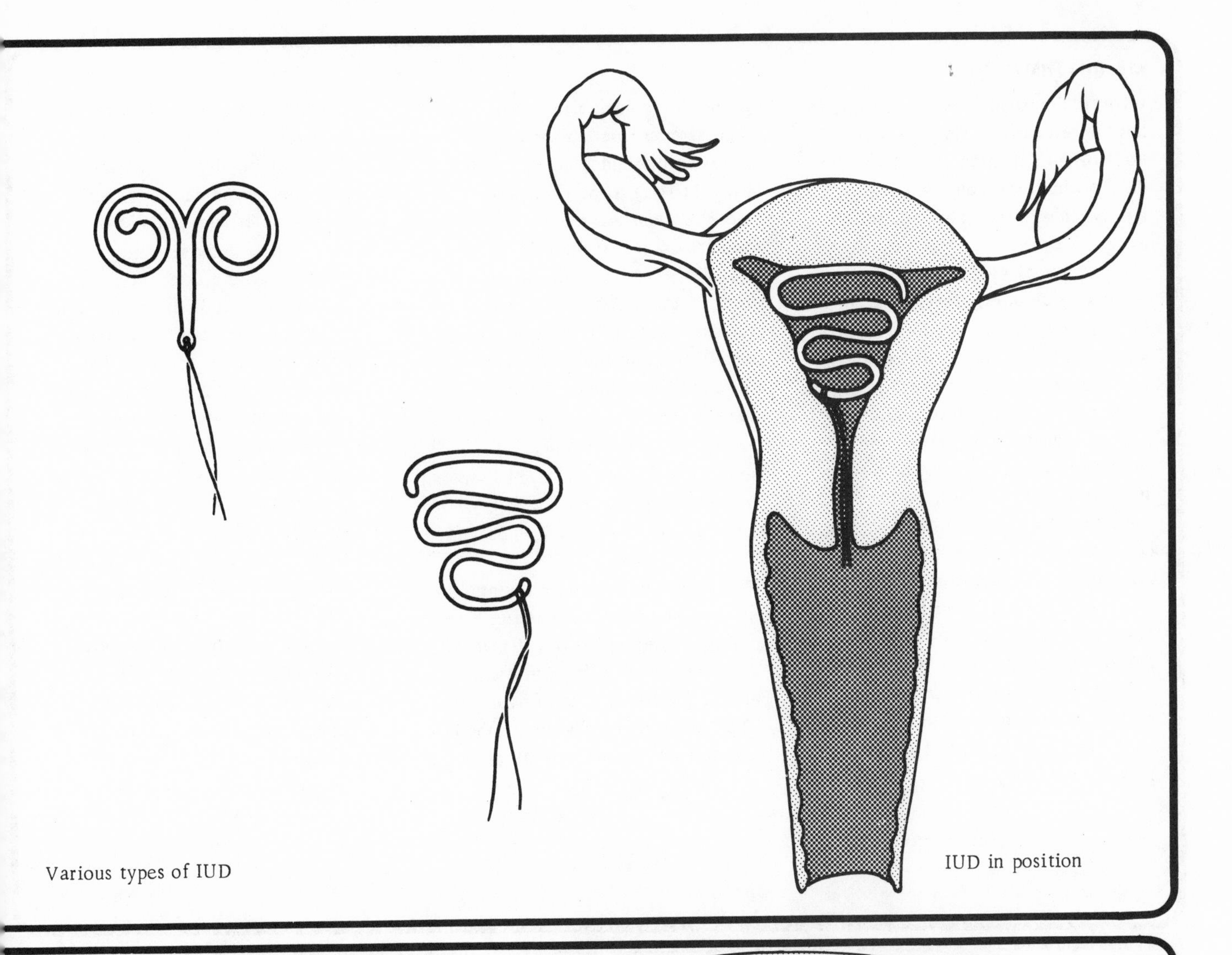

Various types of IUD

IUD in position

intercourse, or sexual enjoyment. But it cannot normally be reversed, which means that the woman can never again have a child. If circumstances change, this may be greatly regretted. It is therefore a very serious step to take.

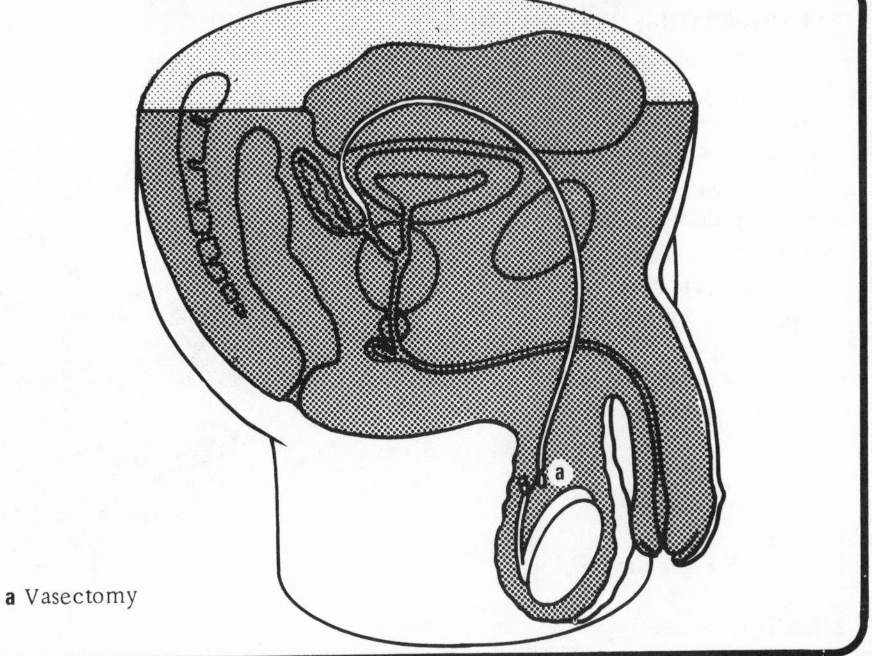

a Vasectomy

CONTRACEPTION 3

K18 RHYTHM METHOD

With this method, a couple do not have intercourse during the part of the woman's menstrual cycle* during which she can conceive i.e. when a fertilizable egg is available.
The menstrual cycle lasts (in principle) 28 days. During this, the egg is available for fertilization for only about 1 day - the 24 hours following ovulation*. However, there is no direct sign of ovulation, only of menstruation. Ovulation typically occurs half-way between menstruations - in fact, on the 15th day. So a woman can count forward 14 days from the start of her last menstruation, to guess when ovulation will occur. But the menstrual cycle is seldom perfectly regular. In most women menstruation is erratic when periods return after the birth of a baby, and in a quarter of women it is always fairly erratic. (Other women may have a record of regular menstruation for years, followed by sudden unexpected irregularity.) Also, even where menstruations are regular, ovulation need not occur at the mid-point, the 15th day. It can occur anywhere from 16 to 12 days before the next menstruation. In fact, ovulation is sometimes induced by the stimulus of sexual intercourse. Finally, sperms can live in the woman's cervix for up to 72 hours and sometimes longer - so even if an intercourse is four days before ovulation it may on rare occasions cause conception.
Therefore the "calendar rhythm method" - just based on dates - is not very effective, even if several days are kept free from intercourse around the likely date of ovulation. The "temperature rhythm method" is better. A woman normally has a sudden rise of several degrees in body temperature during the day of ovulation, due to increased progesterone production. Use of a thermometer and a record chart should show this rise.
By the time the temperature rise is actually recorded, the possible fertilization period is normally over. (Also, the action of the progesterone makes the cervical mucus unfavorable to sperm penetration.) This gives a "safe period" after ovulation, from the temperature rise up to (and including, if desired) the next menstruation. But it gives no safe period after menstruation, since there is no way of telling when the next ovulation will occur. Between menstruation and ovulation, only the calendar method gives any indication of safety.

K19 TEMPERATURE RHYTHM METHOD

The temperature should be taken first thing on waking, before any activity (even getting out of bed). A rectal thermometer is preferable to an oral one.
The circle shows the pattern of temperature during the menstrual cycle. Low temperatures are at the outside, high at the center. There is an abrupt rise at ovulation (about day 14).

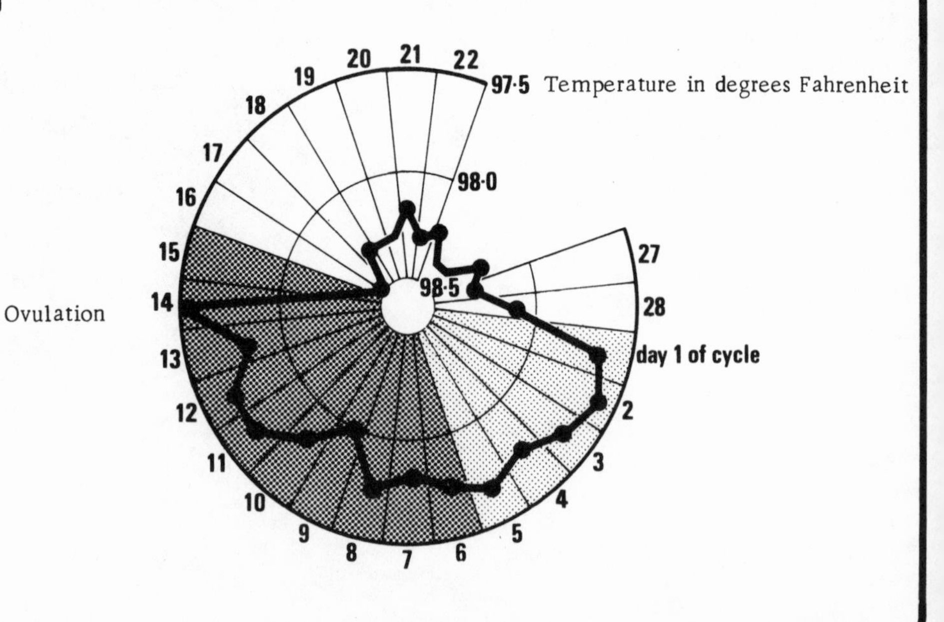

Menstruation

Other safe days

Unsafe days

K20 CALENDAR RHYTHM METHOD

REGULAR MENSTRUATION

Suppose a woman had menstruation regularly every 28 days. Ovulation would be most likely on the 15th day of the cycle, but could happen anytime from the 13th to the 17th - a period of 5 days. Since sperms can live 72 hours and even longer, four days before this are also unsafe. And since the egg may still be fertilizable 24 hours after ovulation, the day after the 5 day period is unsafe too. This gives a total of 10 unsafe days, from the 9th to the 18th days of the cycle inclusive.

Some women have cycles as short as 21 days, others as long as 38 days - but this does not matter if the cycles are still regular. The woman still allows a period of 10 days, beginning 20 days before the next menstruation is expected.

IRREGULAR MENSTRUATION

A woman with irregular menstruation should keep an accurate record of her menstrual cycle for a year beforehand, and note the shortest and longest cycles. She must then calculate as follows:

a) she subtracts 19 from the number of days in her shortest cycle; and

b) she subtracts 10 from the number of days in her longest cycle.

Figure (a) gives the earliest day on which pregnancy can occur, counting from the start of the last menstruation; figure (b) gives the latest.

For example, if the shortest cycle is 25 days, and the longest 29:

a) 25-19=6; and b) 29-10=19

So the unsafe days are from the 6th to the 19th days, inclusive, after the start of the last menstruation. Perhaps 15% of women have menstrual cycles so irregular that the calendar rhythm method cannot be applied.

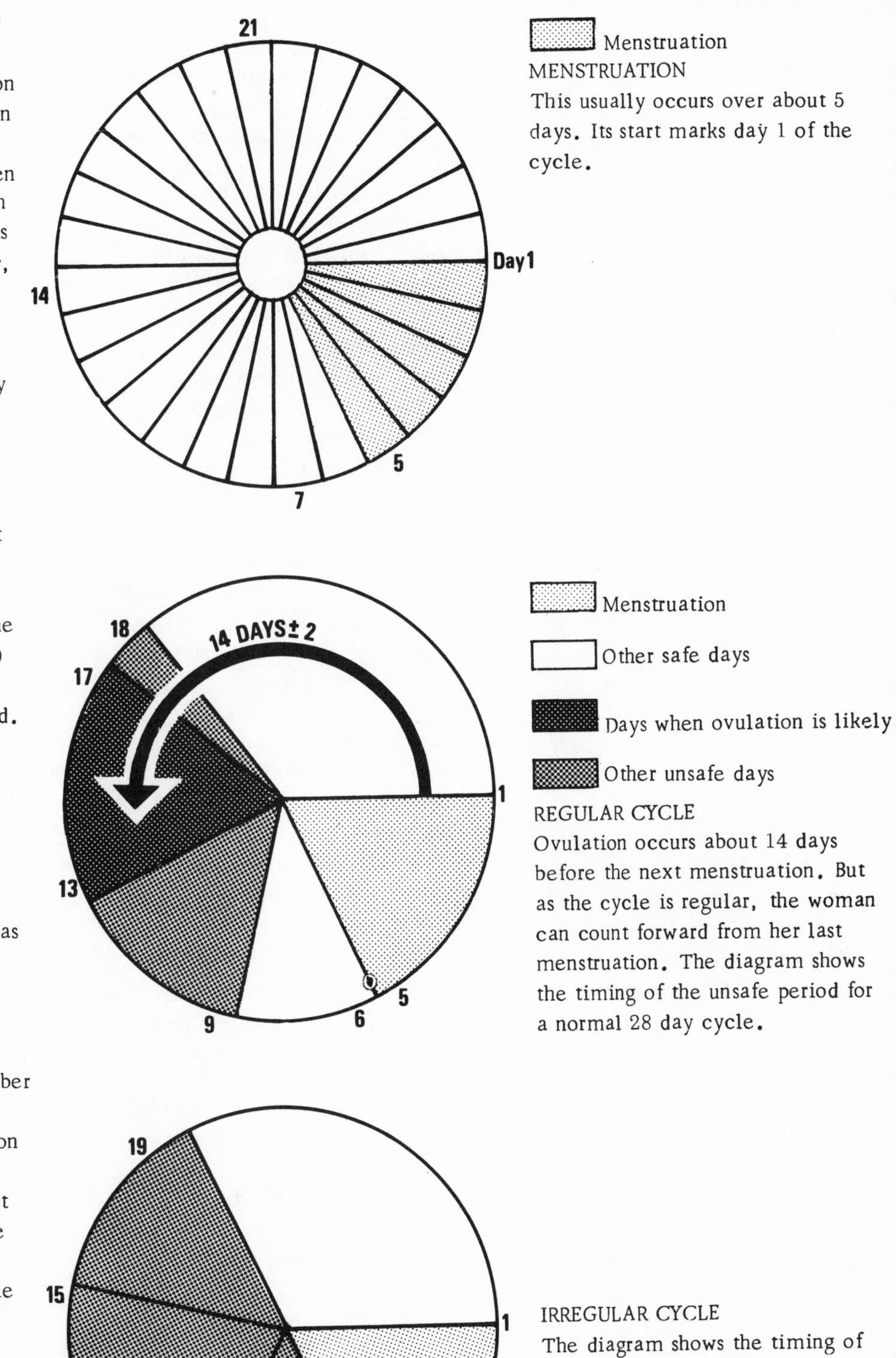

MENSTRUATION

This usually occurs over about 5 days. Its start marks day 1 of the cycle.

REGULAR CYCLE

Ovulation occurs about 14 days before the next menstruation. But as the cycle is regular, the woman can count forward from her last menstruation. The diagram shows the timing of the unsafe period for a normal 28 day cycle.

IRREGULAR CYCLE

The diagram shows the timing of the unsafe period when cycles vary between 25 and 29 days. The unsafe period of the shortest cycle lasts from the 6th to the 15th days; that of the longest from the 10th to the 19th. So the total unsafe period is from the 6th to the 19th days.

K

K21 CONTRACEPTIVE PILL

The standard oral contraceptive ("the pill") is a small pill that a woman swallows once every day for most or all of each menstrual cycle. The pill contains chemicals that produce changes in the woman's body that prevent pregnancy. Sexual intercourse can occur without any restriction.

The chemicals contained in oral contraceptives are synthetic versions of the natural female hormones estrogen and progesterone. These hormones are produced naturally by a woman for several days in the normal course of each menstrual cycle*. Also they are produced continuously during pregnancy, when they have the effect of preventing any output of FSH and LH hormones*. FSH and LH are needed if follicles are to ripen for ovulation, and this is why no ovulation occurs during pregnancy. The contraceptive pill has exactly the same effect; and as no ovulation occurs, no egg is available for fertilization by sperms.

Contraceptive Pills require a doctor's prescription. If a woman is on the pill, she should have a yearly checkup including a Pap test, breast exam and blood pressure test. She should discuss any prolonged side effects with her physician.

Oral contraceptives are normally available in packages of 20 to 28 pills, each package being designed for use during one menstrual cycle. The package indicates which pill should be taken on which day of the cycle.

The combination pill contains both synthetic hormones.

With the combination pill, a woman takes one standard pill each day for 20 to 21 days, beginning on the 5th day after menstruation starts and ending on the 24th or 25th day. There is a gap of 7 or 8 days, during which no hormone is taken, and menstruation occurs (usually 3 days after the last pill). A new package is needed for the next cycle. Some packages include pills for every day of the cycle. But the extra pills are dummies, for the period during which menstruation is to occur. They contain no hormones. The combination pill is easy to use and highly effective because it also makes the cervical mucus less favorable to sperm transport, and the uterus lining less receptive to a fertilized egg, if one does occur. However, the combination pill is also a cause of unpleasant side effects such as nausea, headache, sore and swollen breasts, "fatness" due to water retention, and vaginal bleeding (though all these usually disappear after the first few months). Also there may perhaps be a decrease in sexual desire in some women.

Apart from such side effects, the disadvantages of the pill are:

a) the importance of motivation and memory; and

b) the risk of blood clotting in some women.

Women with a certain blood type run a higher risk than normal of blood clotting from pill use, and the resulting thromboses* can kill. Even so, the normal mortality risks of pregnancy are 10 to 15 times greater - providing that the woman has no history of thrombosis, high blood pressure, diabetes, and certain other disorders; But no woman should take the pill without consulting a physician who knows her medical history.

Re-examination at 6 or 12 month intervals is desirable, and immediate consultation if unusual symptoms occur.

The pill may also be prescribed to make menstruation regular.

Ovulation (and so normal fertility) return 2 to 6 weeks after a woman stops using the pill.

RISK FACTORS FOR WOMEN

Women who take oral contraceptives run a greater risk of incurring a stroke than women of a similar age who are not on the pill. They also run an increased risk of coronary heart disease, which is further aggravated by cigarette smoking. Other risks associated with the pill include high blood pressure and diabetes. All of these risks increase with age.

A recently published study by the Kaiser-Permanente Medical Center at Walnut Creek, California, sponsored by the National Institute of Child Health and Human Development, states that the risks associated with birth-control pills for young, white middle-class American women are low.

Information primarily from the United States Department of Justice, Drug Enforcement Administration.

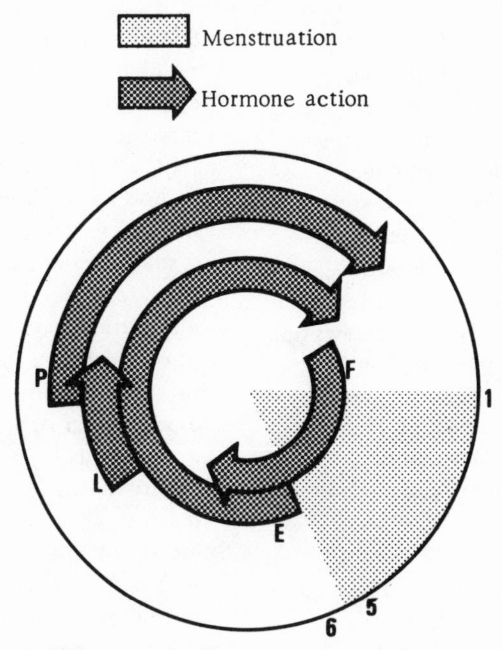

NORMAL CYCLE
For details of the hormones produced by a woman's body during the menstrual cycle, see M06.

F FSH
E estrogen
L LSH
P progesterone

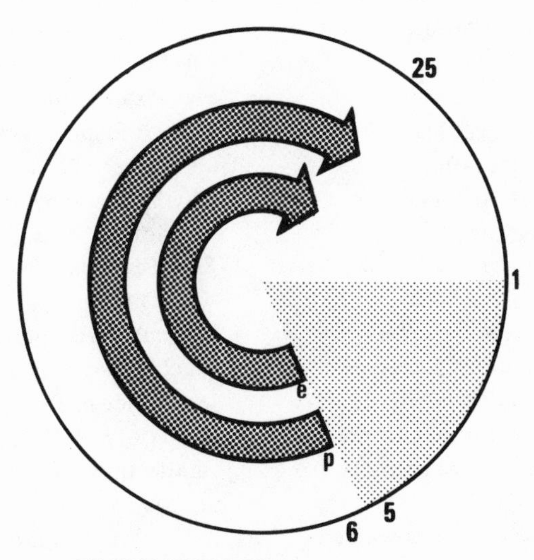

COMBINATION PILL
All active pills taken contain both synthetic estrogen and progesterone.

e estrogen
p progesterone

K22 EFFECTIVENESS OF TECHNIQUES

A contraceptive method can fail to work for any of three reasons:
a) the couple may fail to use it;.
b) they may use it incorrectly;
c) they may use it correctly but the method may fail.
Different methods tend to fail for different reasons. For example, oral contraceptives because the couple fail to use them (usually due due to forgetfulness), spermicides because the method fails. So it is difficult to make strict comparisons. However, the following figures are adapted from G. Pincus in "Science" for July 29, 1966. They measure the likely number of pregnancies occurring in a year, if a method is used for that time by 100 couples. The least effective are at the top of the list.
There are, of course, other factors in the choice of contraceptive, apart from effectiveness.

Method	Pregnancies
douche	31
rhythm	24
spermicide jelly	20
withdrawal	18
condom	14
diaphragm	12
spermicide foam	8 to 12
IUD	5
sequential pill	5
combination pill	0.1
vasectomy	nearly 0

The figures for sequential pills may be too high.

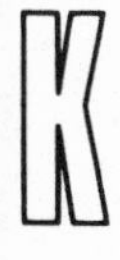

MALE DISORDERS OF INTERCOURSE

K23 DISORDERS

PAIN DURING INTERCOURSE

There are several possible causes:
a) inflammation of the foreskin;
b) chronic prostate infection;
c) scars in the urethra, due usually to untreated gonorrhea;
d) over-tight foreskin, that makes erection painful; or
e) allergy of the penis to vaginal fluids or contraceptive chemicals.
The first, second, and third can be treated by dealing with the infection; the fourth (and again the first), by circumcision; the fifth by use of a condom.

PSYCHOLOGICAL IMPOTENCE

An occasional incident of impotence is quite normal. It should only be thought of as a problem if it is a regular occurrence. The general nature of impotence is dealt with in J12 together with possible physical causes. But 9 cases in 10 are psychological - as is often shown by an ability to have erection (and orgasm) from self-masturbation or during sleep, but not in a sexual relationship. Such impotence typically involves men who have experienced intercourse to orgasm as the norm at a past stage in their lives, and who may eventually return to this. However, in a few cases of deep psychological disturbance, a man may never have had an erection in any circumstances.
The psychological causes of impotence can arise from various levels of motivations. Conscious or nearly conscious causes can be:
a) fear of the consequences of intercourse - pregnancy or venereal disease;
b) feelings of resentment, disgust, or dislike towards the partner; and especially
c) fear of sexual failure - the feeling that one is on trial. For example, fear that one will fail to "perform impressively", or fail to please the partner; especially, fear of premature ejaculation, and of impotence itself. Such fear may be set off by a single incident or particular situation, or by the impact of one's own or one's partner's sexual difficulties.
More deep-rooted causes are usually due to early experience, including especially the relationship with one's parents, or to traumatic experiences when first attempting intercourse. They can result in:
a) distaste for sexual activity;
b) feelings of resentment towards women in general;
c) inability to reconcile sexuality with an idealistic image of women;
d) fear of unacceptable incest fantasies, through failure to progress beyond a childhood "Oedipus complex" (a desire to kill one's father and have intercourse with one's mother);
e) fear of the vagina as a castration instrument (i.e. belief that it could chop off one's penis); and
f) general neurotic personality disorders.
But by far the most common cause is simply the fear of failure. Premature ejaculation, for example, can set up a self-consciousness that eventually ends in impotence. Thereafter, a vicious circle of impotence and fear of impotence may be established.

PREMATURE EJACULATION

This is when the man reaches ejaculation too quickly, for the woman to be sexually satisfied. Occasional premature ejaculation is normal - it can happen simply because of prolonged lack of sexual outlet. Besides, few women are likely to reach orgasm at every intercourse. Consistent premature ejaculation is a serious problem that can lead to partner dissatisfaction, self-consciousness, and impotence.
Sometimes early experiences can set up conditioning in over-rapid ejaculation; for example, intercourse with prostitutes, need for speed in semi-private places such as automobiles, and lack of concern for the partner during one's sexual learning. Even in maturity, possible causes of premature ejaculation can include real lack of consideration for the woman. However, in our culture, and especially in stable relationships, a man is likely to feel that the ability to satisfy his partner is as much a symbol of his sexuality as his ability to reach orgasm.
As a result, the major cause of premature ejaculation is simply anxiety that premature ejaculation will occur. The situation is the same as with impotence. Once there is anxiety about one's sexual performance, a vicious circle is set up ; for anxiety immediately inhibits a true sexual response.
In addition, with premature ejaculation, the situation is likely to be complicated by bitterness between the sexual partners. If the man is impotent, neither partner can find sexual release. But if he ejaculates prematurely, he seems to have found it at the expense of his partner. So lack of consideration may be the accusation, even when it is not the cause.

EJACULATORY INCOMPETENCE

This is more rare. The man has no difficulty with erection, but cannot reach orgasm inside the vagina. As with other difficulties, it can lead to anxiety, self-consciousness, and finally impotence. The cause usually lies in the past, often in particular traumatic incidents, and often against a background of a sexually restricted upbringing. The result is a psychological attitude that sees the woman as repulsive or contaminating or threatening.

K24 TREATMENT

Difficulties that have psychological causes are nevertheless amenable to physical therapy - if this is built on a basis of communication and love. The techniques described here are those developed by Masters and Johnson, the researchers into human sexual biology, and described in their book "Human Sexual Inadequacy". No precis is really sufficient, though, and they are not responsible for the descriptions here.

The techniques for treating these disorders may seem emotionally degrading - to those who do not have the far greater burden of the disorders themselves.

BASIC PRINCIPLES

Masters' and Johnson's basic principles are that sex is a form of communication, and that treatment can only occur in the context of a sexual partnership (typically, the married couple). Successful therapy depends on the goodwill of both partners, their ability to learn to relax, and their realization that sex is not primarily a matter of successful performance.

SENSATE FOCUS EXERCISES

These are simple but vital. The couple lie naked, stroking and feeling each other's bodies - but not the breasts or genitals. No intercourse is allowed. The couple learn to relax and experience sensual pleasure free from any demand (whether of end-point release, self-explanation, reassurance, or immediate return of pleasure received). At first, clumsiness, self-consciousness, and embarrassed humor are likely; but usually genuine enjoyment soon begins. This undermines the crippling tendency to sexual self-evaluation. Later, sexual expression is allowed. Breasts and genitals may be touched, and the couple guide each other and explain what is most pleasurable.

During these exercises a lotion is used to prevent roughness and also help some get more used to genital fluids. Rejection of the lotion (eg, as immature) was found to be a very good guide to who would fail to benefit from therapy.

Later, specific treatment for the disorders begins. Where impotence exists as a result of another underlying disorder, the impotence is treated first.

PSYCHOLOGICAL IMPOTENCE

Here the principles of communication and demand-free activity are especially important. After sensate focus, the couple progress to more specific manual manipulation, with the man guiding the woman's hand. There is still no attempt at intercourse; if erection occurs, it is allowed to go again, then to re-establish itself. Once erection is easily obtainable, the woman uses a position astride the man. First she only tries to keep the penis within her vagina; later she begins gentle, non-demanding thrusting. Finally the man joins in slow thrusting, but with no goal of ejaculating or satisfying his partner. Orgasm is just accepted if it happens.

PREMATURE EJACULATION

Common techniques for this include:

a) distracting the mind with mental tasks or physical pain;
b) avoiding any touching of the male genitals before intercourse begins, while manually stimulating the woman almost to orgasm; and
c) use of anesthetic creams and jellies, tranquilizing drugs, and even excessive doses of alcohol.

None of these necessarily works, and they are anyway hardly symbols of a happy sexuality.

Masters and Johnson found this problem fairly easy to deal with. In their therapy, the couple first use a sitting position - the woman leaning back against the bedhead, the man, between her legs, leaning with his back against her. The woman masturbates the man till he is too near to orgasm to stop it for himself (2 to 4 seconds before ejaculation). At his warning, she presses the penis tip firmly between her thumb and first two fingers for 3 or 4 seconds, and the man loses the urge to ejaculate. This is repeated 4 or 5 times a session. After thorough practice, the couple use a position of intercourse with the woman above. They remain motionless, with the man's penis inside the woman's vagina, and the woman intervenes with squeeze control if necessary. Also the husband thrusts if necessary to maintain erection. Later a lateral position is used, so the woman can still intervene if the man's orgasm begins too soon. Squeeze control is used regularly, for 6 months to a year, before at least one intercourse a week. After that it is used as needed.

EJACULATORY INCOMPETENCE

The Masters and Johnson therapy begins with masturbation of the man's penis by the woman, discovering what the man finds stimulating and bringing him to orgasm. There should be no attempt to hurry this. Once the man can identify the woman with sexual pleasure, the couple use one of the positions with the woman above.

The man is again brought to imminent orgasm manually, and then the woman thrusts to take the penis into her vagina. The technique is repeated until the man gets used to ejaculating into the vagina. Later he also gets used to inserting his penis into the vagina when his sexual excitement is low. Moisturizing lotion prevents irritation during the stages of manual stimulation.

K25 ORAL SEXUALITY

Oral sexuality includes lip kissing, deep kissing (in which the tongue is inserted into the partner's mouth), breast kissing, oral contact with the body in general, and oral-genital contact. All these are common sexual behavior. With some, most of the pleasure may be emotional (eg lip kissing); with others, the pleasure of giving pleasure (eg body kissing). But the mouth also ranks with the genitals as potentially one of the two most erotic areas of the body. This is clearly shown by the practice of deep kissing.

ORAL-GENITAL CONTACT

The term "fellatio" is used for contact between the mouth and a male partner's penis: the term "cunnilingus" for contact between the mouth and a female partner's genitals. Both are increasingly accepted in our society. Both are also a common aspect of sexuality: in other mammalian species; in human civilizations since ancient times; and, unadmitted, in our own society in recent history.

The oral techniques involved include kissing, sucking, licking, and (in the case of fellatio) movement of penis inside mouth and/or mouth around penis in the manner of intercourse. Pleasure is usually felt by both partners. One receives genital stimulation, the other experiences the partner's pleasure and receives oral stimulation.

Mutual pleasure also occurs where there is simultaneous oral-genital contact by both partners. The usual technique for this is for the partners to lie in opposite directions facing each other. Each then has access to the other's genitals.

Both fellatio and cunnilingus may be used as adjuncts to intercourse or as ends in themselves. Both can be very intense sexual experiences, though neither are likely to be very stimulating if done in a haphazard or harsh way. (For example, care must be taken to keep the teeth out of the way. This is mainly a problem with fellatio.) Where fellatio is taken to ejaculation, sometimes the partner chooses to swallow the ejaculated semen, sometimes not.

OCCURRENCE

Fellatio is common in male homosexual activity, and cunnilingus in female. This is simply because no genital connection is possible for homosexuals. There is nothing "homosexual" in these procedures in themselves. Kinsey found that oral-genital contact occurs even among pre-adolescent children, and that 60% of all men are involved in oral-genital contact at some time in their lives. His figures show over 45% of all men receiving fellatio in heterosexual relations, though only about 16% have given cunnilingus.

In marriage, the occurrence of cunnilingus remains about the same, while fellatio falls drastically. All these heterosexual contacts are much more common the higher the education level.

As for homosexual oral-genital contact, Kinsey suggests that 30% of all men have experienced this at some time. Interestingly, only about 11% have given fellatio, while nearly 30% have received it. All these figures were probably underestimates for their time, and the true incidence may be even higher today.

OBJECTIONS

Some people object strongly to oral-genital contact. It remains a state offense in many parts of the USA, and desire for such contact in marriage has sometimes resulted in divorce and even murder. Objections have been that is is unnatural, sinful, unhygienic, or simply unpleasant. However:

a) Its widespread practice in many human societies makes it hard to dismiss it as unnatural.

b) Its sinfulness must be a matter for the individual conscience. Some religions have included oral-genital contact in their ritual.

c) If the genitals are kept clean (which is wise even if no sexual activity occurs) there are fewer and less harmful bacteria there than in the mouth. There is no reason to be concerned about the association with urination, or the nearness of the anal opening. In fact, communication of disease is no more likely than through genital contact and (outside sexual infections) less likely than through kissing. Finally, no harmful effects have ever been known from swallowing semen, except in the very rare case of someone with a skin allergy to it.

d) The unpleasantness of oral-genital contact must be a matter of personal judgement. But genitals do not smell, if clean, and vaginal fluid and semen are just body fluids and often tasteless. Violent reaction to the thought of oral-genital contact only suggests, in fact, that a basic urge is being psychologically blocked.

Nevertheless, such contact should never be forced on an unwilling partner - any more than any other sexual behavior. If offered with love as an expression of love, it will usually be accepted as such in the end.

It has been suggested that the recent emphasis on oral sexuality reflects male fears of heterosexual intercourse, in the face of the sexual and psychological liberation of women. This is possible, but it is more likely that it reflects the media's search for subject matter.

K26 HOMOSEXUALITY

Homosexuals are men and women who are emotionally and physically attracted to their own sex.

In our society, conventional images of male homosexuals are that they are in some way "feminine", or perhaps that their sex interests make them a danger to children. The vast majority of homosexuals fit neither of these ideas. They are just ordinary people - not identifiable by body type, mannerisms, dress, or occupation. Most non-homosexual people will, without realizing it, have friends and relatives who are homosexual. However, today many homosexuals do declare themselves openly, and refer to themselves as "gay".

INCIDENCE

It is very difficult to state the number of homosexuals in a population. Because of guilt and secrecy, surveys need not reveal the truth. Also it is important to distinguish between occasional incidents and a real preference. "Homosexual" activities can occur in preadolescent sex play, while homosexual feeling, perhaps accompanied by mutual masturbation and group masturbation, is typical of one stage of adolescence.

Perhaps ⅓ of all men have at least one homosexual experience to orgasm between adolescence and old age. But only perhaps 2 to 4% of adult males in western society are exclusively homosexual. Between these numbers are those who have considerable adult experience of both heterosexuality and homosexuality - whether in the same or different periods of their lives. Many such individuals may be married and have children. There is more homosexuality in all-male societies such as the armed forces, prisons, and single-sex schools, where heterosexual outlet is denied.

K27 HOMOSEXUAL ACTIVITY

There is still considerable ignorance and fear among non-homosexuals about homosexual procedures. However, apart from the impossibility of genital intercourse and the changes of emphasis this causes, homosexual activity is basically parallel to heterosexual. Many techniques are are common to both, and in both there are mutual kissing and caressing, and the general processes of getting used to one another and giving affection.

The main sexual techniques used include mutual masturbation*, fellatio*, anal intercourse, and interfemoral intercourse (where the penis is stimulated by being moved between the partner's thighs). The first two of these are quite common in heterosexual activity, while anal and even interfemoral intercourse do also occur.

Most non-homosexuals also think that homosexual partners take on exclusively passive (female) or active (male) roles. In reality, the roles often alternate.

ANAL INTERCOURSE

This involves inserting the penis into the partner's anus. Normally some kind of artificial lubrication is used.

Two rings of muscles, called sphincters, are sited at the opening to and inside the anus. They are normally closed, to prevent waste products coming out involuntarily. The outer sphincter can be relaxed or tensed at will, but the inner is less under conscious control. However, homosexual men have to learn to relax both these muscles, to avoid pain during anal intercourse. A dilator can be used, which will gradually stretch them, but most men find that both these muscles do relax if they are at ease with their partners.

When the penis has passed through the two sphincters it reaches the rectum, which is wide and does not register pain.

The passive partner in anal intercourse often experiences intense pleasure. This is partly because of the erotic sensitivity of the anus (which is familiar to heterosexuals too), but also because his partner's penis tends to rub against his prostate gland, which is sited near the rectum. Stimulation of the prostate seems to produce an especially prolonged and intense orgasm.

During orgasm the anus automatically tightens and puts pressure on the penis inside it, so intensifying the pleasure of the active partner.

One objection to anal intercourse is a hygienic one. But the rectum is normally free of waste products, and contains only about as many bacteria as the mouth. These are of a different kind, though, and the genitals should be washed carefully after anal intercourse (and especially before any oral-genital contact or heterosexual intercourse). Objections to being the passive partner in homosexual intercourse include the fear of pain and of "subjection" and "femininity". Anal intercourse can in fact be very painful if the sphincters are not properly relaxed. But the usual exchange of roles between partners prevents the development of superior/inferior roles or psychological typecasting.

INCIDENCE OF TECHNIQUES

Temporary adolescent homosexuality does not usually go beyond mutual masturbation. When fellatio or anal intercourse occur, it is a likely sign that a homosexual preference will continue in adulthood. Among adults, mutual masturbation and fellatio are common to both incidental and preferred homosexuality, but anal intercourse is usual only where homosexuality is preferred.

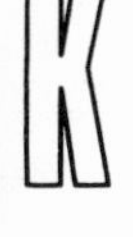

K28 ATTITUDES TO HOMOSEXUALITY

Human societies have shown a tremendous range of attitudes to homosexuality. In most European countries homosexuality was given the death penalty in the Middle Ages. More recently, homosexuals were sometimes charged with indecency if found holding hands. Yet in some societies (such as the Mohave tribes of North America) homosexuals have been allowed to "marry", and have had their needs tolerated. In other cases (as in Arab countries and traditional Samoan society), homosexual feeling has not even been defined as unusual, but simply treated as a part of one's normal sexuality.

Finally, at least one society - ancient Sparta - tried "state-fostered homosexuality" as part of a male military cult. However, most societies have regarded a homosexual preference as abnormal.

MODERN LEGAL ATTITUDES

Over the world these range from tolerance to extreme opposition. Many countries now have laws permitting homosexuality in private between consenting adults (France introduced this in 1810). But the age of consent varies considerably. In the USA it is 16 in most states, but in Delaware it is 12, Hawaii 14, and Illinois 17.

In the UK, France, Scandinavia, Japan, and China, the age of consent is 18.

In Spain, in contrast, all homosexuality is persecuted and treated as socially dangerous. Imprisonment for up to 8 years can be imposed on suspicion of homosexual tendencies, and compulsory "therapy" electric shock treatment and drugs.

In general, all countries also have laws against indecency, soliciting, abuse of the young, and sexual misuse of a position of authority. Sentences vary from probation to life imprisonment.

K30 THEORIES

Homosexuals themselves may articulate reasons for their preferences; but society in general tends to see homosexuality as an abnormal state needing explanation in terms of some physical or psychological defect. Physical theories put forward include:

a) neurophysiological - in which homosexual behavior is due to malfunction or stimulation of certain parts of the brain;

b) hormonal - in which it is due to hormone imbalance (eg, in a male homosexual, a lack of male hormones or an excess of female ones); and

c) genetic - in which some inherited defect is blamed.

Bits of evidence for each of these include:

a) a recent very experimental technique of transforming homosexuals into heterosexuals by using tiny electric shocks to knock out certain cells in the brain.

b) evidence of hormone imbalance in a few homosexuals; and

c) evidence that homosexuals tend to have been born to elderly mothers, a situation that is known to be one in which chromosome abnormality often occurs.

But research findings for all these theories are mainly ambiguous or contradicted by other studies, and there is no scientific agreement about any of them.

PSYCHOLOGICAL FACTORS

Even if physical factors are involved, psychological ones seem more important. It is significant that the potential for homosexuality seems to exist in all men; and that homosexual feeling is typical of one stage of early adolescence, and only unusual if prolonged.

This prolongation seems to happen, in our society, when certain family emotional patterns have occurred in childhood. In particular, combination of an unaffectionate, even hostile, father, with an emotional, over-intimate mother, may mean that a growing boy lacks or reacts against identification with a male model, and is drawn into his mother's femininity.

The situation may be made worse if the mother accompanies her mother-son intimacy with subconsciously ambiguous physical caresses, out of frustration or resentment against the father.

The child's sexuality may be awakened; but as he cannot imagine himself taking a sexual initiative in relation to his mother, women may come to seem unobtainable or alarming.

Even where a firm break with the mother is made, a fear of her power may remain as a fear of the power of women in general. This is especially true where the mother's force is not one of intimacy compared with a distant father, but of outright dominance compared with a weak one. This is another situation in which homosexuality can arise, for the growing boy sees no advantage in becoming "male".

All this depends, though, on a pervasive influence of the traditional roles of men and women.

K29 PROBLEMS OF HOMOSEXUALITY

These mainly arise because society treats homosexuality as abnormal. First, homosexuals have difficulty admitting their sexual preference even to themselves. On average, it takes 6 years from the first feelings of homosexual attraction to outright self-admission of "being homosexual" - and some may avoid it for a lifetime, suffering instead a lingering dissatisfaction with heterosexuality.
Second, self-admission is often followed by acute depression and shame. However militant some "gays" may now be, the typical features of "psychological coming out" in the past have been suicide attempts and psychiatric treatment.
Third, self-admission often leads to fear of the opinion of others, if they find out. In particular, fear of parental knowledge may produce acute guilt feelings.
Fourth, the homosexual will often need to suppress ordinary expression of his sexuality (eg, in most jobs heterosexual flirting is acceptable, but homosexual is not.)
Fifth, the homosexual may find it hard to meet others like himself. Homosexual organization is more common now, in big cities, but many individuals remain isolated.
Sixth, homosexual alliances tend to be fragile and transient, because:
a) the inability to reproduce removes the binding purpose of raising another generation, and leaves an empty sexuality;
b) the partners are often guilty and insecure; and perhaps
c) any alliance suffers the less clearly defined the partner's separate roles.
Finally, alliance instability, lack of reproduction, and a resulting inevitable emphasis on sexuality and youth, leave many older homosexuals to face years of appalling loneliness - which may lead to the desperation of a sexual offence.

K31 "CURES"

Because homosexuality is generally seen as abnormal, it is also seen as something requiring treatment. Many homosexuals themselves look on it in this way. Here are some of the methods attempted, and the difficulties or misconceptions involved.

HORMONE TREATMENT
This tries using doses of male or female synthetic hormones.
However:
a) male hormones, far from making male homosexuals more "masculine", simply increases the desire for whatever sexual activity they are used to; and
b) female hormones (used to control sex offenders) reduces all sexual desire in men, eventually produces impotence, and has such side-effects as breast development.
In any case:
a) the ethical justification for interfering with the hormone balance of a physically healthy person is extremely doubtful; and
b) only a very small proportion of homosexuals suffer from hormone abnormality. It may be that they tend towards homosexuality because of this, but it has not been proved even for this small category.

BEHAVIORAL THERAPY
Behavioral therapy rests on the assumption that homosexuality is a bad habit with no really deep significance, and that it can be easily changed to another habit. This is attempted in several ways. A homosexual may be introduced to female seduction in an "anxiety-free atmosphere" with the aid of drugs to inhibit the usual response. Alternatively, in "aversion therapy", a patient may be shown pictures of nude men and given an electric shock or an injection inducing nausea. He may also be given a sexual stimulant while looking at pictures of nude women.
All these procedures are crude and treat people as sex objects rather than as human beings with complex feelings. It is very doubtful if they change a homosexual into a well-adjusted heterosexual. It is more likely that those "effectively" treated in this way simply become so guilt-ridden that they abstain from homosexual activities and struggle to find pleasure in heterosexual ones.

PSYCHOANALYSIS
Psychoanalysis uses regular long sessions between a patient and a trained analyst, in which the conflicting emotions, fantasies, and inner conflicts of the patient are revealed. Psychoanalytic theory believes that uncovering these conflicts itself sets off their resolution.
However:
a) the process is immensely costly;
b) it demands great patient motivation;
c) as a procedure for dealing with mental conflicts, it has not been finally proved to be any more effective than the passage of time; and
d) any one therapist's theory of homosexual causation is unlikely to to be universally valid.

K

K32 LONE SEXUALITY

"Masturbation" means stimulation of the genitals other than by intercourse - usually with the hands, but sometimes with other parts of the body or with objects, and usually with the intention of achieving orgasm. It usually means self-stimulation - but not always. It also includes stimulation of a partner's genitals, whether or not the couple also experience sexual intercourse, and whether in heterosexual or homosexual circumstances. So its uses range from the first experiments of schoolchildren to the mature relations of lovers.

But here we are concerned only with those techniques people use in lone situations, when there is no-one to share sex with, or simply when they choose an experience of self-stimulation ("auto-eroticism"). It is in this sense, of a lone sexual activity, that the term is used in surveys of sexual behavior, and in this book. Such masturbation occurs throughout society, and masturbation to orgasm is experienced at some time in their lives by about 93% of all men (and by over 60% of all women).

TRADITIONAL ATTITUDES

In our society, masturbation has has been a subject more taboo than interpersonal sex. There were, perhaps, three reasons for this. First, masturbation is the way in which the sexuality of their offspring forces itself on parents' attention. Second, for most people masturbation seems an admission of failure, compared with finding sexual expression in a relationship with another person. (This is especially true whenever sexuality is dominated by concepts of male "conquest" of the female.) Third, acceptance of masturbation means recognizing the power of the sex urge - beyond (if need be) both social pretense and human communication.

So the traditional attitude was one of disapproval, reaching psychotic levels in the later 19th century. Children were terrified with stories that masturbation would bring physical and mental illness. Some were even forced to wear physical contraptions designed to prevent the wearer ever "abusing himself".

MODERN ATTITUDES

First, it is now generally recognized that masturbation causes no special physical or mental deterioration. Physically, excessive masturbation can cause prostate gland trouble - but so can excessive intercourse, or total abstinence. Mentally, excessive masturbation may well form a part of some failure to face up to reality - but so can excessive eating. Masturbation is here a sign of failure, not a cause; at most, it reinforces the sense of failure. Second, past masturbation is not a cause of difficulty when interpersonal sexual relations begin. There may be fears about sex, which express themselves in a preference for masturbation. But the cause of these lies in personality disorders, due to childhood experience, bad sexual education, a traumatic incident, or or a repressive family atmosphere. The masturbation is not the cause.

Nowadays masturbation - though still little talked about - is more generally accepted for what it is: part of our normal sexual experience. First, it has functioned (especially before the development of the pill) as a way of diverting some of the sexual drive that otherwise would result in immature partnership commitments. Second, it releases acute tension due to an unsatisfactory sexual life or the temporary absence of a partner. Third, it alleviates the sexual loneliness of old age. Certainly, it is not something that parents should try to create guilt feelings about, in their offspring.

WHEN MASTURBATION BEGINS

Some kind of stimulation of the genitals occurs in many infants only a few months old. One survey found that genital play, or rocking to and fro, on the genitals, occurred in more than half of infants under one year old. Some such cases have been reported in which stimulation was even carried to orgasm (though not, of course, ejaculation): the youngest a boy of 5 months and a girl of 3 months. More conscious auto-eroticism can begin at any age from 5 years on, but for most men it begins sometime between the ages of 9 and 18, with the great majority in the time just after puberty (i.e. for most men, 13 or 14). For in men, with the onset of puberty, masturbation becomes a necessary release of sexual tension and sperm production, rather than just a pleasant sensation. Masturbation, in fact, provides the first experience of ejaculation for ⅔ of all boys. The average age of this is 13.9 years. Thereafter, masturbation is normally the main sexual outlet of early adolescence. Those women who masturbate before adulthood tend to start a little earlier than men. But by the age of 20, only 40% have tried masturbation, compared with 92% of all men. Masturbation provides the first orgasm for only just over ⅓ of women.

MASTURBATION IN ADULTHOOD

Male masturbation frequencies range from once a month or less to two or three times a day or more. (Women, on average, masturbate much less frequently.) The average male frequency, among those who do masturbate, is about twice a week at the age of 15. Thereafter, it declines throughout adulthood. (With women, it increases up to middle age.) The importance of masturbation as an outlet varies greatly with age, education level, and, of course, marital status: see K38. Masturbation is responsible for between 5 and 10% of the outlet of married men, depending on age. It is mainly accounted for by temporary absence of the partner, conflicts, or psychological difficulties. Among single men, it varies from as low as 20% to as high as 80%. It is highest in the young and the highly educated.

SEXUAL PROCESS

Masturbation is identical with other forms of penis stimulation, in the sequence of changes it produces in the sexual system. However, in feeling, intensity and psychology, its orgasm may well seem different to that of intercourse (as well as varying considerably from occasion to occasion).

Techniques of masturbation vary considerably between different people: especially in the part of the penis stimulated, the speed of hand movement, the hardness of touch, and whether stimulation continues during ejaculation.

OTHER SOURCES OF ORGASM

Other forms of deliberate self-induced orgasm are rare. Only 2 or 3 men in a 1000 are able to suck their own penises. Very few men can reach orgasm by stimulating other parts of the body. Only 3 or 4 men in every 5000 can achieve orgasm by fantasy alone. But involuntary orgasm, during sleep, accompanied by a sexual dream, is fairly common in men from adolescence on. Almost every man experiences it at some time (and about ⅔ of women). As a source of orgasm in men it typically varies between 2 and 8% of total outlet (2 to 3% in women). It tends to happen more frequently when masturbation is the main form of sexual outlet.

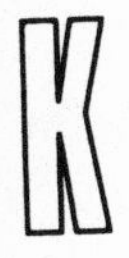

AVERAGE MALE EXPERIENCE 1

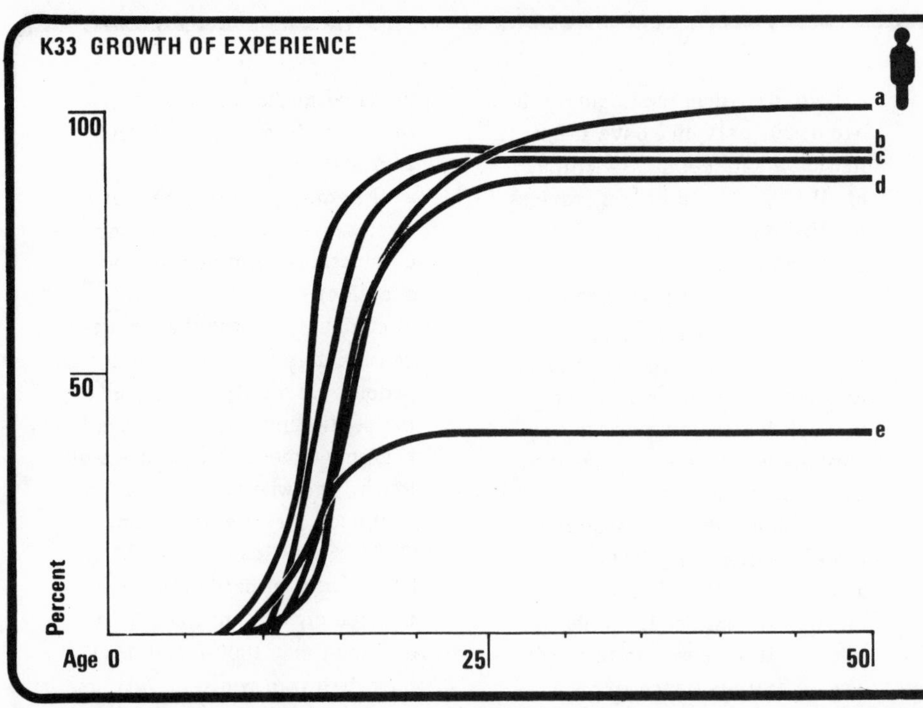

We have numerous scientific studies on the sexual life of remote tribes - and almost none on our own society. The data on these four pages is taken from the classic work by Kinsey and his associates. Their surveys of American men and women are over 30 years old now, but are still the only precise studies we have, on the sexual life of modern man. These first two tables look at different kinds of sexual activity, and show what percentage of the population have experienced them at least once, by a given age. All material K33-41 by permission Institute for Sex Research Inc. See "Sexual Behavior in the Human Male" (W B Saunders Co, Philadelphia).

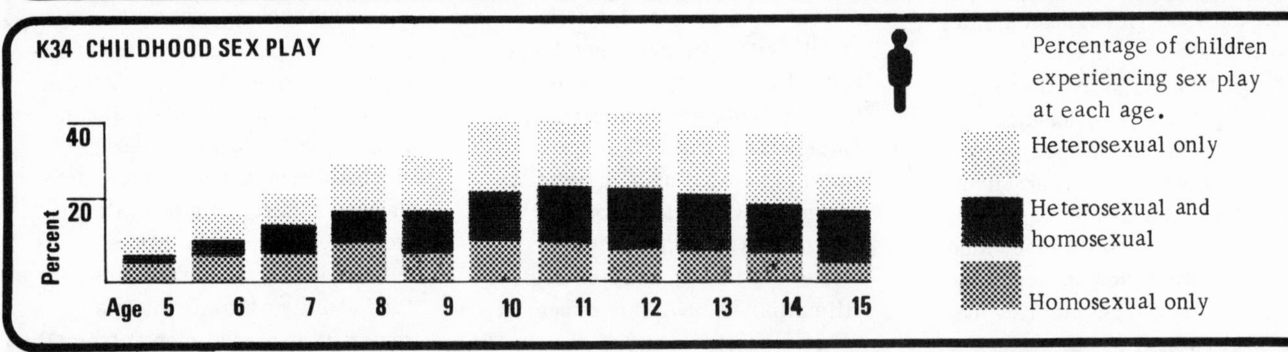

Percentage of children experiencing sex play at each age.

Heterosexual only

Heterosexual and homosexual

Homosexual only

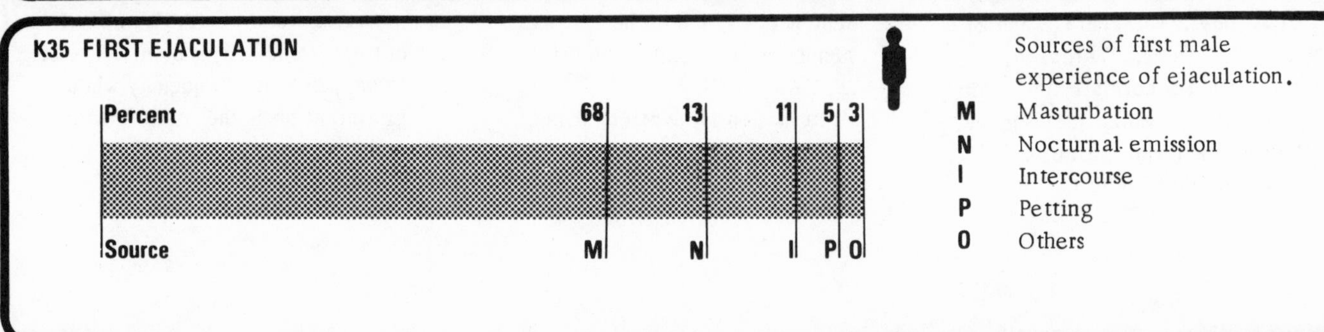

Sources of first male experience of ejaculation.

- **M** Masturbation
- **N** Nocturnal emission
- **I** Intercourse
- **P** Petting
- **O** Others

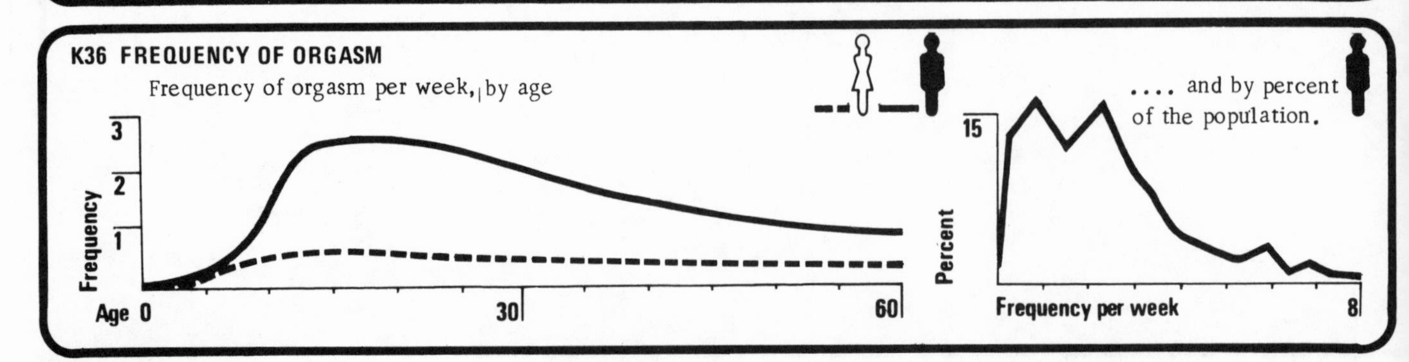

Sexuality

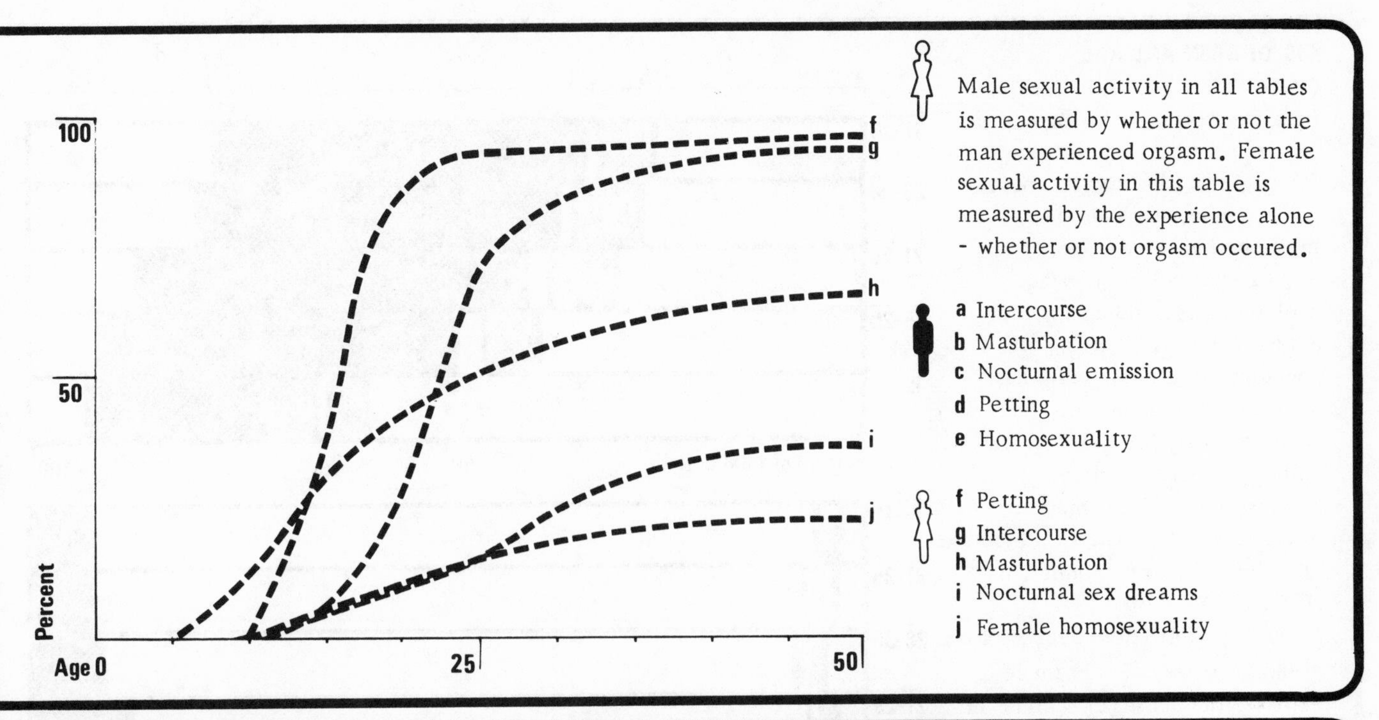

Male sexual activity in all tables is measured by whether or not the man experienced orgasm. Female sexual activity in this table is measured by the experience alone - whether or not orgasm occured.

K37 SOURCES OF ORGASM

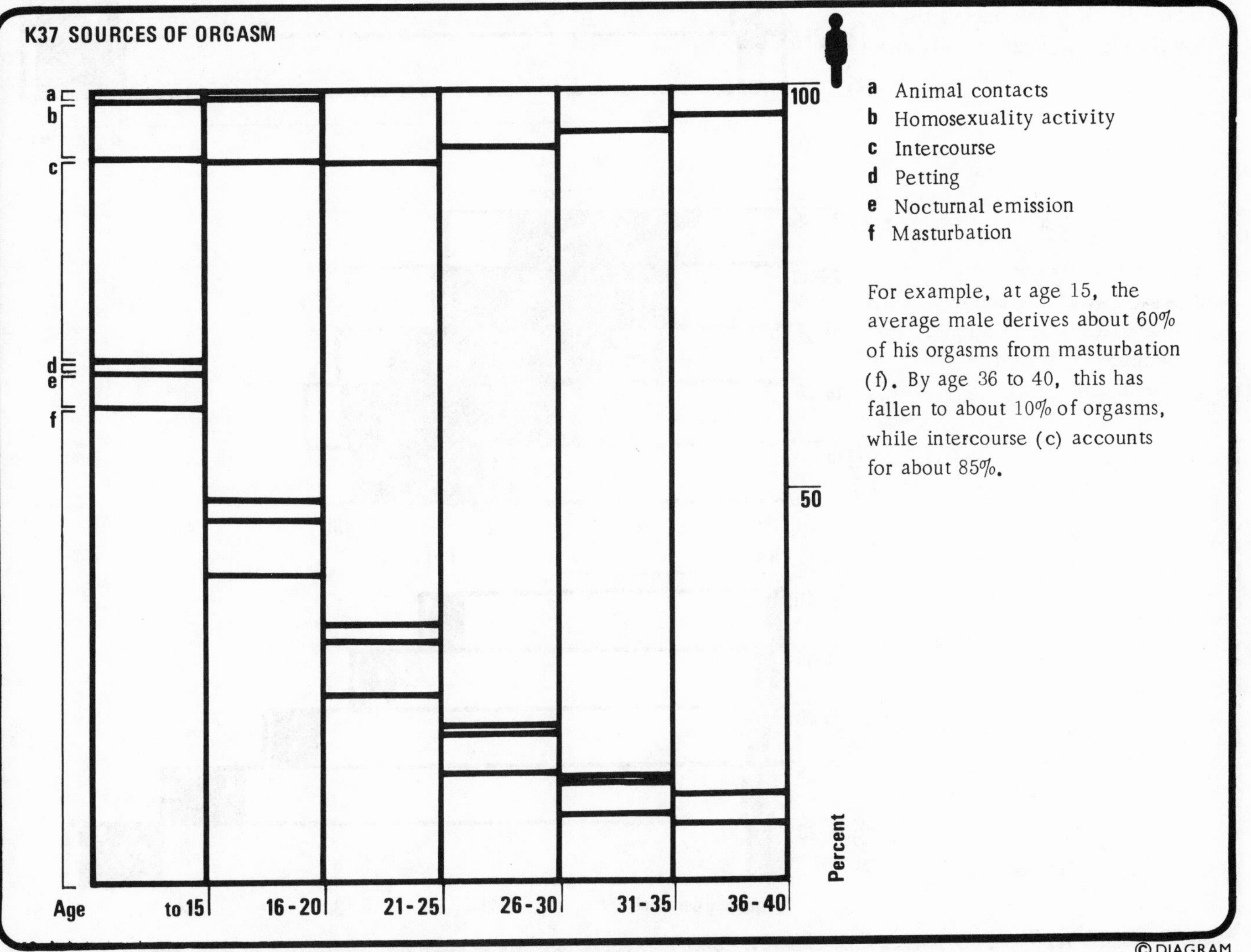

For example, at age 15, the average male derives about 60% of his orgasms from masturbation (f). By age 36 to 40, this has fallen to about 10% of orgasms, while intercourse (c) accounts for about 85%.

K

AVERAGE MALE EXPERIENCE 2

K38 ORGASM AND AGE

SOURCES

Here we show how the sources of orgasmic outlet vary with age, for single and for married men. For example, in single men, masturbation (a) averages about 60% of total outlet in young adolescents (15 and under), but only 25% by age 31 to 35, when non-marital intercourse (d) has become the main outlet. Homosexuality (e) also increases with age - because more heterosexual men get married. In married men, marital intercourse (g) is by far the main outlet.

FREQUENCY

Frequency of different outlets varies in the same way. For example marital intercourse (c) declines in married men from almost 4 times a week (age 16 to 20) to only about twice a week (age 36 to 40).

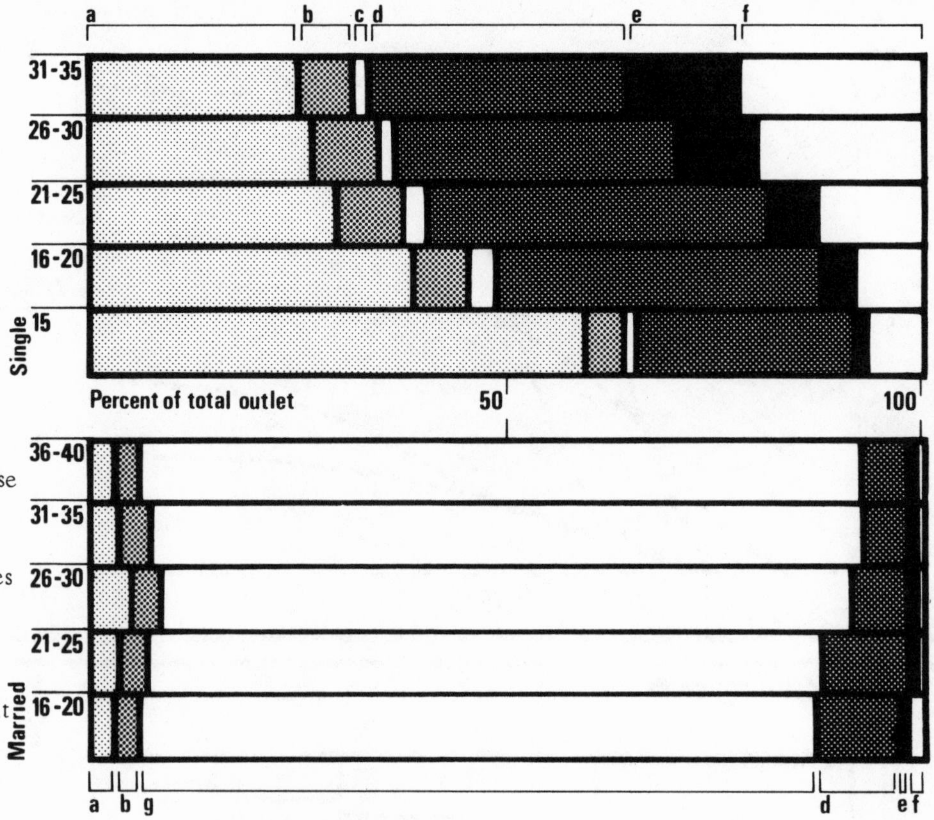

- **a** Masturbation
- **b** Nocturnal orgasm
- **c** Petting to orgasm
- **d** Non-marital intercourse
- **e** Intercourse with prostitutes
- **f** Homosexual activity
- **g** Marital intercourse

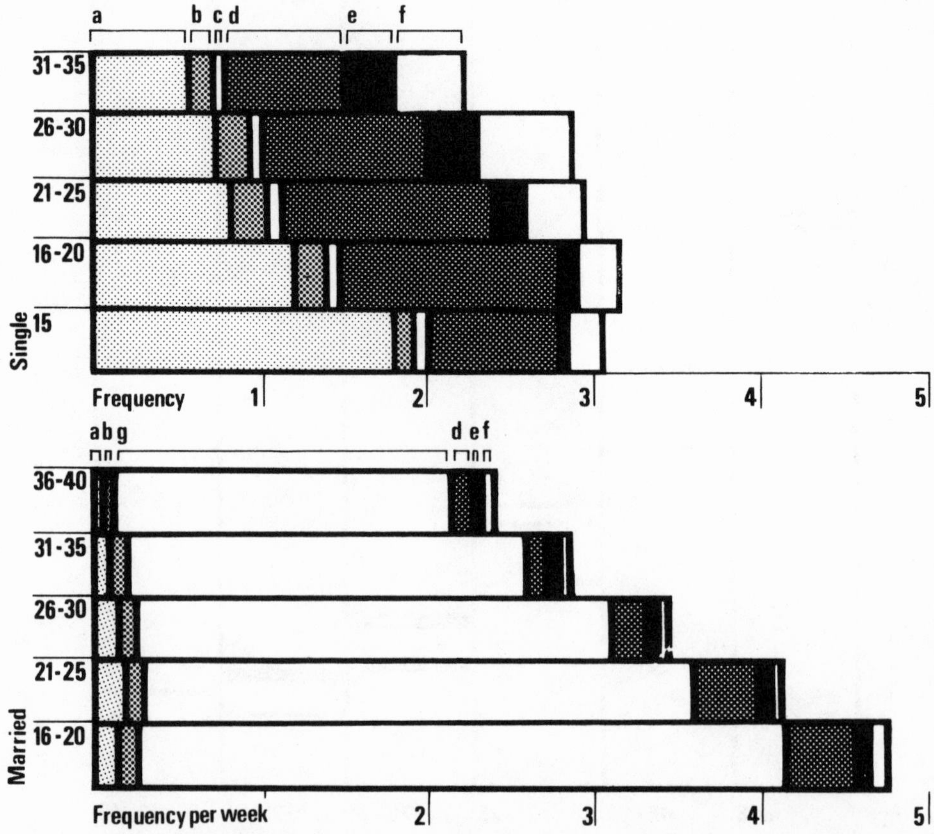

K39 SEXUAL RESPONSE

Here we show how sexual response changes with age. For example, the percentage lacking all sexual response declines from almost 100% at age 5 to almost 0% at 35, and then begins to rise again.

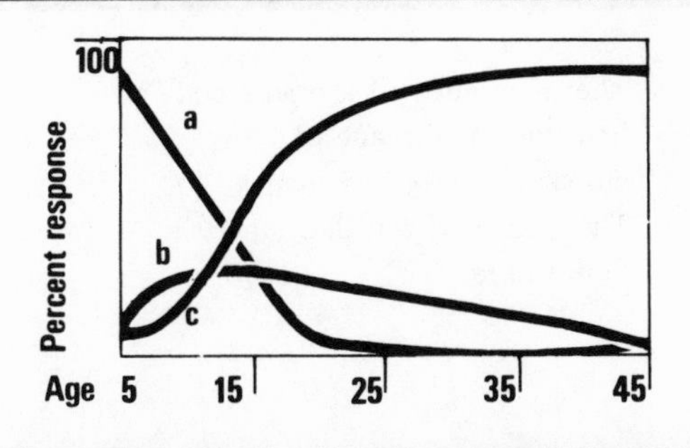

Sexual response in men
a No sexual response
b Homosexual response
c Heterosexual response

K40 CAPABILITY AND AGE

Morning erection

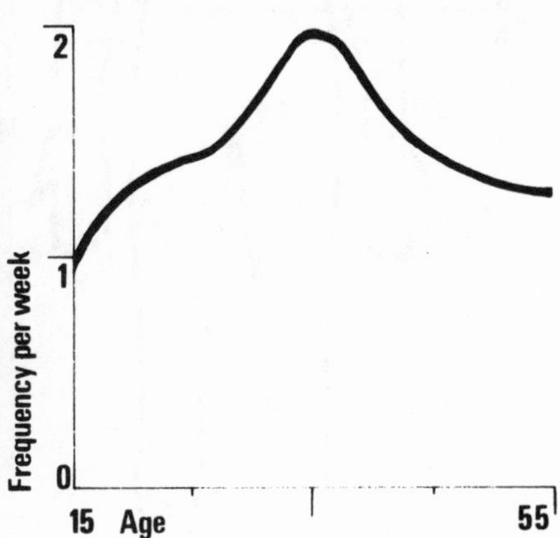

Duration of erection

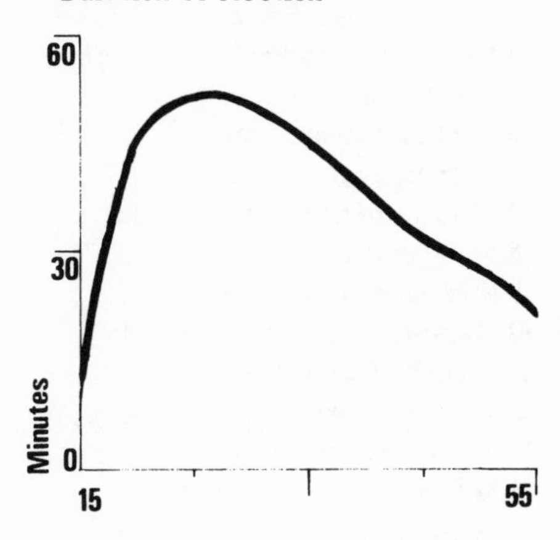

Angle of erection

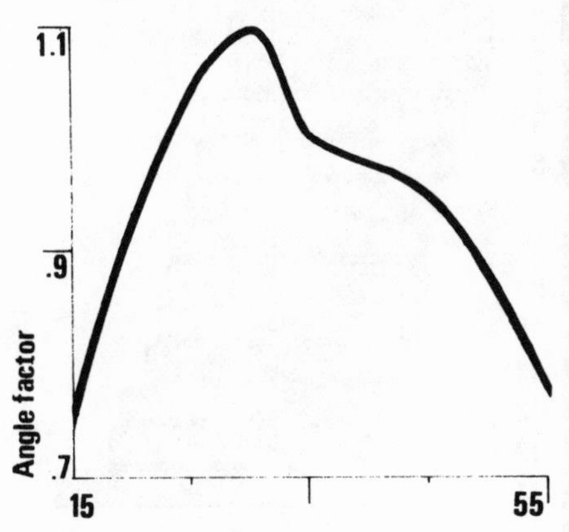

With age:
a) the experience of waking with an erection becomes less frequent;
b) the length of time for which an erection can be maintained shortens; and
c) the angle of the erect penis becomes less steep.

K41 MULTIPLE ORGASM

This compares, for different ages, the percentage of men and women who can reach orgasm more than once during a single session of intercourse. The numbers are calculated as percentages of all those who have intercourse at each age. (For example, at age 10, of the very few males who have intercourse, more than half can have multiple orgasm.) In men, the percentage declines with age - falling rapidly from puberty to 25. In women, it rises between 25 and 30, because for them multiple orgasm is partly a learned response.

Ability to have multiple orgasm

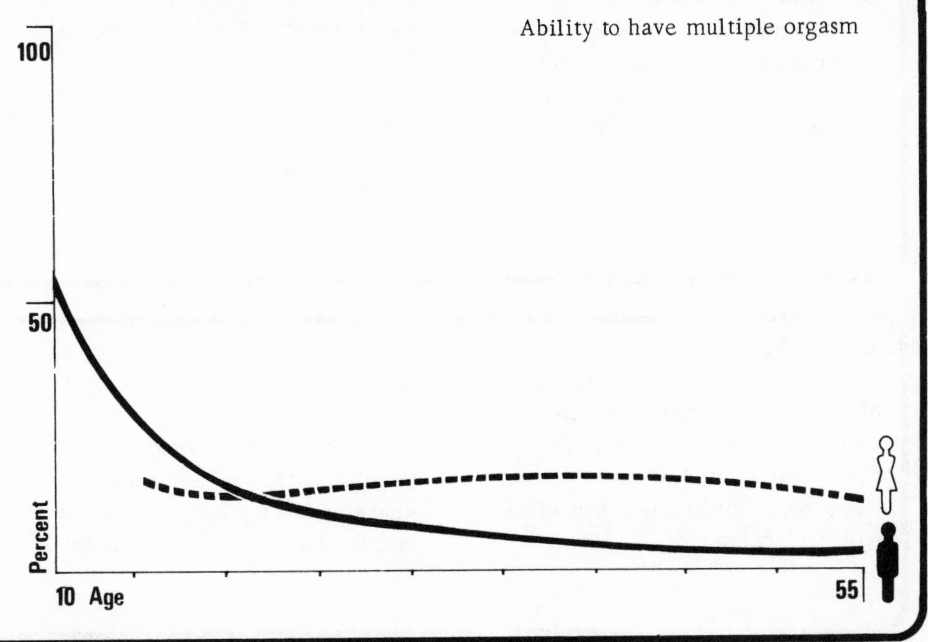

K

THE PROCESS OF AGEING

L01 AGEING

The process of ageing begins in the middle to late twenties, and continues until death. No one escapes its effects; but there are often great differences in its degree of impact on people of the same age.

The efficiency of a man's body functions at the age of 75 is proportionately less than at 30. The extent of this decline is shown here.

Decline in body functions

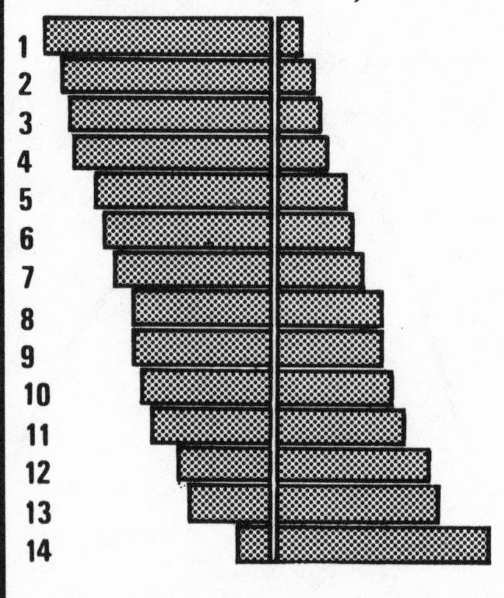

1 Body weight
2 Basal metabolic rate
3 Body water content
4 Blood flow to brain
5 Cardiac output at rest
6 Filtration rate of kidneys
7 Number of nerve trunk fibers
8 Brain weight
9 Number of kidney glomeruli
10 Maximum ventilation volume
11 Kidney plasma flow
12 Maximum oxygen uptake
13 Number of taste buds
14 Return of blood acidity to equilibrium

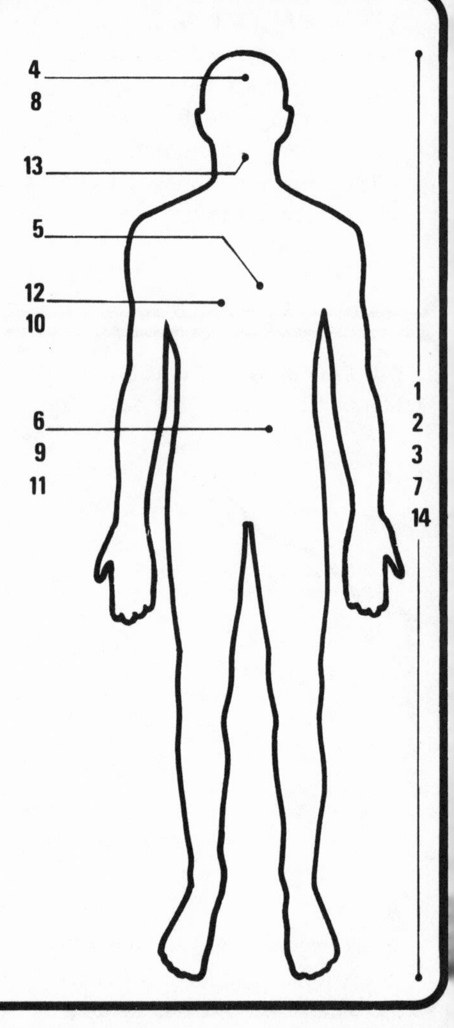

L02 FACIAL APPEARANCE

Changes in facial appearance come about in adulthood through atrophy of the facial bones, recession of the gums, and loss of teeth.
The skin becomes dry and loses its elasticity, taking on a wrinkled appearance. This deterioration is speeded by the loss of fat deposits from under the skin surface.
Hair becomes grey as pigment ceases to be produced. Also both sexes undergo loss of hair, though actual balding is much more common in men.

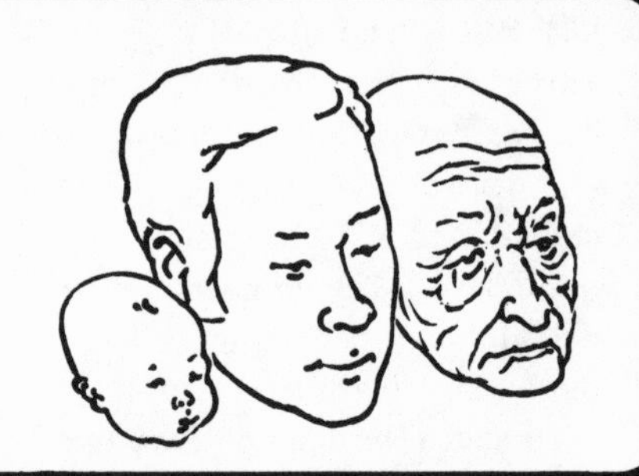

L03 STATURE

Full stature is reached by the age of 20 or shortly afterwards. After that there is little change in the size of any individual bones. However, adult height does decline with the ageing process. This is partly because the vertebral discs in the spine deteriorate, causing the spine to shorten slightly. But more important is the gradual weakening of the body muscles, so that the spine is not held so erect.

L04 POSSIBLE CAUSES OF AGEING

Medical science can prolong the life span - but it cannot yet prolong youth. Gerontology - the serious study of ageing - is still a new science, and even the process and causes of ageing are not yet properly understood.

CELL MUTATION

This is currently thought of as the main cause of ageing.

Most cells in the body reproduce to replace cells that have died. They do so by "somatic division," i.e. by dividing into two. In this way the exact characteristics of the original cell are preserved.

However, it is possible for mutation to occur in a cell. This is any form of damage affecting the chromosomes,* which are the code system built into the cell that decides how it operates.

Mutation can be caused by the gradual exposure over a lifetime to natural radiation (from the sun or from naturally occurring isotopes). Less normally, it may also be caused by: disease; chemical action; or radiation from nuclear activity, exposure to X rays, etc.

When mutation occurs, a cell may become inactive, or do its job badly, or be actively dangerous (as in the case of cancer).

Moreover, because chromosomal damage is involved, the distortion is passed on whenever the original cell reproduces. Somatic division means that the number of mutated cells increases in geometric progression (1, 2, 4, 8, 16, 32, 64). In this way, areas of the body's activities become inefficient or disrupted. The effect is increased when the process occurs in certain organs, eg in the endocrine glands, which form the body's chemical control system.

NERVE CELL LOSS

From the age of about 25, there is a continuous loss of nerve cells ("neurons") from the brain and spinal cord. These cells cannot be replaced once lost; and the rate of neuron loss is accelerated in age by the onset of arteriosclerosis.

L05 OTHER FACTORS

Some other factors have been seen to play a part in ageing - but they are not "causes" in the same sense as cell mutation and nerve cell loss are thought to be.

STRESS

Psychological stress often has physical manifestations, and it has been noticed that stress of all sorts (physical danger, pain, mental strain, etc) can cause premature aging. However, the biological process whereby this happens is not known.

METABOLISM

As a person grows older, there is a drop in his basal metabolic rate: that is, the energy production of his body at its lowest waking level. For example, the body temperature of an old man is on average 2°F less than that of a 25-year-old.

Metabolic decline is a sign of the ageing process, rather than a cause, but it has a wide impact on the body's functions and abilities.

HORMONE PRODUCTION

During the female menopause, the ovaries stop producing estrogen, and male production of testosterone also declines after the middle years (though it never reaches zero level). It was therefore natural for gerontologists to consider using injections of the appropriate hormone to make up the body's failing supply.

However, although injections of these hormones can reduce some physical signs of ageing (smooth out wrinkled skin, for example), they do not seem to prevent the basic physiological process of ageing going on.

In general, hormonal decline seems to be one of the ways in which ageing expresses itself, but not a basic cause.

L06 THE BODY

Muscles lose strength, shape, and size. Joints become worn and lose their ease of articulation.

Combined with the degeneration of the nervous system, ease and confidence of movement is lost.

Loss of bone tissue makes the skeleton brittle. As calcium is lost from the bone, it tends to be deposited in other areas - especially the walls of the arteries and the cartilage of the ribs. This causes loss of elasticity. One effect is a lowering of lung capacity.

Most internal organs - such as the liver, heart, and kidney - become reduced in size and function.

The arteries harden and narrow ("arteriosclerosis"). This increases the normal rise in blood pressure, which goes up about 0.5mm Hg a year from the onset of ageing. The speed of blood flow also rises - though usually not excessively. When arteriosclerosis is combined with atheroma (degeneration of the arteries inner lining) the condition is known as atherosclerosis

These disorders of the vascular system speed up tissue decay, through inadequate blood and oxygen supply. This especially affects the heart and brain.

L

L07 DECLINE IN ABILITIES

Physical abilities

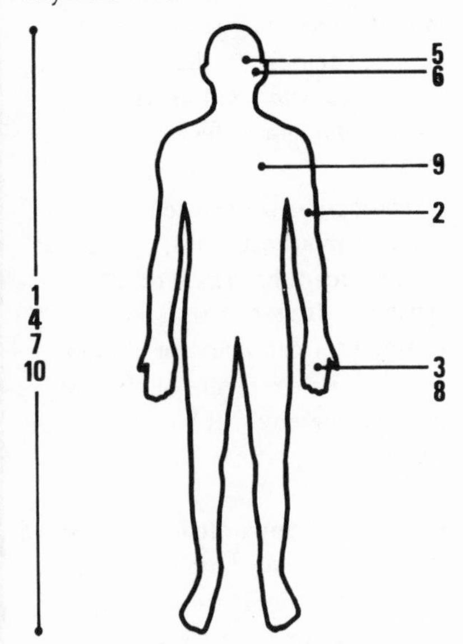

The decline in the efficiency of the body also affects an ageing person's physical strength, conscious capabilities, nervous control, and mental powers (maximum measures in these are mostly reached at different ages from 20 to 30).

1 Nerve conducting velocity
2 Circumference of biceps
3 Persistence of grip
4 Maximum work rate
5 Visual acuity at 20ft
6 Hearing
7 Reaction time
8 Hand grip
9 Maximum breath rate
10 Maximum work rate (for short periods)

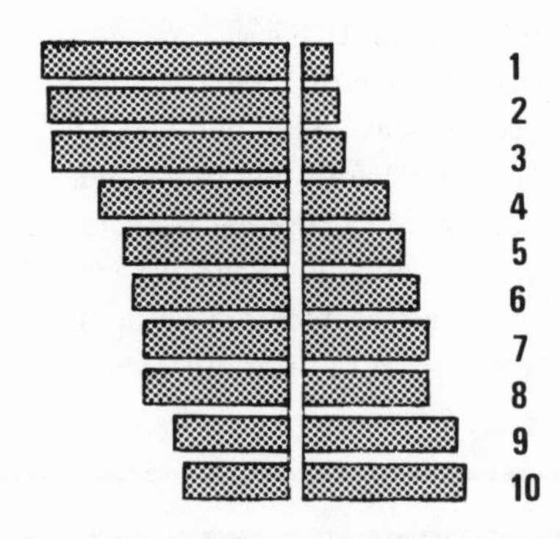

Mental abilities
1 Vocabulary
2 Information
3 Verbal intelligence
4 Comprehension
5 Arithmetic
6 Non-verbal intelligence
7 Intellectual efficiency

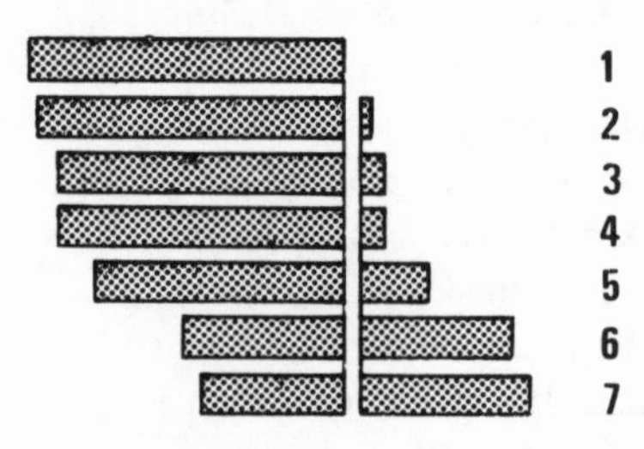

L08 AGEING AND SOCIETY

Changes in temperament and behavior in old people may be accepted as inevitable. But how far they are really due to neurological and mental deterioration is often hard to judge. The changes may rather be a psychic reaction to the person's social, psychological, and physical situation. Old age often brings with it a dramatic change in a person's experience of life. Declining physical ability and efficiency, perhaps involving being looked after by others; the end of the working life; and isolation, due to the disappearance of work contacts, family mobility, and death of friends - all these can affect an old person's self-esteem, and lead to depression and melancholia. Old people find that they have no role to fulfil, and no social label or way of identifying themselves other than by that term "old person" - the associated stereotypes of which are not inspiring. Society's subtle message can seem the same: you are no longer really useful, and though you are enjoying the deserved fruits of your labor, your difficulties and incapabilities are something of a problem for us. Of course, many old people keep up a wide range of active interests - but for others it is difficult, due to lack of finance, isolation, physical incapacity, and lack of mental stimulation. The rate of change in modern society adds to their disorientation; and the way of life in many old people's homes does little to help. All this can result in apathy, listlessness, resentment and mental stagnation, which others then dismiss as inevitable senility.

L09 THE NERVOUS SYSTEM

In man, as in all vertebrates, different levels of organization can be seen in the nervous system. The reflexes of the lowest level (the spinal cord and oldest parts of the brain) are present in the fetus. Those of the forebrain and cerebral hemispheres develop after birth. With the onset of ageing, the course of development is reversed. First, the higher levels are affected: memory, thought, and complex mental functions become slower and less reliable. Eventually the individual may pass through a second childhood, with, finally, only basic reflexes remaining, such as eating, walking, coughing. On average, by the age of 70, the brain has lost 50% of its weight.

CHARACTER CHANGES

The frontal lobes of the brain - the first part to deteriorate - are less concerned with intelligence and intellectuality than with general personality, interest in life, deliberation, and consideration. Moreover, these higher functions often bear a repressive relationship to the lower, so that as the higher deteriorate the lower are released, in what appears to be an exaggerated form. Social inhibitions are removed in the same way as they were originally formed: the person becomes increasingly selfish, inconsiderate, obstinate, and emotional.

L10 TYPES OF DISORDER

About 10% of people over 65 show some signs of organic brain disorder. Such mental illnesses due to old age were originally undifferentiated under the term "senility" - the loss of mental faculties with age. However, four main conditions are now recognized.

ACUTE CONFUSION

This is one of the commonest mental disorders in old people. It is a disturbance of the brain due to physical illness elsewhere in the body, and is also known as "acute brain syndrome". Strange surroundings and other psychological factors may also play a part.

The symptoms are confusion, delirium, and disorientation in time and place. Perception is dulled, and the sufferer is frightened, often reacting violently to situations that he has completely misinterpreted. Speech becomes incoherent and rambling. The outcome depends on the pre-existing mental state and the original causal illness, but complete recovery is rare.

SENILE DEMENTIA

This is the disorder that links most directly with the slow process of natural nerve cell loss. It usually begins to be noticeable between the ages of 70 and 80, and primarily affects the memory. It begins gradually with recent memory, and may proceed to the point at which the patient forgets his relations and even his own name.

This forgetfulness leads to incompetence in personal care and management: the person needs more and more attention as time goes on.

Disorientation in time and place also occur. Emotions are blunted, and there is an increasing lack of consideration for others. Whether the course of the illness is rapid or slow, it is irreversible, and deterioration continues until death. As the numbers of old people rise, so inevitably do the cases of senile dementia. At present it is more common in women than men.

ARTERIOSCLEROTIC DEMENTIA

This is also due to the death of brain cells, though in this case the cells die because blockage in the arteries impairs their blood supply. The onset may be gradual, or follow suddenly upon a major stroke*. In either case the effects, in an old person, are irreversible. Because the brain damage is restricted to the areas affected by the blockage, the basic personality may remain more intact than in senile dementia. The person usually retains more awareness and insight into his condition - though this can result in depression and fear.

DEPRESSIVE ILLNESS

This is a mental illness, but organic nervous decline plays a part in its appearance. It is characterized by acute feelings of sadness, inadequacy, anxiety, apathy, guilt, and fear. It may be triggered off by internal factors of mental make-up (endogenous depression), or by external events such as bereavement or knowledge of an incurable disease (reactive depression). It often results from a combination of both.

The illness manifests itself in moods ranging from apathy to despair, and in delusions, loss of appetite and weight, and a preoccupation with thoughts of suicide. It is, in fact, a major cause of suicide in the elderly. Although treatment may produce a cure, the chances of relapse are very great.

AGEING AND THE SENSES

L11 THE SENSES IN AGEING

The physical atrophy that occurs with age also affects the five senses. As the nervous system degenerates through neuron loss*, touch, taste, and smell become less sensitive. This does not affect the body's physiological functioning, but may have dangerous consequences (eg an impaired sense of smell may mean that escaping gas is not detected). More serious sensory loss, though, comes from some illnesses brought about by, or occurring in, old age, and affecting the more complicated sense organs such as eye and ear.

L12 HEARING

PRESBYACUSIS is the term for hearing loss as a direct result of old age. It is due to a combination of loss of elasticity and efficiency in the actual hearing mechanisms, and the slowing down of mental activities that old age brings. Mechanical losses especially affect the ability to detect high frequency sounds. By the age of 60 years, hearing of these has been reduced by 75%, though normal conversation and most other everyday sounds can still be distinguished with only slight distortion.

OTITIS EXTERNA* (infection of the outer ear) is especially common in the aged, due partly to hearing aid earpieces that fit badly and are too infrequently cleaned.

L13 SEEING

PRESBYOPIA is the term for the natural changes in the eye* that result from old age. The most common (apart from the general loss of efficiency with age) is hardening of the lens. From the age of about 10 years onward the lens gradually loses its elasticity, and so its ability to adjust focus. As a result, by the age of 60 years the eye is often unable to focus on objects close at hand. Spectacles with convex lenses are then needed for close work such as reading.

CATARACT This is an opacity in the lens of the eye. It is caused by deficiencies in the lens proteins, resulting in a special type of hardening and shrinkage at the center of the lens. The lens cracks and disintegrates, so losing its transparency. The process spreads from the center outwards, and impairment of vision increases as the opaque area (the cataract) spreads. Cataracts occur in most people over 60 years of age, though they are usually too small to have a significant effect on sight.

GLAUCOMA occurs most frequently after the age of 50 years. It is caused by a build up of the fluid pressure in the eye. The fluid that fills the eye (the aqueous humor) is normally being continually drained away and replaced by fresh. Drainage takes place along the "canal of Schlemm", which lies at the junction of the iris and cornea. But sometimes the canal becomes blocked, through inflammation of the eye or swelling of the lens pushing the iris forward. The amount of fluid in the eye then increases as secretion of fresh fluid continues. Pressure builds up, damaging the optical disk and the visual fibers of the retina.

Loss of vision is first experienced in the peripheral field, and it spreads gradually to the whole visual field. There is no pain in the early stages, and the process is so slow it goes undetected. But early treatment is vital, as lost vision cannot be replaced. Yearly pressure check-ups for those over 40 are recommended. (Note that the usual watering of the eye with tears has nothing to do with the drainage of aqueous humor; so continued tear production does not prove that all is well.)

Treatment is largely with drugs, to control aqueous humor production and/or drainage. If this fails, surgery may be used.

SENILE MACULAR DYSTROPHY The macular lutea is a small yellowish area of the retina, and the fovea* lies at its center. Here visual perception is most perfect, and differentiation of minute objects takes place (for reading, etc). Senile macular dystrophy is a degeneration of this area due to impaired blood supply as a result of age. It is the most common eye disorder in the old. But affected people can be taught to use their remaining vision so as to read and function almost normally.

L14 DISORDERS IN AGEING

The atrophy of age reduces the body's efficiency, creating greater vulnerability and likelihood of malfunction. The body is still susceptible to all the usual disorders, while its maintenance, defense, and repair processes are all much weaker. Respiratory and heart disorders, for example, occur with much more frequency and intensity, skin wounds are more liable to infection, and bone fractures more difficult to heal. But in addition the deterioration of the body and its functions produces ailments rarely found at a younger age.

L16 INCONTINENCE

This is the inability to control the emptying of bladder and bowels. Incontinence of the bladder is usually due to infection of the urinary tract, or to damage to the controlling nerves. Atrophy of the muscles concerned also contributes. As senility and mental damage associated with old age progress, the person may lose awareness of his bladder, so conscious control is finally lost and it empties automatically. Restricted mobility, emotional insecurity, and abdominal stress (caused by laughing, coughing, lifting, etc) also play their part in precipitating incontinence.

Fecal incontinence is most often due to fecal impaction - the accumulation of a mass of feces in the rectum too bulky to be passed. This mass then acts as a ball valve, with fresh feces trickling round it and escaping in a continuous flow. In other cases it is due to the continual overflow of the original mass. It is occasionally due to diarrhoea*, as might occur in gastro-enteritis* and rectal prolapse*.

L15 NERVOUS DISORDERS

The nervous system of an old person is likely to be affected by degeneration, since nerve cells cannot be replaced. Also he is more susceptible to strokes*, and liable to falls which may damage spinal cord or brain. All these may impair movement, and ability to think, see, hear, and express himself.

PARKINSONISM occurs fairly often in old age, and more often in men than in women. It is due to degeneration of the nerve cells in one part of the brain, usually as a result of arteriosclerosis. It manifests itself in trembling and muscular rigidity, and often begins in one hand and then spreads to other parts of the body. The body's rigidity interferes with all movement, from facial expression to locomotion, and brings increasing discomfort as the disease progresses.

L17 SPINAL DISORDERS

SLIPPED DISK is the common name for a prolapsed intervertebral disk. The spine is built up of a column of bones (vertebrae) separated by disks of cartilage which act as shock absorbers. (The inside of the disk is made of spongy but firm elastic tissue, held in place by the strong fibrous tissue of the outer layer.) In a prolapse, one of these disks, in the lower part of the spine, slips out of position, impairing mobility and exerting painful pressure on the nerves of the spinal cord.

CERVICAL SPONDYLOSIS affects the upper part of the spinal column. Degeneration of the spine shortens the neck, forcing the vertebral artery to concertina, and so impairing the blood supply to the spinal cord and brain. Also pressure is exerted on the nerves of the spinal cord, so their functioning and that of all connected nerves is affected.

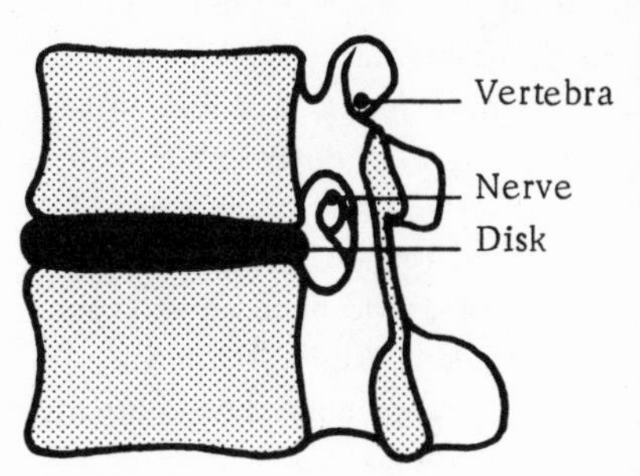

Normal disk

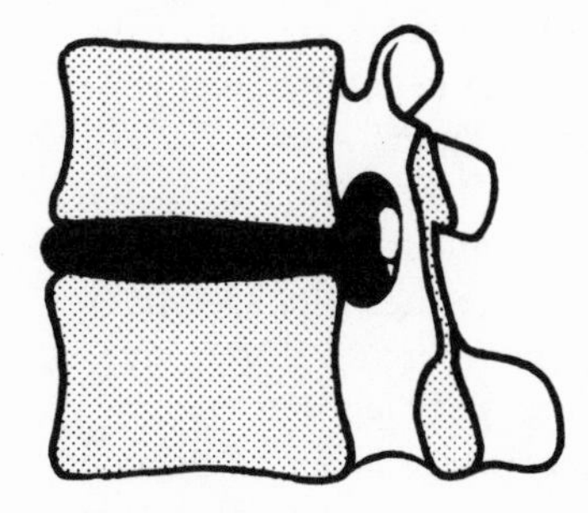
Prolapsed disk

L

L18 HYPOTHERMIA

This is when body temperature falls below 95°F. It mainly occurs in old people who cannot afford adequate heating, food, or winter living conditions. The patient becomes increasingly apathetic and lethargic. Below 90°F coma usually occurs. Treatment does not involve applying direct heat - but the surroundings of the patient should be warmed and a blanket laid over him to prevent further heat loss.

L19 JOINTS

Degeneration in the joints is reinforced by the constant wear and tear they receive throughout life. Also injuries often accentuate and accelerate the disorders.

OSTEOARTHRITIS occurs to some degree in 80 to 90% of people over the age of 60, and in men more than women. It originates from loss of elasticity in the cartilage around the joint. The cartilage breaks up with the joint's movement, and loose bits of cartilage are deposited in the joint itself. These may grow and become calcified, increasing discomfort. The bone around the joint hardens, and cysts may develop, with spurs of bone around the joint's edges.

The knee, hip, and hands are most commonly affected. The process cannot be reversed, but can be delayed by gentle, regular exercise, to loosen the joint and strengthen the muscles.

RHEUMATOID ARTHRITIS usually begins in middle age, but its severity increases with age. It affects more women than men. The tissues of the joints thicken, so the cartilage becomes ulcerated and is eventually destroyed. There is over production of connective tissue, and ultimately the joint is swollen and may be fused solid. The muscles waste with disuse. Special exercises, and rest in serious cases, are the main forms of treatment. Use of the drug cortisone is now thought to cause many problems, though it does give temporary relief.

CONTRACTURES These are deformities of the joints due to shortening (contraction) of the surrounding muscles and ligaments. They are caused by arthritic or neurological disorders, or simply by prolonged inactivity. If untreated they become permanent and cause severe disablement. Treatment is with muscle-relaxing drugs, and physical manipulation.

OSTEOPOROSIS is increased porousness of the bone, usually from unknown causes, but sometimes due to severe nutritional deficiency of calcium salts. The skeleton becomes brittle and prone to fracture. The vertebrae are the bones most affected. They may collapse as they become weaker, and as they lose weight and size the vertebral discs expand, producing increasing curvature of the spine. The condition may be triggered off by prolonged immobilization in bed. It is more common in women than in men.

L20 DIET

NUTRITIONAL NEEDS

The main difference between the nutritional needs of old people and those of younger age is simply a matter of quantity. As a person ages, decrease in physical activity, coupled with a fall in the metabolic rate, lowers his food energy needs. Because of this, the calorific intake of an ageing person should be gradually reduced (see G17). Otherwise, the kind of food needed remains basically the same at any age, though in old age there is rather less need for protein, fat, thiamin, glucose, and also calcium (but see osteoporosis). More foods may cause digestive problems, because of slowing of the speed and completeness of digestion and absorption.

POOR NUTRITION

Old people often eat badly: more dietary disorders are found than in any other age group.

There are several reasons. The lonely, impoverished and neglected may eat badly through apathy, poverty, lack of facilities, buying and eating the wrong foods, and general lack of physical and mental ability. Even the reduced calorific needs may not be obtained.

In other cases, where economic and other practical factors are not restrictive, there may be overeating of such foods as pastries and cakes which supply calories but little else. This replaces muscle tissue with fat, as activity is reduced, and lays down additional fatty tissue elsewhere. The resulting excess weight greatly affects health.

Finally, unhealthy teeth and badly fitting dentures can also affect eating habits, encouraging the old to choose comfortable rather than nutritional food.

L21 PHYSIOLOGICAL FACTORS

Sexual activity declines with old age. But is this because of lack of ability, or lack of opportunity?

HORMONE PRODUCTION

The decline in testosterone production is quite steady, from the age of 20 onwards - there is no sudden point at which old age takes effect, and in fact after the age of 60 the rate of decline eases off.

The decline of sexual activity does seem to follow the same kind of pattern. But there are so many other factors affecting sexual performance in the older male that it is unlikely that the testosterone level exercises a major influence. The amount produced, even right to the end of life, is usually adequate for sexual activity.

In fact, at any time after puberty, sexual response and activity probably come to depend more and more on the higher centers of the brain (the hypothalamus) and on the automatic nervous system, rather than on testosterone production.

GENERAL PHYSICAL DECLINE

The physical degeneration of ageing naturally slows down the processes of sex. Semen production, erection, and ejaculation all take more time and more stimulation. The need and ability for orgasm declines. All this continues the decline observable in men from an early age. But in old age, some new factors appear. Poverty may lead to poor nutrition - with a resulting loss of energy, and specifically sexual energy. And decline or disease in non-sexual bodily functions may make it difficult to perform sexual roles.

Nevertheless, a healthy and fit person should be capable of some sexual activity at any age.

L22 PSYCHOLOGICAL FACTORS

The main causes of declining sexual activity may often be psychological.

PSYCHOLOGICAL IMPOTENCE

The percentage of men suffering from total impotence increases slightly through the middle years, and more rapidly as old age is reached. In old age, physical factors are certainly involved. Yet one major cause of total impotence, at any stage of life, seems to be psychological. It occurs more often in those who have been sexually anxious, and for whom age provides a safe and valid excuse for ceasing sexual activity. In addition, the psychological trauma experienced by a male in middle age, when coming to terms with his life's work and expectations, may lead to depression, disappointment and self doubt, and this can sometimes affect future sexuality.

PARTNER PROBLEMS

The availability and attitude of, and the feeling for, a sexual partner will also increase or lessen desire. Again, age may give an excuse for ending sexual relations that have been merely dutiful.

SOCIAL NORMS

The prevalent attitudes of an individual's social surroundings - his national culture, religion, social contacts and intimate friends - can all impinge on the individual's attitude and thereby his performance. Many people, for example, end their lives in institutions in which any continued interest in sexuality is looked on as obscene.

L23 EVIDENCE OF DECLINE

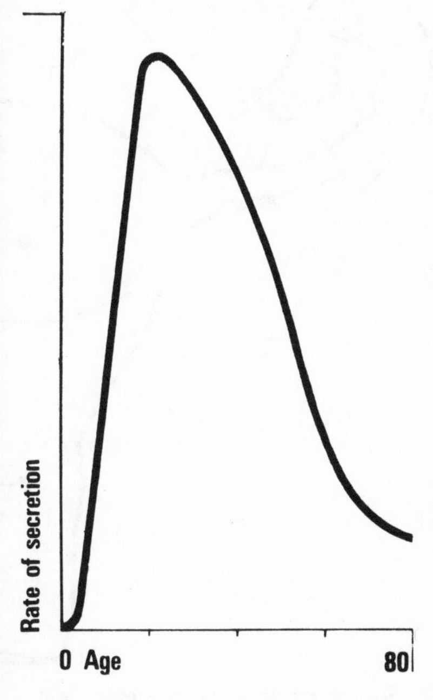

Above we show the pattern of testosterone production in the life of a typical male. It rises steeply until age 20, and declines thereafter. By 60, it has fallen to the level of a 9 or 10 year old.

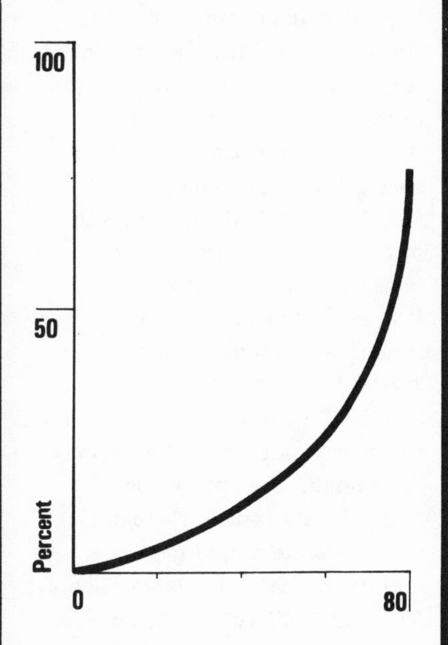

The above graph shows the percentage of the male population impotent at each age.

FEMALE SEX ORGANS

M01 THE SEXUAL ORGANS

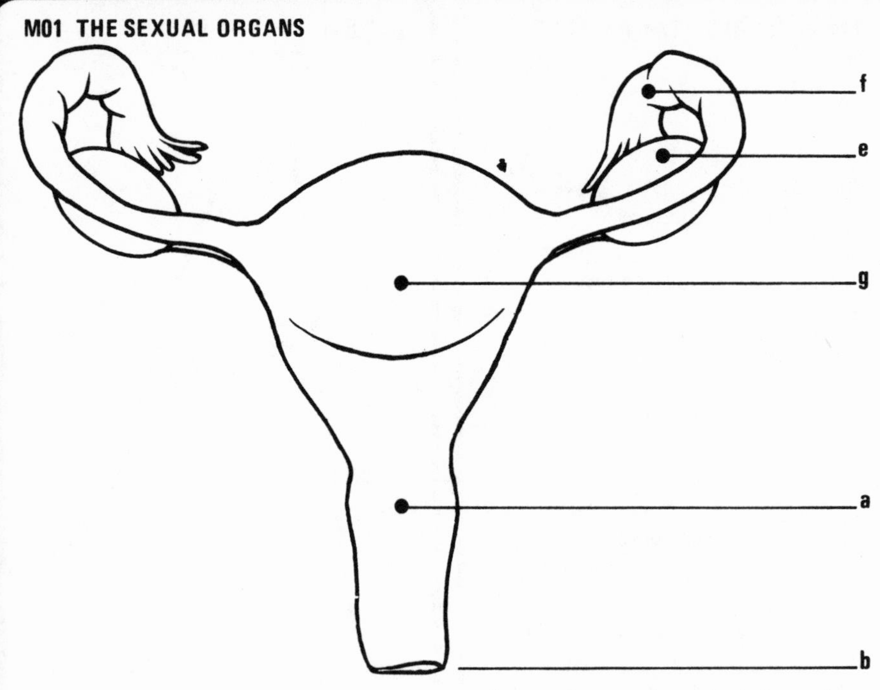

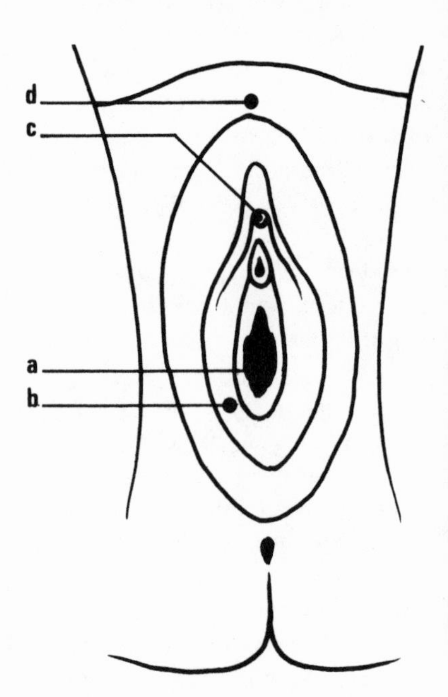

A woman's sexual organs include some concerned mainly with sexual activity, and others concerned only with creating a new life from that activity.

THE VAGINA (a) is a hollow muscular tube, which opens onto the outside between the woman's legs. It is lined with folds of tissue, and is normally 3 to 5in long, but it is capable of great expansion. It is into the vagina that the male's penis is inserted during sexual intercourse.

The "hymen" is the name given to a ring of flesh tissue, just inside the vaginal entrance. It is usually found intact in a woman who has never had sexual intercourse (see K04).

THE LABIA (b) are the two sets of lips that protect the entrance to the vagina. They are made of folds of fatty tissue. The outer, larger lips are called the labia majora, the inner the labia minora.

THE CLITORIS (c) is a bud or projection of sensitive tissue, located just above the entrance to the vagina, at the point where the labia minora join. It is very responsive to sexual stimulation. The length of the clitoris varies greatly in different women, from a fraction of an inch to, in very rare cases, several inches. Under $\frac{1}{4}$in is normal. The average clitoris is often hidden beneath the hood of flesh called the prepuce.

The "vulva" is the name sometimes given to all the external female genitals, i.e. the labia and the clitoris.

THE MONS PUBIS (d), or mons veneris, is a pad of fatty flesh located above and in front of the labia. After puberty it is normally covered with pubic hair.

THE OVARIES (e) are two glands that produce the human eggs (ova) and also certain female hormones. They are located in the cavity inside the hip girdle (pelvis), and each is attached to the uterus by a cord of tissue.

THE FALLOPIAN TUBES (f) are each about 4in long. Their fringed ends pick up the eggs released from the ovaries, and the tubes channel the eggs down into the uterus. The eggs are pushed along by contractions in the walls of the tubes, and by the movement of thousands of tiny hairlike structures projecting from the tubes' linings.

THE UTERUS (g), or womb, is a hollow organ, sited inside the pelvis, and suspended loosely in place by cords of tissue. Its lower part (the cervix) projects down into the vagina. It is in the uterus that a fertilized egg develops into a baby during pregnancy, stretching the uterus from about 3in long to over 12in. At birth, the child passes out of the women's body through the vagina.

In women, the urinary and reproductive tracts are not combined, as they are in men. The urethra, down which urine passes from the bladder, has its opening between the clitoris and the vaginal entrance, but has no sexual or reproductive function.

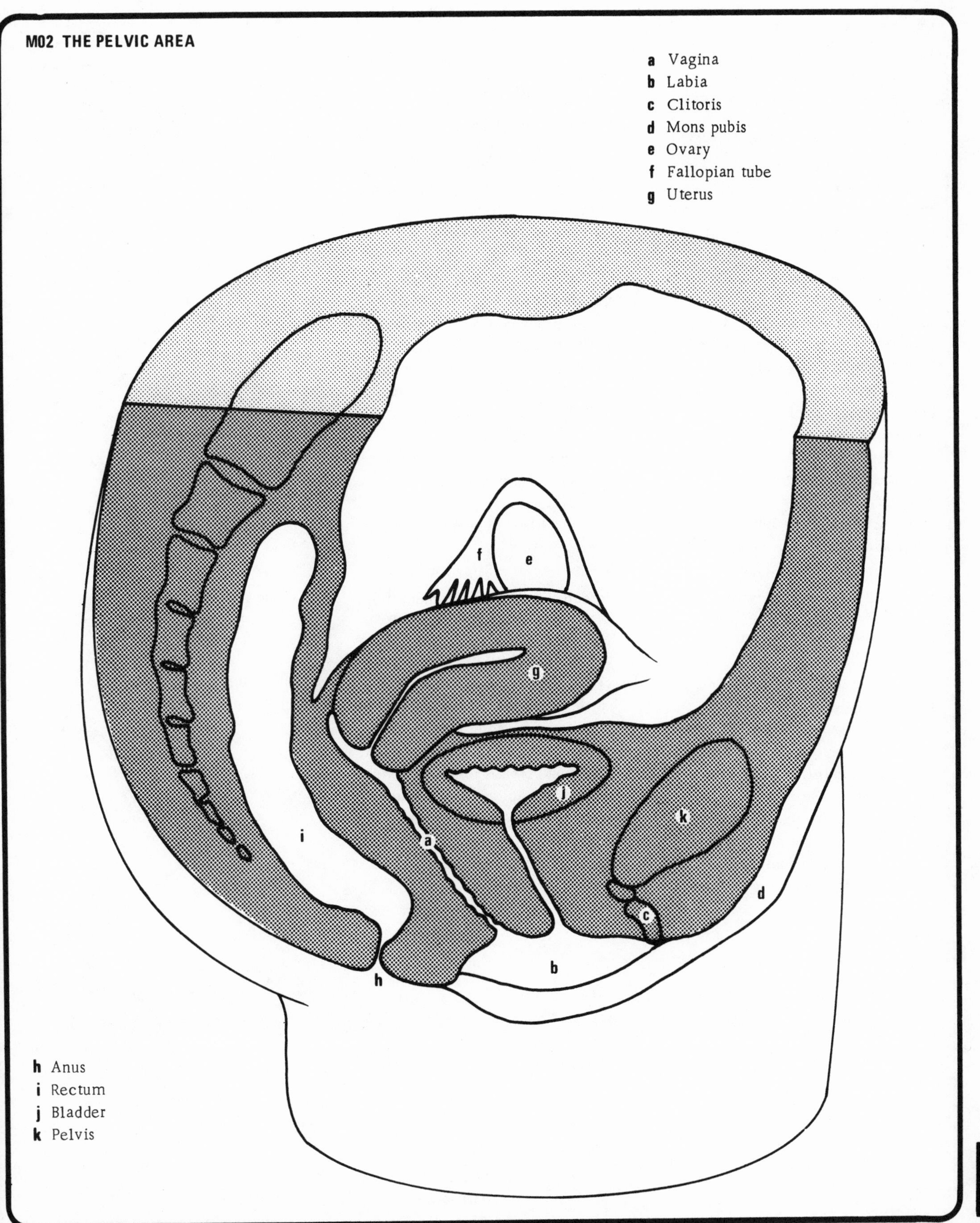
M02 THE PELVIC AREA
a Vagina
b Labia
c Clitoris
d Mons pubis
e Ovary
f Fallopian tube
g Uterus
h Anus
i Rectum
j Bladder
k Pelvis
a
b
c
d
e
f
g
h
i
j
k

M03 BASIC SEX PROCESS

Ideally, the sexual process takes a woman's sexual system from its normal, inactive state to orgasm. Her responses can be divided into the same four distinct stages as in men, and they come about for the same two simple reasons: muscular tension, and the swelling of certain tissues with blood. The patterns of heartbeat, blood pressure and breathing are also very similar.

EXCITEMENT PHASE The vagina becomes lubricated, as moisture "sweats" through its walls. The clitoris lengthens. Breast nipples become erect, swollen and sensitive. Later the breasts themselves swell, and also the areolas (the dark rings around the nipples). The labia majora open and spread flat. The labia minora swell and extend outwards. The inner $\frac{2}{3}$ of the vagina expands, and the uterus moves up away from it. (This occurs whether or not the penis has yet entered the vagina.)

Parts of the body may flush darker in color.

PLATEAU PHASE Swelling of nipples and areolas, expansion of vagina, and lifting of uterus, all continue. The clitoris shortens and lifts, may disappear under its hood, and in any case often becomes too sensitive for direct touch. The outer $\frac{1}{3}$ of the vagina contracts, gripping the penis. The labia majora may swell further. The labia minora change color, from pink to bright red, or, in a woman who has had children, from bright red to deep wine color; this is a certain sign that orgasm will occur within 1 to $1\frac{1}{2}$ minutes if stimulation continues.

ORGASM The outer $\frac{1}{3}$ of the vagina contracts rhythmically, 3 to 5 times in a mild orgasm, 8 to 12 times in an intense one, beginning with one contraction every 0.8 seconds and tapering off. The uterus also contracts rhythmically, and muscular spasms close the anus and distort the face. There is no fluid ejaculation.

RESOLUTION Three things happen very rapidly:

a) the areolas subside, so the nipples are more prominent (this is one sign that there has been an orgasm);

b) any body flush vanishes;

c) a film of perspiration appears on the soles and palms, and sometimes over the whole body.

More slowly, the clitoris, vagina, uterus and breasts return to normal shape, size and position. There is muscular and psychological relaxation. After half an hour the body has returned to its unstimulated state.

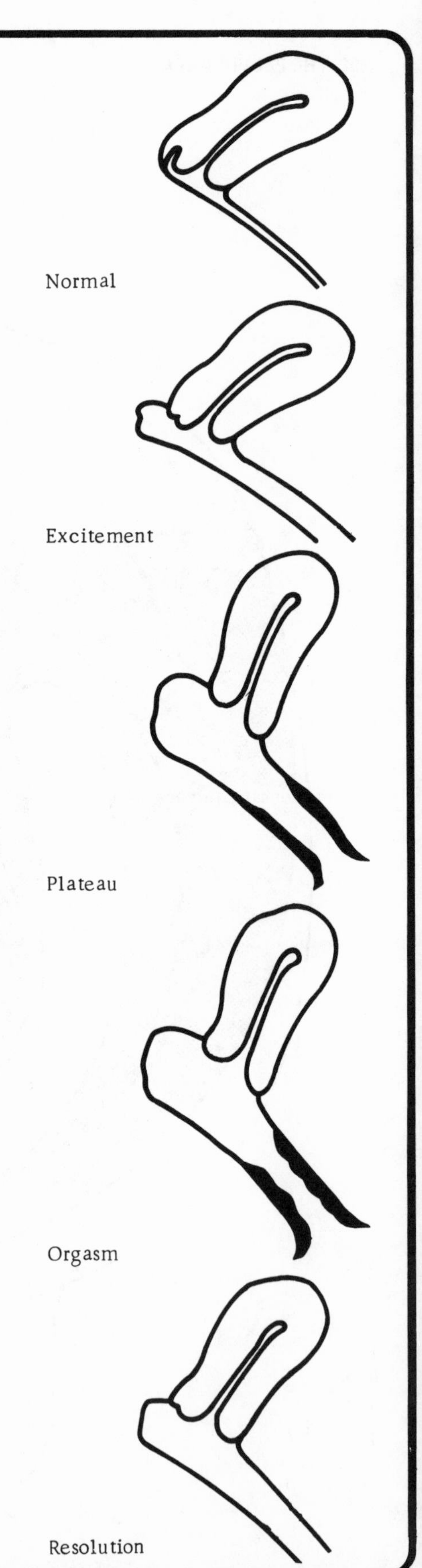

Internal sex organs during sexual process

M04 ORGASM

EXPERIENCE OF ORGASM

Probably all women are capable of orgasm. Few, though, expect to experience orgasm every time they make love, and some never do so at all (in fact, 1 in 14 women, in a recent survey). Yet others can experience many more orgasms that their male partners when making love; and, from 20 to 35, a woman's capability rises with age.

Absence of orgasm can occur for many reasons, temporary and permanent, to do with circumstances, partners, and basic feelings, and fears, conscious or unconscious, about sex and life. In the long term it almost inevitably creates psychic tension. Individual incidents may cause dissatisfaction and irritability - but it seems a woman can sometimes derive sufficient physical or emotional satisfaction from the sensation of the man ejaculating into her vagina.

REACHING ORGASM

Women vary greatly in what they respond to sexually. Many orgasms are caused by emotion, or awareness of the partner's pleasure, rather than by the direct physical impact of sex. Physically, a woman's responsiveness is often linked diffusely with sensations throughout her body; but the vaginal entrance, labia minora, clitoris, prepuce, and mons pubis are almost always important. In intercourse the penis normally stimulates all these as a unit. Other areas of especially erotic sensation can include the anus, the area between anus and genitals, and often, but not always, the breasts (all these are often important in men too).

The special role of the clitoris is confirmed by female masturbation and lesbian techniques. But a woman who has had her clitoris surgically removed can still experience orgasm, if she did before. Moreover, direct stimulation of the clitoris can often be less pleasurable to a woman than general manipulation of the genital area and mons pubis.

The time needed to reach orgasm varies from woman to woman and occasion to occasion. In masturbation, a woman can reach orgasm as rapidly as a man; in intercourse, she is usually slower. In fact, achievement of orgasm in women is closely related to the duration of intercourse, and of foreplay. One survey found that 95% of women had orgasm if intercourse continued for over 16 minutes, and 92% if foreplay continued for over 20 minutes.

REPEATED ORGASM

After a man's orgasm there is always a "refractory period", in which he cannot reach orgasm again. This is not true for a woman: she can have another orgasm immediately if stimulation continues. Some women can experience 3 or 5 within a few minutes, and 10 to 12 in an hour have been recorded. In the more extreme cases, the woman returns directly to the plateau level of arousal after orgasm; she has successive peaks without ever passing through the resolution phase.

THE FEELING OF ORGASM

A man's idea of orgasm is dominated by the experience of ejaculation. For a woman, the main sensations are:

first, a moment of suspense, with acute sensual feeling, usually centered on the clitoris but spreading through the pelvic area;

second, a rapid spread of warmth through the pelvis and the whole body;

third, the sensation of throbbing in the pelvis, as the muscular contraction occurs.

Orgasm is usually followed by feelings of relaxation and peace.

TYPES OF ORGASM?

Women's orgasms vary in intensity, just as men's do. They can be localized tremors, or convulsions of the entire body. Also, different orgasms may seem to be centered on different parts of the genitals. But the distinction between clitoral and vaginal orgasm is a myth. As a bodily process, all orgasms are identical.

Physical intensity of orgasm for a woman is, on average, highest in masturbation, next highest in genital manipulation by a partner, and lowest in sexual intercourse. Men have to hope that some aspects of sexual satisfaction are linked to other things.

M

MENSTRUATION AND CONCEPTION

M05 MENSTRUATION

Around every 28th day, from when she is about 12 to when she is about about 47, a woman - if she is not pregnant, and has not recently had a baby - has a discharge of blood, mucus and cell fragments from her vagina. The discharge, occurring over 2 to 8 days (usually 4 to 6), is more likely to be liquid than clotted, and totals about 2 to 4 tablespoonfuls of blood. The process means that she has to wear pads or tampons (absorbant tubes placed in the vagina) if she wants to stop blood soiling her clothes; and before the days of discharge she may be irritable, and have headaches, tiredness and nausea. All this is menstruation (or "the period") - the outward sign of the routine cycle of egg production and hormone change in a woman's body.

EGG PRODUCTION

Each ovary contains groups of cells called follicles, and these in turn contain immature eggs. When the woman is about 12, these eggs begin to mature, at the rate of one every 28 days or so - usually alternating between the two ovaries. (At birth, a female child's ovaries contain perhaps 350,000 immature eggs. Between puberty and menopause, only 375 ever mature.)

As each egg matures, it bursts from the ovary ("ovulation") and passes into the fallopian tube leading down from that ovary to the uterus.

FERTILIZATION

When a man and woman have sexual intercourse, the man's ejaculation deposits live sperm in the woman's vagina - perhaps 200 million of them. Many of these move up into the uterus, and towards the fallopian tubes, swimming in the semen and the fluid on the uterus' walls. Perhaps 100,000 will enter one fallopian tube - the rest having died, or stayed in the uterus, or taken the wrong tube. If ovulation has just occurred, and there is an egg in the tube, then perhaps 100 may reach it - if they blunder into it (for there is no process of attraction).

If they do meet an egg, the sperms release enzymes to digest its outer layer. One sperm then manages to be first to enter it - and immediately the egg's surface hardens, to prevent more sperms from entering. The nuclei of the egg and sperm unite*, creating a fertilized egg, a single, unique, independent, living cell.

IMPLANTING

This single cell divides several times, as it moves slowly down the fallopian tube. By the time it reaches the uterus, after about 2 to 3 days, it is a hollow ball of over 100 cells. It floats free in the uterus, still increasing in size, until about 7 days after fertilization it sticks itself to the uterus wall. This happens because the wall of the uterus is now ready to receive it - for by about this time in every menstrual cycle, the latest in the succession of hormones has stimulated the uterus to produce a thick lining, into which the young embryo can be "implanted".

MENSTRUATION

But if there are no sperm in the fallopian tubes, when the egg travels down it, then no fertilization occurs. The egg begins to degenerate 24 to 48 hours after leaving the ovary. By the time it has reached the uterus, it is useless.

The egg - a tiny object - passes unnoticed out of the body, in the normal discharge from the vagina. Then the cycle of hormones moves on, and with the next hormone to appear, the wall of the uterus - which was thick, ready for a fertilized egg - degenerates again. So blood and mucus, and bits of discarded cell lining, appear as a discharge: "menstruation".

Only if a fertilized egg gets implanted does the cycle change - but not because the body "knows" what has happened. It is because the developing embryo, once implanted, quickly takes over the job of producing the right hormone, to maintain the thick uterus lining - which will eventually develop into the mother's half of the placenta*, through which the embryo will be fed.

Then the next menstruation does not appear - and the woman can begin to wonder if she is pregnant.

IRREGULARITY

But menstruation can cease for other reasons too. For example, emotional stress may disrupt the proper production of hormones.

Many women sometimes find they miss a menstruation, and then start again. Others find their menstrual cycles are shorter than normal (down to 19 days) or longer (up to 37) or irregular. (Sometimes the contraceptive pill is prescribed to regularize menstruation.)
Also, menstruation does not begin again immediately after a pregnancy. Sometimes - but not always - it does not recommence as long as the mother is breast feeding her child.
Finally, at about the age of 47 (but varying in different women, even from the 30s to the 50s in a few cases), menstruation stops completely ("menopause") because ovulation has stopped: the woman is no longer capable of having children.

DAYS FOR CONCEPTION

The cycle of ovulation and menstruation means that a woman can calculate when it is possible for her to conceive a child. About 14 days after her last menstruation, a new egg will have ovulated - and about 2 days after that it will have degenerated. Allowing for the time a sperm can survive in her reproductive tract (perhaps even up to 4 days in rare cases), and - especially - for variations in the exact date of ovulation, this gives her a period of up to 10 days, in which conception can occur, beginning on the 9th day after the last menstruation. It also gives her a "safe" period outside of that, if she does not want to conceive. However, the more irregular the cycle, the more uncertain such prediction is: see K18-20.

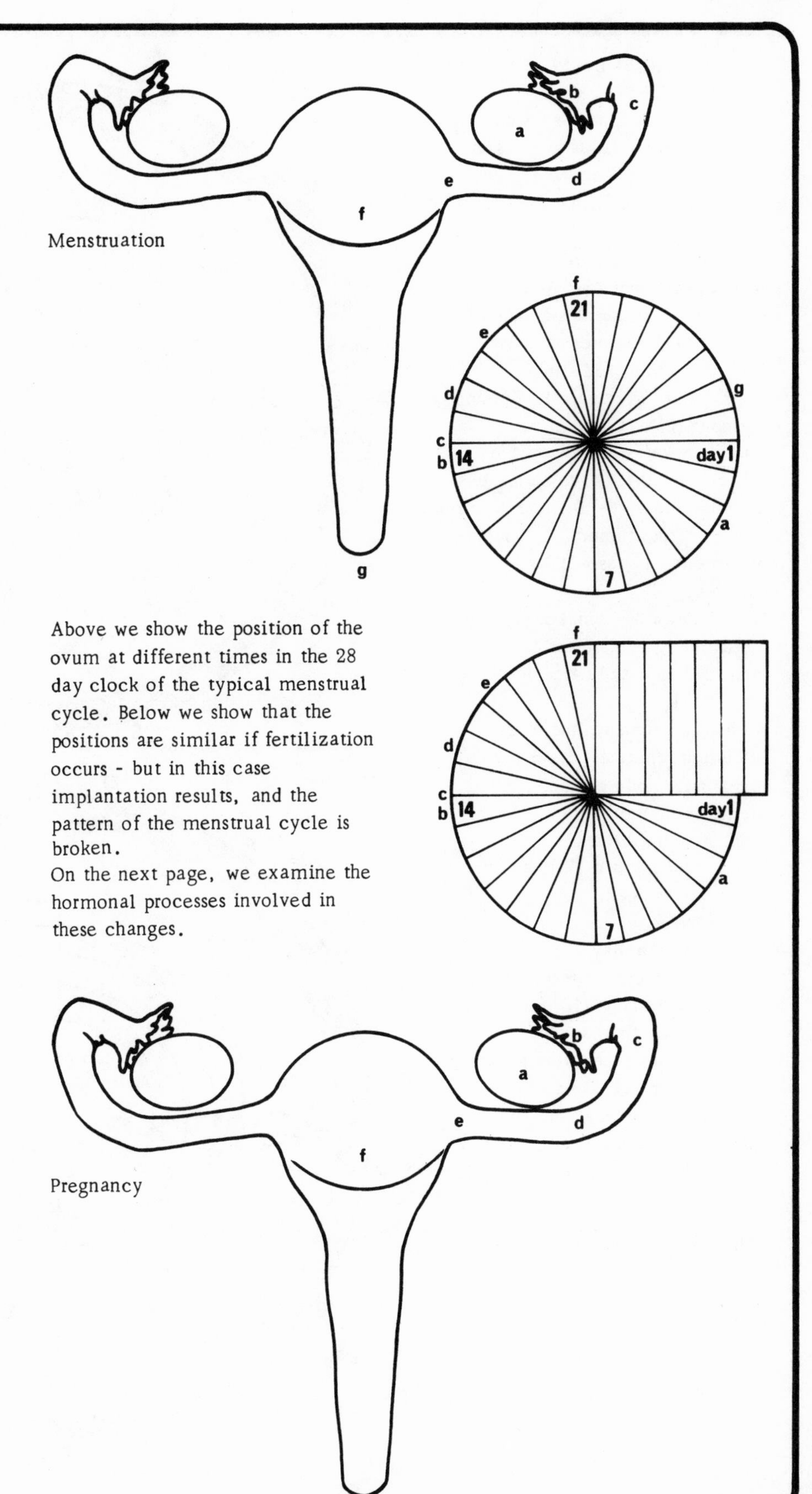

Above we show the position of the ovum at different times in the 28 day clock of the typical menstrual cycle. Below we show that the positions are similar if fertilization occurs - but in this case implantation results, and the pattern of the menstrual cycle is broken.
On the next page, we examine the hormonal processes involved in these changes.

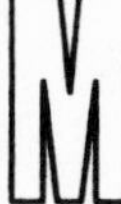

M06 MENSTRUAL CYCLE

NORMAL MENSTRUAL CYCLE

Day 1 onwards: pituitary is already producing the follicle stimulating hormone (FSH) - a new egg begins to mature in one of the follicles (a).

Day 4 onwards: the follicle produces estrogen (E). As this builds up it: stimulates growth of uterus lining and breasts; halts FSH production; and stimulates the pituitary to release luteinizing hormone (LH).

Day 12 onwards: LH causes the follicle to burst, (b) releasing the egg; and makes the follicle develop into a "corpus luteum", producing progesterone (P) as well as estrogen.

Day 14 onwards: P makes the uterus lining prepare for a fertilized egg; and halts LH production.

Without LH support, the corpus luteum degenerates (c), E and P levels fall, and eventually the uterus lining breaks up - menstruation (day 28).

E no longer inhibits FSH, and the cycle begins again.

PREGNANCY

As before up to day 21.

Day 22 onwards: the fertilized egg secretes a hormone (H) resembling FSH and LH. This prevents the corpus luteum degenerating - it goes on secreting E and P, preventing menstruation.

The corpus luteum lasts for 2 to 3 months, till its hormonal function is taken over by the placenta.

FSH Follicle stimulating hormone
E Estrogen
LH Luteinizing hormone
P Progesterone
H Hormone from fertilized egg

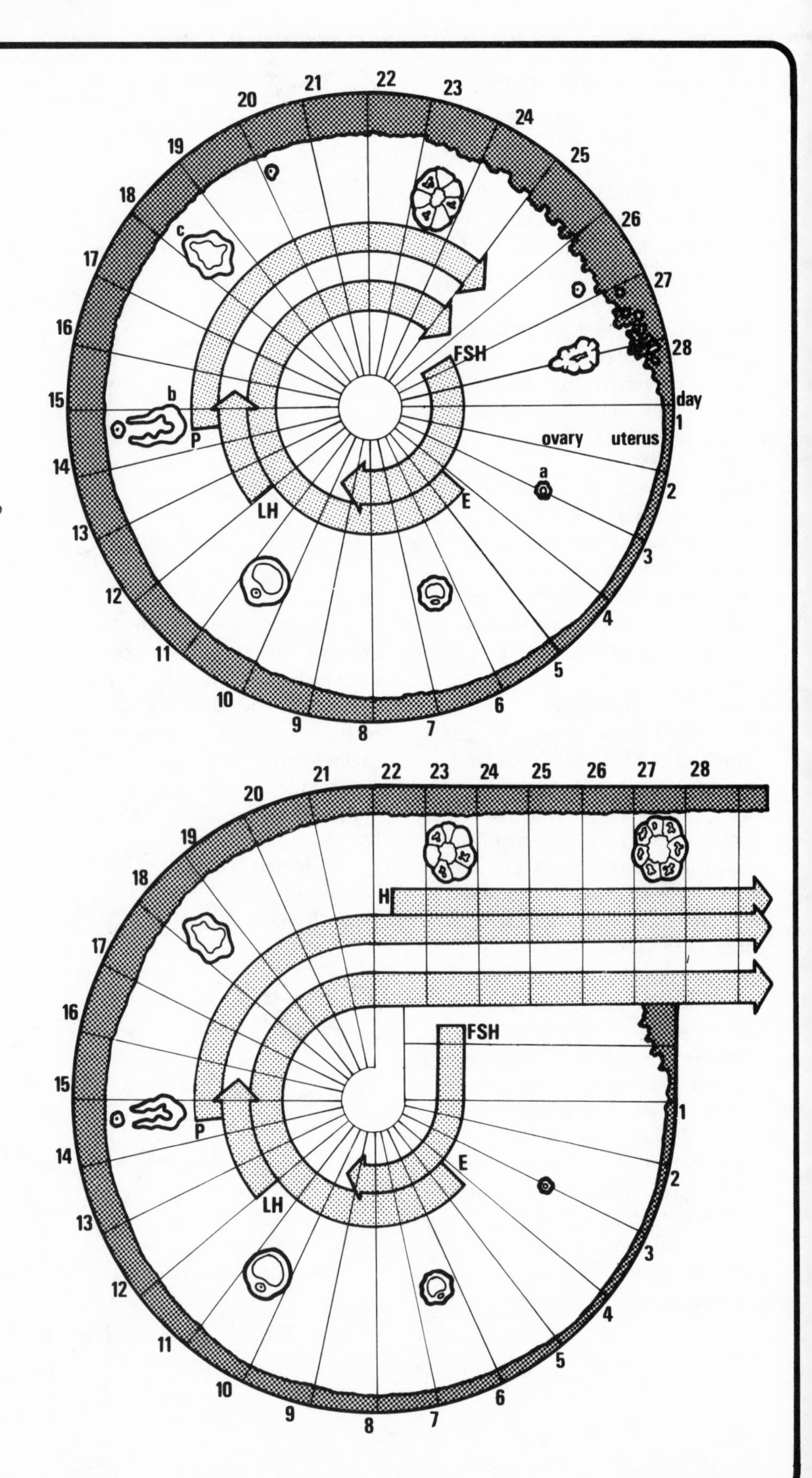

M07 PUBERTY

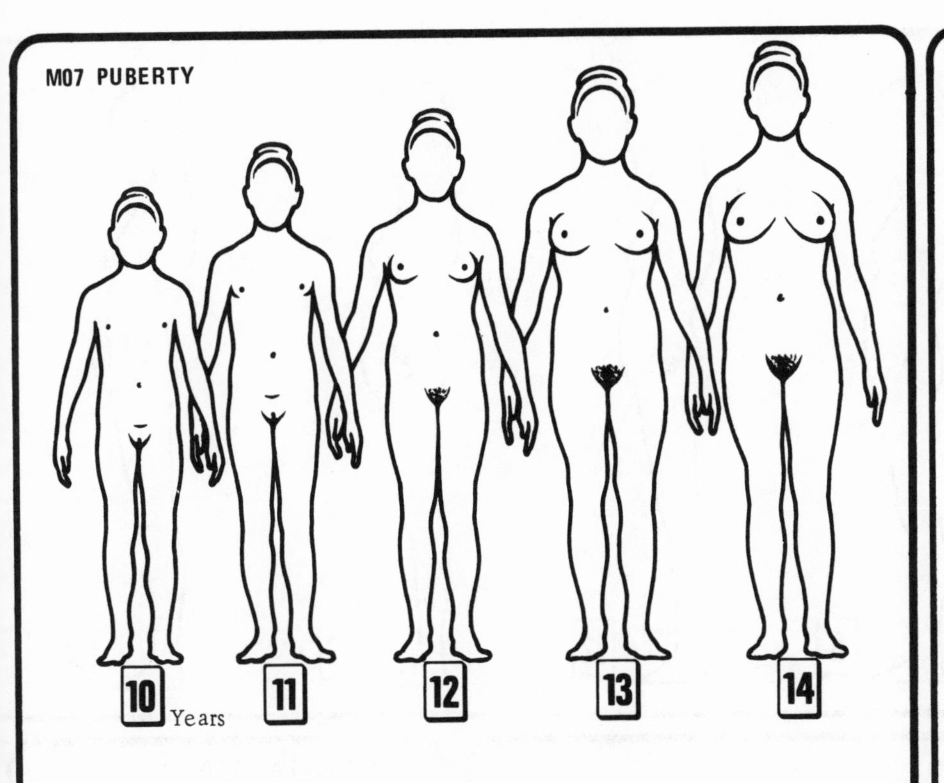

As in boys, puberty shows the impact of changes in hormone production.

TIMING

The changes of puberty usually start earlier in girls than in boys. The typical age is 11 rather than 12. (It can begin, quite normally, as early as 7 - or as late as 15.) More important, the changes happen more rapidly and more simultaneously. They are spread over only about $2\frac{1}{2}$ to 3 years, rather than 4 or more, and have already reached a peak between $11\frac{1}{2}$ and 12. For all these reasons, girls mature earlier. An average girl, 1in shorter than an average boy at 9 years, is $\frac{1}{2}$in taller than him at 12 - but her growth stops at about 16.

SEQUENCE

There is even more variation in the sequence of events than in boys. But four things do tend to happen in set order:

1) the hip bone widens;
2) the nipples, and then the breasts, begin to grow;
3) the sex organs, both internal and external, start to enlarge; and
4) menstruation occurs.

The other main events, jumbled in with these, are:

a) a rapid increase in body height and weight (the "adolescent spurt");
b) growth of pubic hair and hair in the armpits; and
c) laying down of fat on the thighs, breasts, hips and buttocks, further changing body shape.

M08 HORMONAL MECHANISMS

PUBERTY

As in boys, at puberty hormones produced outside the sex organs trigger off production of another hormone in the sex organs themselves. Also the trigger hormones are the same as in boys: FSH and LH, produced by the pituitary gland. FSH stimulates growth of ovaries and follicles, and, with LH, sets off estrogen production. The estrogen then causes the growth sequence involving hip bone, breasts and sex organs. Finally, all three hormones are involved in the rhythms of the menstrual cycle. In addition, there is in girls a second, "masculinizing" hormone, released from the adrenal gland under stimulation from the pituitary. This causes growth of body hair, and certain changes in the external genitals.

MENOPAUSE

In middle age, the FSH level falls and the LH level rises: the follicles are less stimulated, and ovary hormone production falls. This causes irregular and infrequent ovulation, and reduced progesterone production, resulting in menstrual irregularities. Later, as the ovaries responsiveness to hormones declines, estrogen production falls. This disturbs the hormone feedback mechanism, so FSH increases to a very high level. But this fails to stimulate the aging ovaries. The remaining follicles decay, and estrogen level goes on falling until menstruation finally ceases (the menopause).

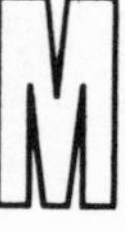

M09 PREGNANCY

HOME PREGNANCY TESTS

Since 1978, a woman using a simple kit has been able to perform a pregnancy test at home about nine days after she expected her period to begin. The results of the first test are about 97% accurate if the result is positive, and about 80% accurate if the result is negative. If the result is negative and woman does not begin menstruating in a week, she should repeat the test or make an appointment with her physician. The kits are readily available in most pharmacies without a prescription for as little as $10 to $12. Each kit can be used only once. The procedure is simple.

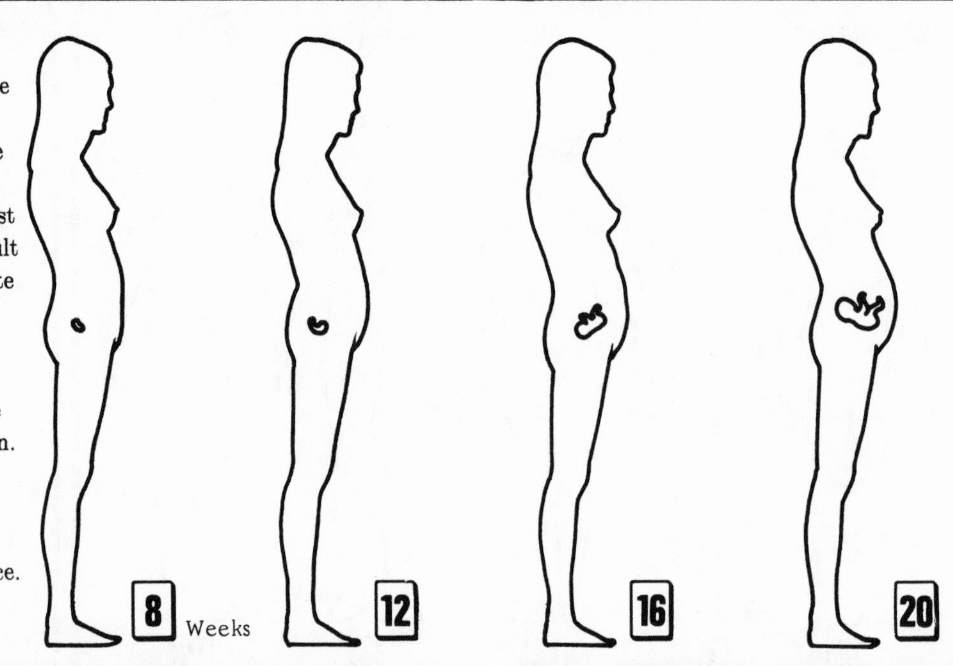

M10 SIGNS AND SYMPTOMS

Menstruation ceases (though this can, of course, happen for other reasons).

About ⅔ of women experience "morning sickness", from the date of the first missed period until the second or third month after conception. Sometimes there is only nausea, but often vomiting too.

The woman begins to tire more easily and sleep longer.

Pressure of the uterus on the bladder makes urination more frequent.

The breasts first itch and tingle, then become enlarged and sensitive. Eventually they start to secrete a thin fluid from the nipples.

After the third month the fetus is large enough for the abdomen to show signs of swelling, as the uterus extends beyond the pelvis.

The face, the external genitals, and the areolas* of the breasts all darken, and a dark line may appear running downwards from the navel. Also the veins in the breasts become visible.

Appetite and liquid intake often increase. There may be cravings for certain foods.

The mother's weight increases - eventually, on average, by 27½ lbs. Her posture changes, as she has to lean back to balance the baby's weight. Eventually she may have to walk with a waddling movement, with her legs slightly apart.

Between the fourth and fifth month, "quickening" occurs i.e. the mother feels for the first time the movements of the fetus.

From the fifth month of pregnancy on, the heartbeat of the fetus can be heard with a stethoscope, and the fetus can be seen to move from the outside.

Common difficulties can include: more serious morning sickness; constipation and diarrhoea; hemorroids; varicose veins; and, eventually, continual weariness.

Incidentally, sexual intercourse is usually not advisable in late pregnancy (the 32nd week can be used as a guide, but there is no general rule).

M11 THE PLACENTA

The baby grows inside a bag made of membrane and filled with fluid. It is linked to the mother by the umbilical cord - a tube carrying blood vessels.

Where the cord reaches the wall of the uterus, is the placenta - a "frontier custom's post", through which oxygen and nutrients pass from the mother's blood supply to the baby's, while carbon dioxide and other waste products pass in the other direction to be carried away. The two blood supplies do not mix. Already, by the second week after conception, the embryo's own blood supply is being pumped around by a tiny primitive heart.

The bag surrounding the baby, and the baby's side of the placenta, grow from the cells of the fertilized egg.

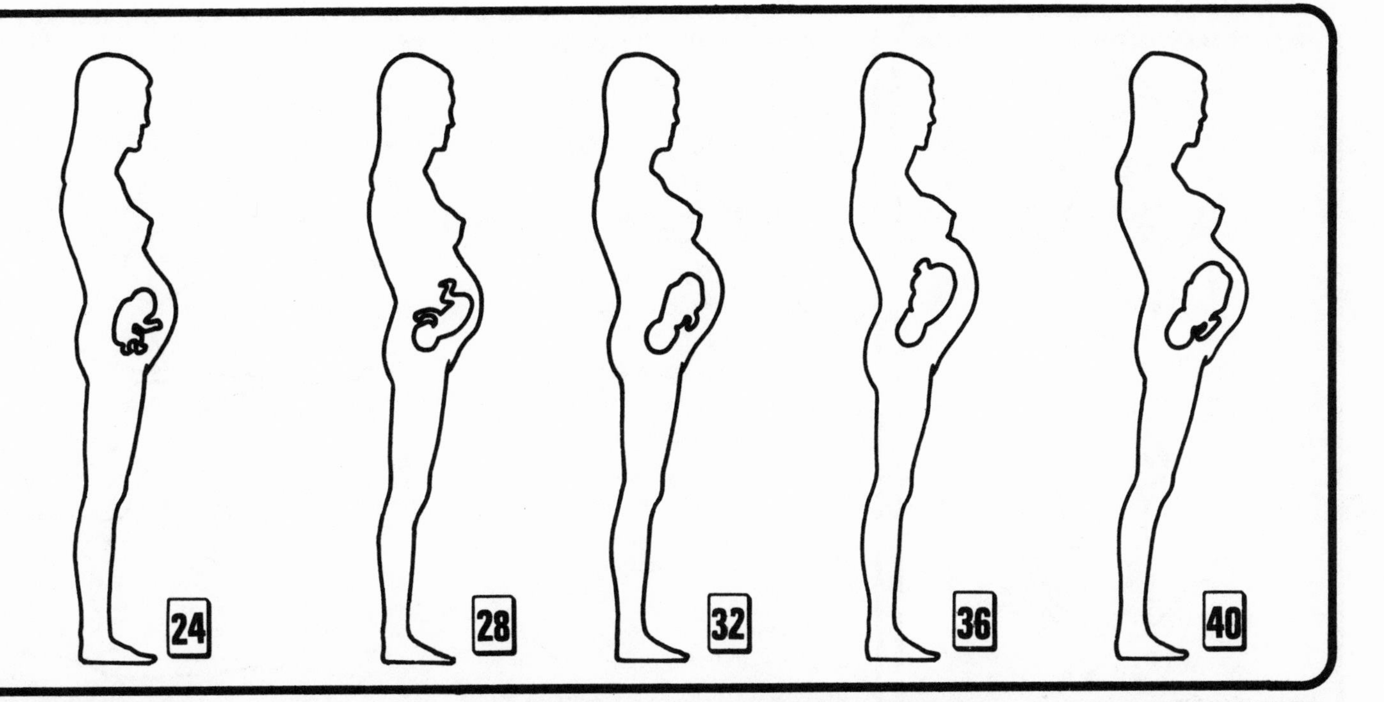

M12 THE BREASTS

The female breasts, which start to develop just before puberty, consist mainly of the fat which gives them their shape, and muscle and connective tissue. But each breast also contains a number of milk ducts, running back from the nipple and branching out into clusters of small glands, grouped in 12 to 20 different compartments.
During pregnancy the breasts enlarge steadily, starting at an early date. Eventually a thin yellowish fluid seeps from the nipples. Shortly after the baby's birth, milk production can begin in most women. The ability disappears if the baby is not fed from the breast; but, if it is, milk production in some women can go on almost indefinitely (hence the "wet nurses" in traditional society, who hired out their ability to produce milk).
In most human societies, the baby is taken off a milk diet (weaning) at about 7 to 9 months.

M13 MISCARRIAGE AND ABORTION

MISCARRIAGE
Called medically a spontaneous premature termination, miscarriage occurs most often at the 6th or 10th week of pregnancy. It is due to major abnormality in the fetus, death of the fetus, hormonal failure, or defect in the uterus. The fetus detaches from the uterus, and passes out of the mother's body. Perhaps 1 in 10 pregnancies end this way.
ABORTION
Medically, any termination before the 28th week is called an abortion; but in popular use this means deliberate destruction of the fetus. Possible reasons for abortion include:
danger tc the mother's life if pregnancy continues;
or, similarly, danger to the mother's physical health;
or, danger to her mental health;
or likelihood that the baby will suffer from mental or physical abnormalities (as when the mother has contracted german measles in the 2nd or 3rd month of pregnancy); or simply the desire of the mother not to have a baby. Which reasons are legally accepted varies greatly from country to country, and depends partly on interpretation, (for example, whether any unmarried pregnancy is seen as threatening the mother's mental health).
In the USA the situation varies from state to state. In 1967 in the UK there were 5 legal abortions abortions per 100 live births, in Sweden 7.9, Poland 32, Japan 38.5, Czechoslovakia 44, and Hungary 126, i.e. more abortions than live births.
Legal abortion is preferably only carried out in the first three months of pregnancy.
ECTOPIC PREGNANCY
Sometimes the fertilized egg implants itself elsewhere than the center of the uterus. If so, complications occur and abortion is usually necessary. Possible sites for implantation are the fallopian tubes (most common), the bottom end of the uterus (very rare), the ovary itself, and even within the abdomen.

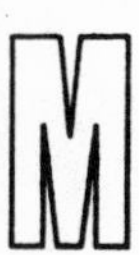

M14 FETAL POSITIONS

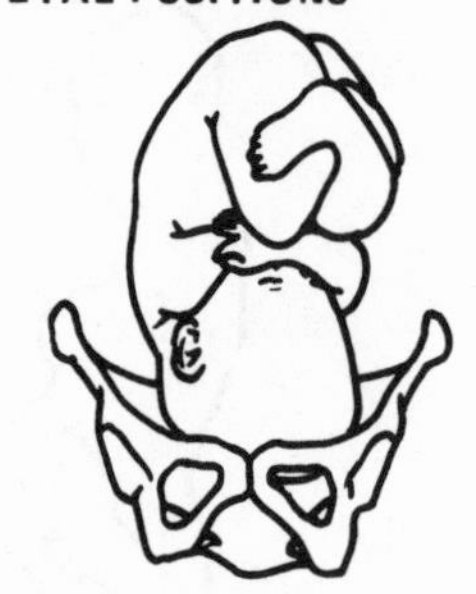

Vertex: head down, 95%

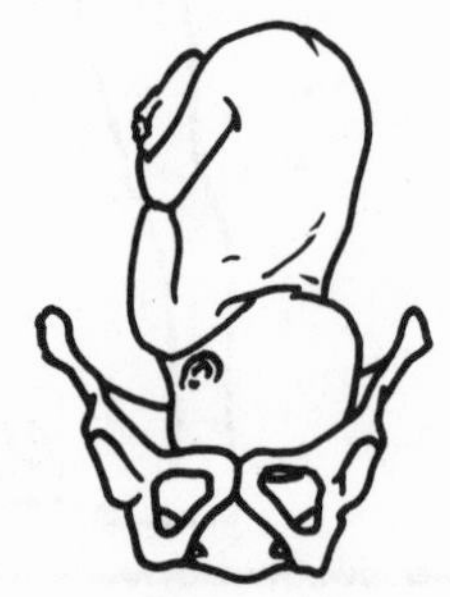

Vertex: face down, 0.5%

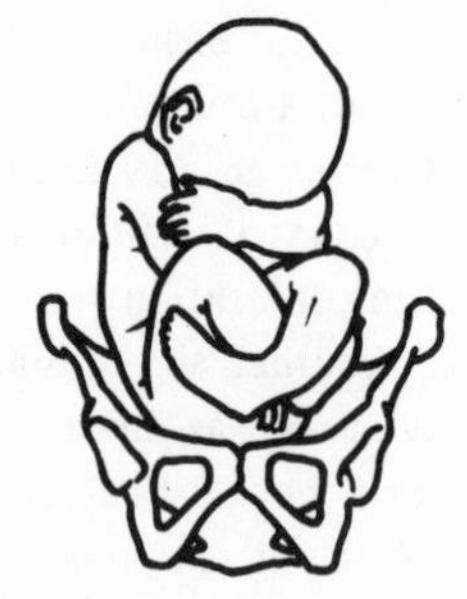

Breech, 3.5%

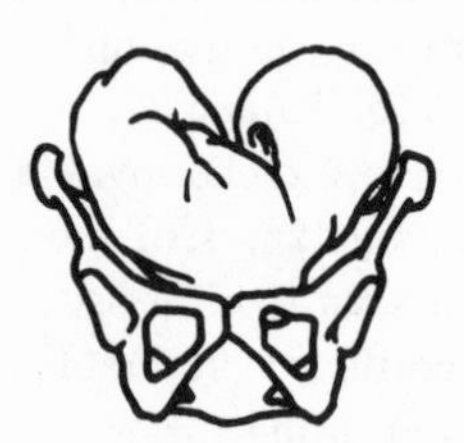

Transverse, 1.0%

These are the positions in which the baby can lie in the mother's womb just before labor begins. The face down position may cause remolding of the skull. A transverse lie can usually be manipulated into another position; uncorrected, it requires a cesarian birth.

M15 LABOR AND DELIVERY

Birth occurs about 38 weeks after fertilization. "Labor" is the process by which a woman's muscles contract and force the baby out of her body.

a) Labor contractions begin. They grow in regularity from every 20-30 minutes to every 3-5 minutes, and in intensity until each may last up to 1 minute. Discomfort begins in the small of the back and moves round to the front of the abdomen. This stage loosens and stretches the cervix.

b) The baby's head passes through the cervix. Contractions occur every 2-3 minutes, and last up to 100 seconds. The mother "bears down" with her muscles to help move the baby. There may be a tightening feeling and a low backache. A small plug of mucous slightly marked with blood may slide out of the vagina.

c) Contractions and the use of voluntary muscles continue. The baby's head rotates 90° to squeeze through the pelvis. The bag of fluid around the baby bursts, giving a water discharge.

d) The baby's head is born, and rotates back to its previous position. The baby's shoulders begin to rotate to pass through the pelvis.

e) The rest of the body is born. The baby breathes spontaneously or is helped by slapping. The umbilical cord is tied and cut. Within 20 minutes after this the placenta, womb membranes, and remaining fluid have been expelled as "afterbirth."

Stage a) lasts usually between 6 and 24 hours: 13 hours, on average, for a woman's first birth, and 7 for subsequent ones.
Stages b) to e) usually last 1 hour for a first birth and ½ hour for a subsequent one.

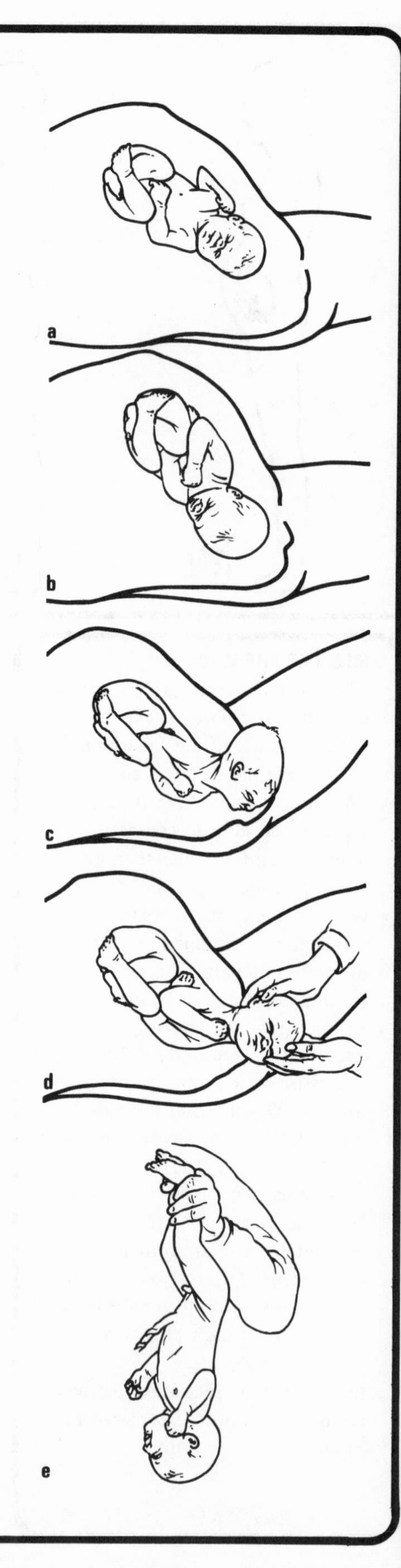

M16 PREMATURE BIRTH

Premature birth occurs when the fetus is born before it is fully grown. A baby weighing less than 2,500gm is defined as premature; but more significant is any underdevelopment of its internal organs. This reduces its chances of survival, though babies born as early as their 24th week have been known to live.

About 5-9% of births are premature. Causes, where understood, include high blood pressure or diabetes in the mother, and multiple pregnancy. Most premature babies eventually catch up in size and development.

M17 MULTIPLE PREGNANCY

Multiple pregnancy can occur either from the fertilization of two or more ova, or from the division of a single ovum. In the first case there is a placenta for each baby (a); in the second, only one, shared between them (b).

On average, twins occur about once in 85 births, triplets 1 in 7500, quadruplets 1 in 650,000, and quintuplets 1 in 57 million But these ratios vary greatly from country to country.

In multiple birth, labor begins earlier and takes longer. The death rate among mothers is 2-3 times greater. In 1 in 14 twin births, one twin dies, and with larger multiple births the likelihood of death rises steeply.

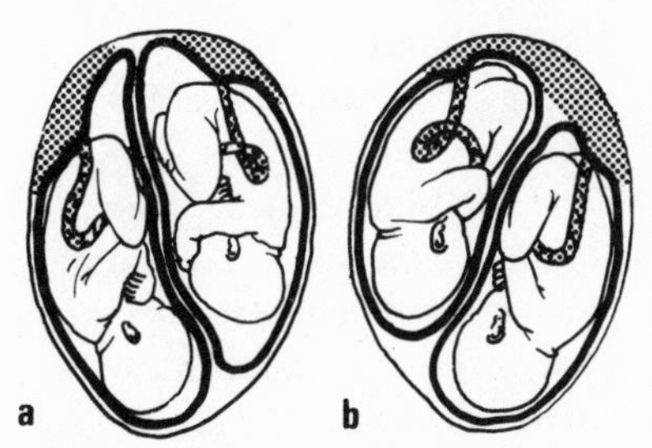

Multiple births need not occur together - the record for twins is a month between their appearance!

Positions of twins in the womb: both in vertex position, 30-45% of cases; one vertex, one breech, 35-40%; both breech, 8-12%; one vertex, one transverse, 4-12%.

M18 INDUCED LABOR

Labor is artificially induced if the health or life of the mother or baby is in danger, eg if the mother has high blood pressure, or rhesus blood conflict with the baby; or if the fetus has died or is overmature. Induction is rarely done before the 35th week of pregnancy.

Techniques include injection to stimulate contraction, rupturing the fetal membranes, or dislodging the membranes from around the cervix.

In some countries births are increasingly induced merely for convenience of timing.

M19 CESARIAN SECTION

Cesarian section is delivery of the baby by an abdominal operation that cuts directly into the mother's womb and removes the fetus.

This may be done to deliver a baby from its dead mother; or to save both mother and child where some difficulty prevents normal birth. Cesarian section is usually needed if the baby is in a transverse position; also if the mother's frame is too small compared with the fetus's size.

One woman in Ireland is said to have had 13 successful cesarian births.

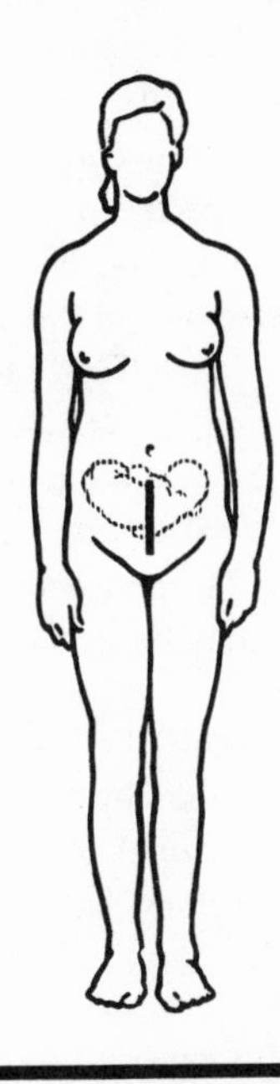

M20 SUDDEN INFANT DEATH SYNDROME

Sudden Infant Death Syndrome, known as SIDS or crib death, affects from 7,500 to 8,000 infants in the United States each year. Usually it strikes an apparently healthy infant between four weeks and seven months old. The child is put to bed, and some time later is found dead. There is often no evidence that the baby struggled. Sometimes the autopsy reveals an inflammation of the upper respiratory tract; sometimes there is no evidence of illness. The disease is not hereditary and has no symptoms.

The National Sudden Infant Death Foundation, Inc. is a national organization with chapters in cities throughout the U.S. It helps parents cope with the tragedy, educates a community, and promotes SIDS research. The organization's headquarters are in Chicago at 310 South Michigan Avenue, Chicago, Ill. 60604. Information from the U.S. Department of Health and Human Services, National Institutes of Health.

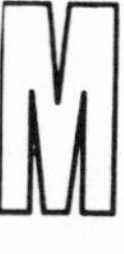

M21 MENSTRUAL DISORDERS

AMENORRHEA is the absence of menstrual periods. (It can date from the beginning of puberty, in which case menstruation never begins.) Causes include anemia, hormone imbalance, congenital defects of the genitals, tumors or cysts, excessive dieting, and emotional stress. Absence of periods is normal before puberty, after the menopause, and during pregnancy and breast feeding.

DYSMENORRHEA is menstruation that is uncomfortable or painful. There are two types.

a) Primary or spasmodic. This is linked directly with the uterus: spasmodic pain lasts up to 12 hours after the period starts. Half of all women have some experience of it, especially between the ages of 18 and 24, but it usually disappears after childbirth or if the contraceptive pill is used.

b) Secondary or congestive. This occurs before the period begins - usually a few days before. There is a dull aching in the abdomen and lower back, and often also constipation, headache, irritability, lethargy, and depression. The symptoms usually end when the period occurs. The problem may be due to a hormone imbalance.

OTHER DISORDERS include: excessive bleeding at periods; abnormal vaginal bleeding between periods; and abnormal vaginal discharges caused by infection.

EARLY MENOPAUSE The menstrual cycle usually ceases in the late 40s, but can stop earlier. Causes are unknown, but possibilities include: frequent abortions and miscarriages; prolonged nursing of a baby; too many babies in succession; very poor general health, overproduction of the thyroid gland, coupled with serious obesity; and others.

M22 THE WOMB

PROLAPSE OF THE WOMB is a not uncommon condition, in which the uterus sags down into the vagina, and may even protrude out between the legs. The symptoms include frequent and difficult urination; incontinence; low backache; a feeling that something is coming out of the vagina; and, especially, that all the above symptoms immediately disappear on lying down.

The condition is produced by weakening of muscles that support the uterus.

The cause is usually damage done in childbirth, though the symptoms do not appear till later; but aging and heavy physical activity can also contribute. The necessary operation is safe and normally successful.

HYSTERECTOMY is the surgical removal of the uterus, or of all the reproductive organs ("total hysterectomy"). It can be carried out via the vagina or the abdomen. Total hysterectomy is followed by the usual symptoms of menopause, unless hormone treatment is prescribed. Most hysterectomies are performed because fibroids are growing in the uterus. These are benign tumors, but may cause bleeding, and can grow to an enormous size. After hysterectomy, a woman cannot have children, but sexual enjoyment is unaffected.

M23 INFERTILITY

There are many possible causes of female infertility. The most common is failure to ovulate, due to failure in hormone production. This can be due to actual disorders of the hormone mechanism, or it may result from emotional stress and other psychological factors. Hormonal imbalance can also prevent a fertilized egg attaching itself to the wall of the uterus, while emotional stress may also operate directly by setting up spasm in the fallopian tubes and preventing the movement of the egg.

Another group of causes are congenital, including:
deformity of the sex organs (eg in extreme cases, absence of a vagina);
tilting of the cervix, so that the sperm do not normally find their way in;
possession of a hymen or vagina too tight for penetration;
and excessive acidity of the vaginal fluid, so that sperms are immobilized and die.

A third group is linked with other disorders in the sex organs, infection with venereal disease, cystitis, etc;
growth of fibroids, polyps, cysts or cancer;
and the effects of exposure to high doses of radiation.

These can affect the functioning of the ovaries, block the fallopian tubes, etc.

M24 CANCER

Cancers peculiar to women are those of reproductive organs and breast. BREAST CANCER accounts for 20% of all cancer in women. It is not fatal if caught early, but growth is very rapid and may not be noticed immediately, because it is painless. Usually the entire breast and surrounding tissues must be removed - through radiotherapy, drugs, or a more limited operation may be sufficient. (But only a quarter of breast tumors are malignant (see B32).

CANCER OF THE CERVIX occurs in 1% of women (usually between 45 and 50), and half of these die from it; however it is now on the decline. It is associated with general bad health and chronic vaginal and cervical infection. The smegma* of uncircumcised males may be responsible. A routine test (Pap test or cervical smear) can be made for it, once or twice a year being adequate. Treatment of an advanced case may require total hysterectomy.

OTHER REPRODUCTIVE SITES may also require hysterectomy. Cancers of the vagina and vulva are rare, and usually due to spreading cervical cancer. Cancer of the ovaries is also rare, but more often fatal. It can occur at any age, and affect the production of male and female hormones in the body.

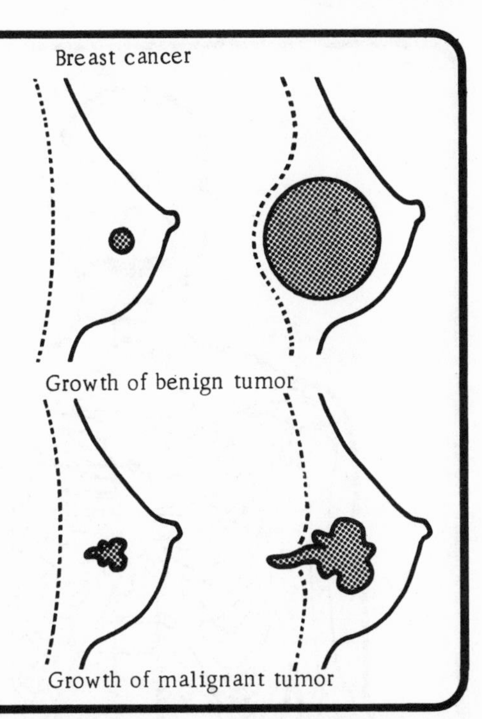

M25 CANCER-RELATED CHECKUP GUIDELINES

Guidelines for the early detection of cancer in women with no symptoms follow. Speak with your doctor about how these guidelines relate to you. Checkups should include the listed procedures plus health counseling (such as tips on quitting cigarettes) and examinations for cancers of the breast, thyroid, mouth, ovaries, skin, and lymph nodes. Some women are at higher risk for certain cancers and may need to have tests more frequently.

Reprinted with permission by the American Cancer Society.

AGE 20-40: CANCER-RELATED CHECKUP EVERY 3 YEARS

BREAST
- Exam by doctor every 3 years.
- Self-exam every month.
- One baseline breast X-ray between ages 35-40.

(Higher Risk for Breast Cancer: Personal or family history of breast cancer, never had children, first child after 30.)

UTERUS
- Pelvic exam every 3 years.
- Cervix: Pap test - after 2 initial negative tests 1 year apart - at least every 3 years, includes women under 20 if sexually active.

(Higher Risk for Cervical Cancer: Early age at first intercourse, multiple sex partners.)

AGE 40 & OVER: CANCER-RELATED CHECKUP EVERY YEAR

BREAST
- Exam by doctor every year.
- Self-exam every month.
- Breast X-ray every year after 50 (between ages 40-50, ask your doctor).

(Higher Risk for Breast Cancer: Personal or family history of breast cancer, never had children, first child after 30.)

UTERUS
- Pelvic exam every year.
- Cervix: Pap test - after 2 initial negative tests 1 year apart - at least every 3 years.

(Higher Risk for Cervical Cancer: Early age at first intercourse, multiple sex partners.)
- Endometrium: Endometrial tissue sample at menopause if at risk.

(Higher Risk for Endometrial Cancer: Infertility, obesity, failure of ovulation, abnormal uterine bleeding, estrogen therapy.)

COLON & RECTUM
- Digital rectal exam every year.
- Guaiac slide test every year after 50.

(Higher Risk for Colorectal Cancer: Personal or family history of colon or rectal cancer, personal or family history of polyps in the colon or rectum, ulcerative colitis.)

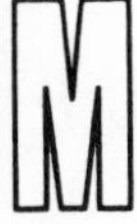

REFERENCE MAN 1

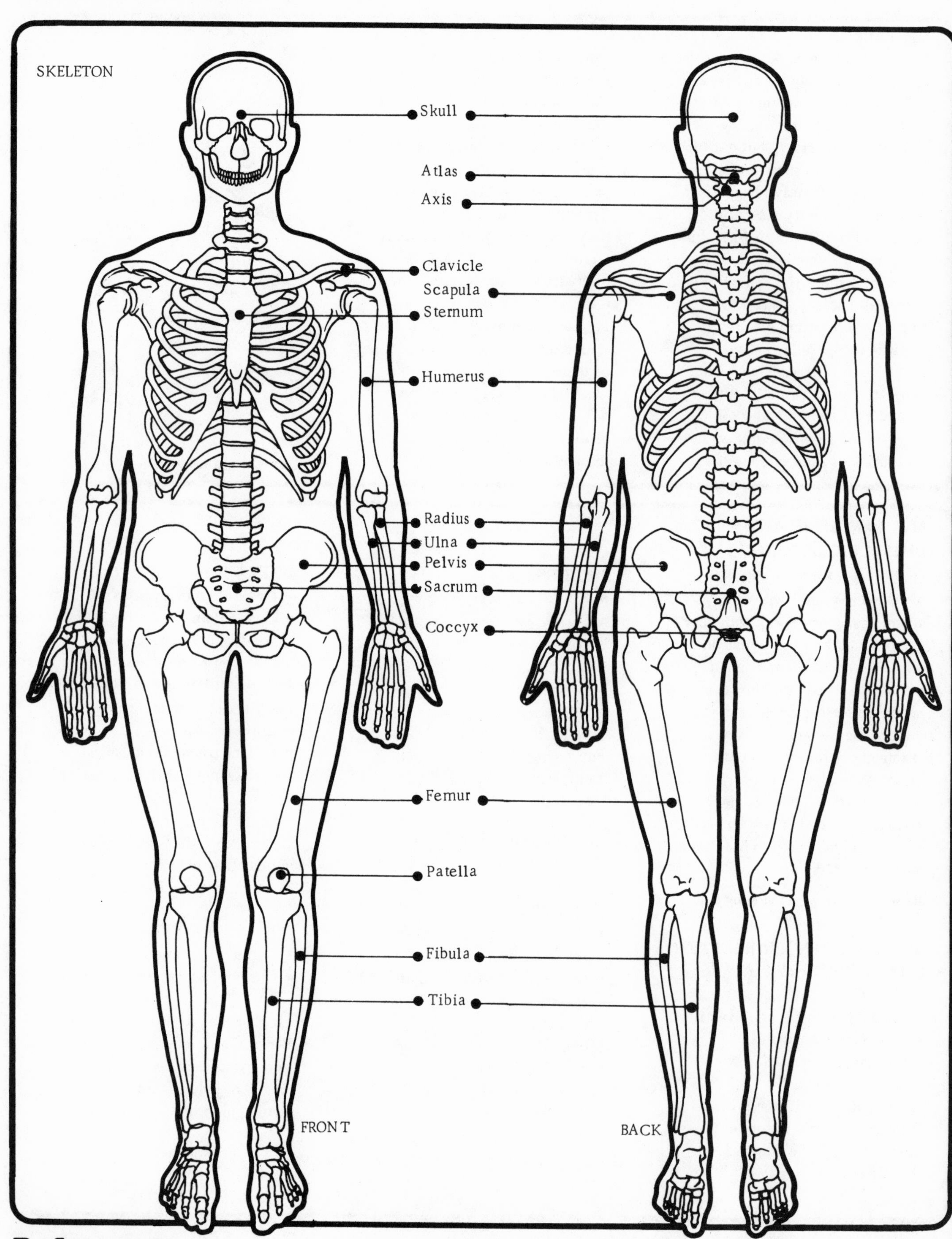

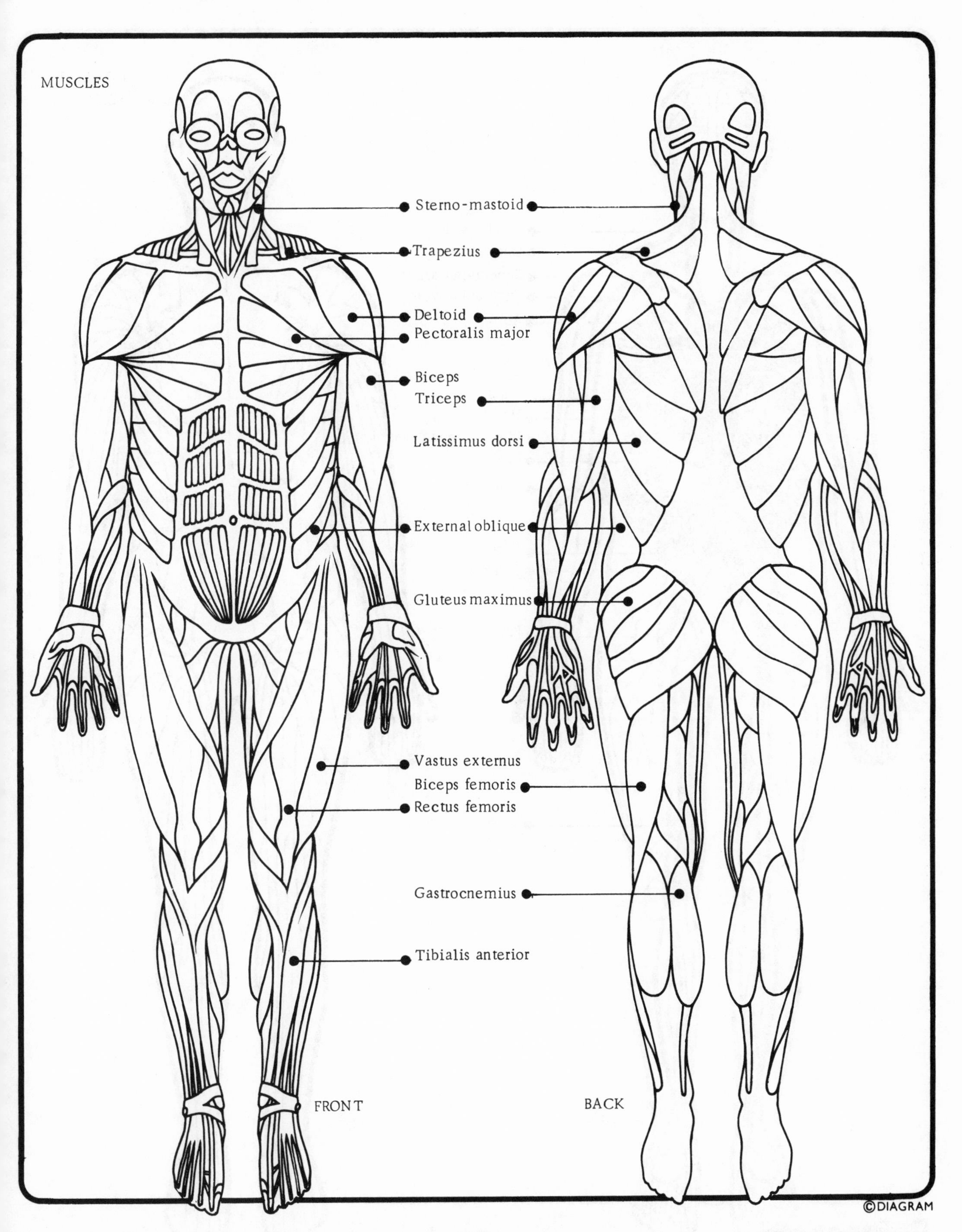
MUSCLES
Sterno-mastoid
Trapezius
Deltoid
Pectoralis major
Biceps
Triceps
Latissimus dorsi
External oblique
Gluteus maximus
Vastus externus
Biceps femoris
Rectus femoris
Gastrocnemius
Tibialis anterior
FRONT
BACK

REFERENCE MAN 2

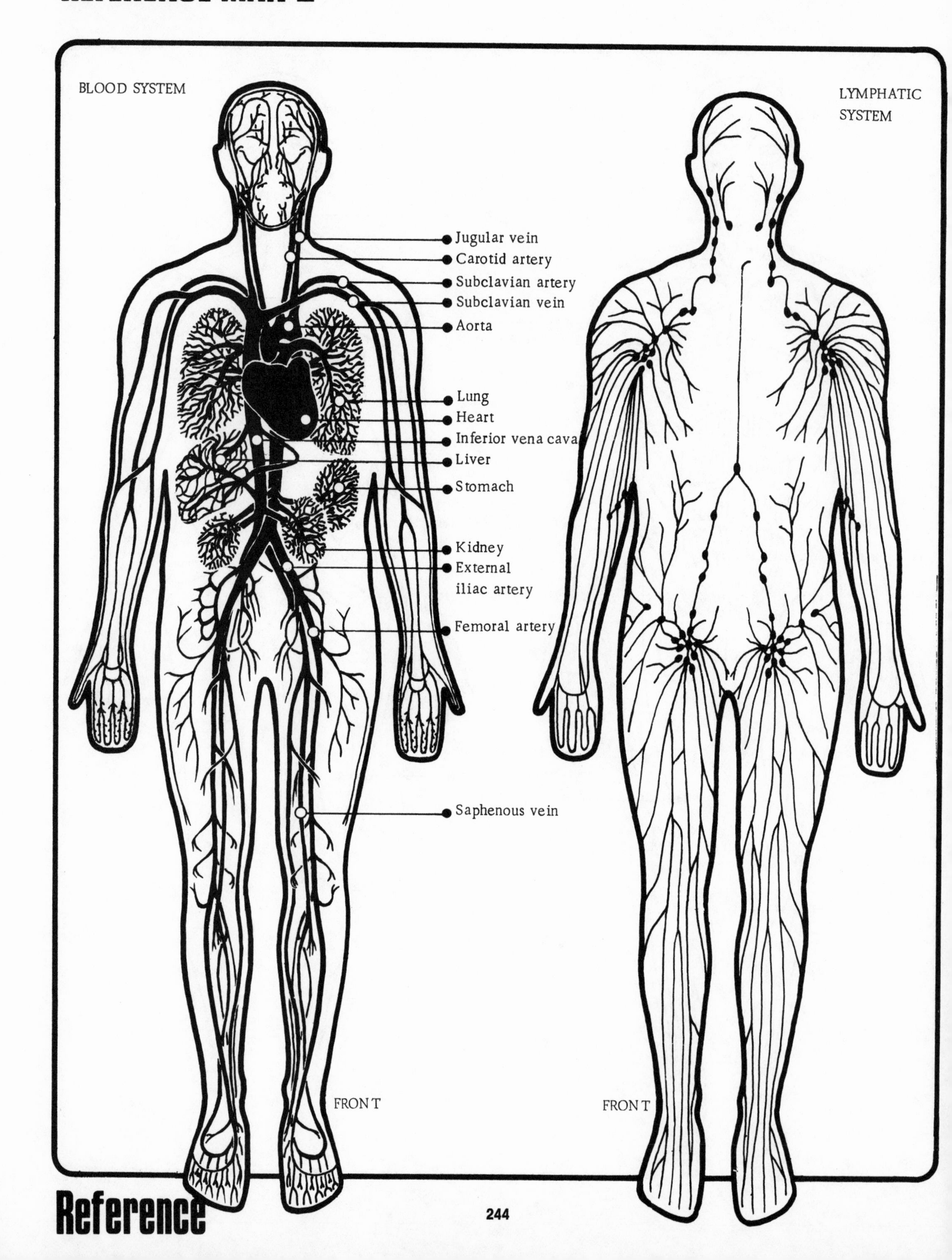

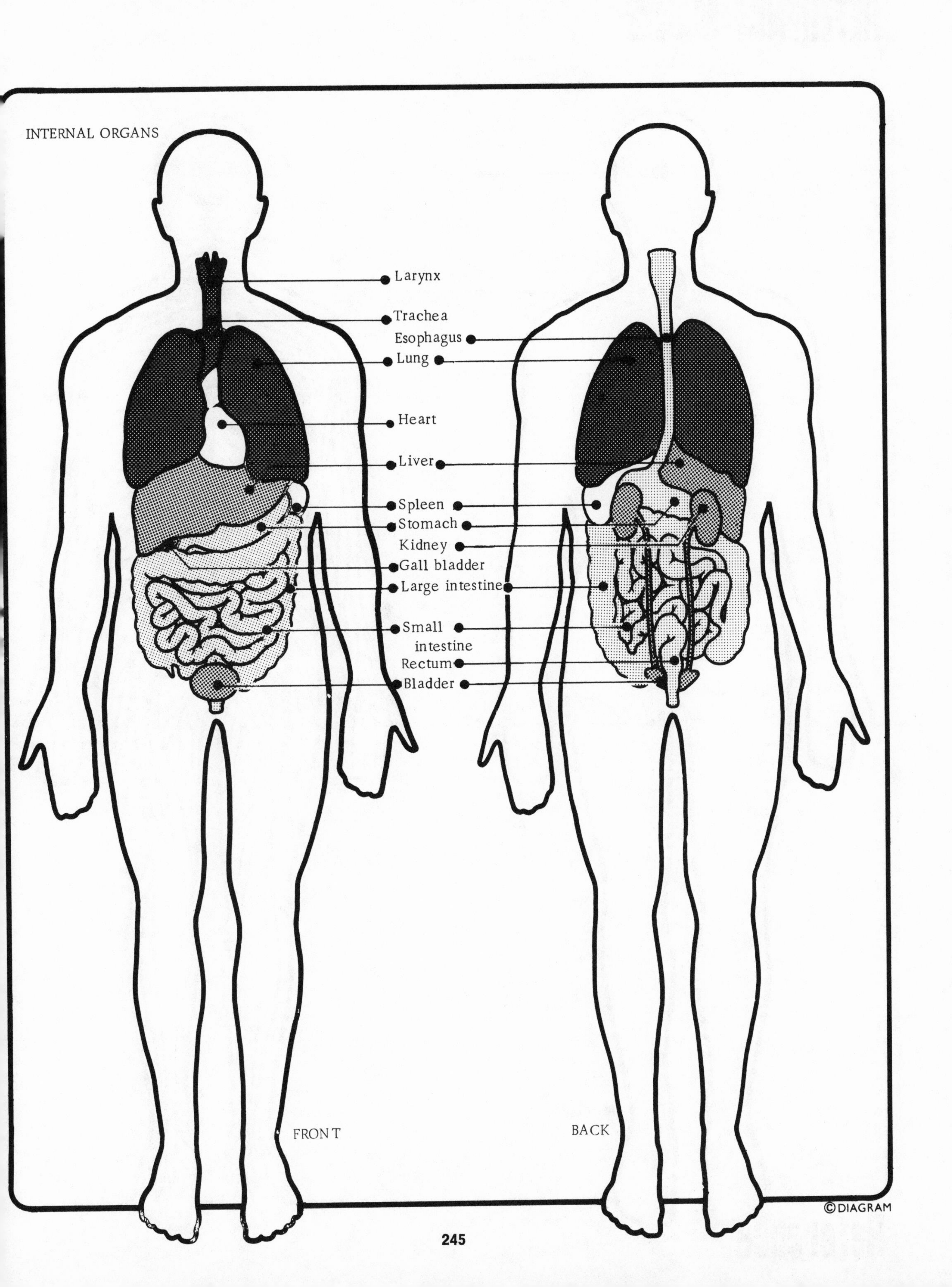
INTERNAL ORGANS
Larynx
Trachea
Esophagus
Lung
Heart
Liver
Spleen
Stomach
Kidney
Gall bladder
Large intestine
Small intestine
Rectum
Bladder
FRONT
BACK
©DIAGRAM

REFERENCE MAN 3

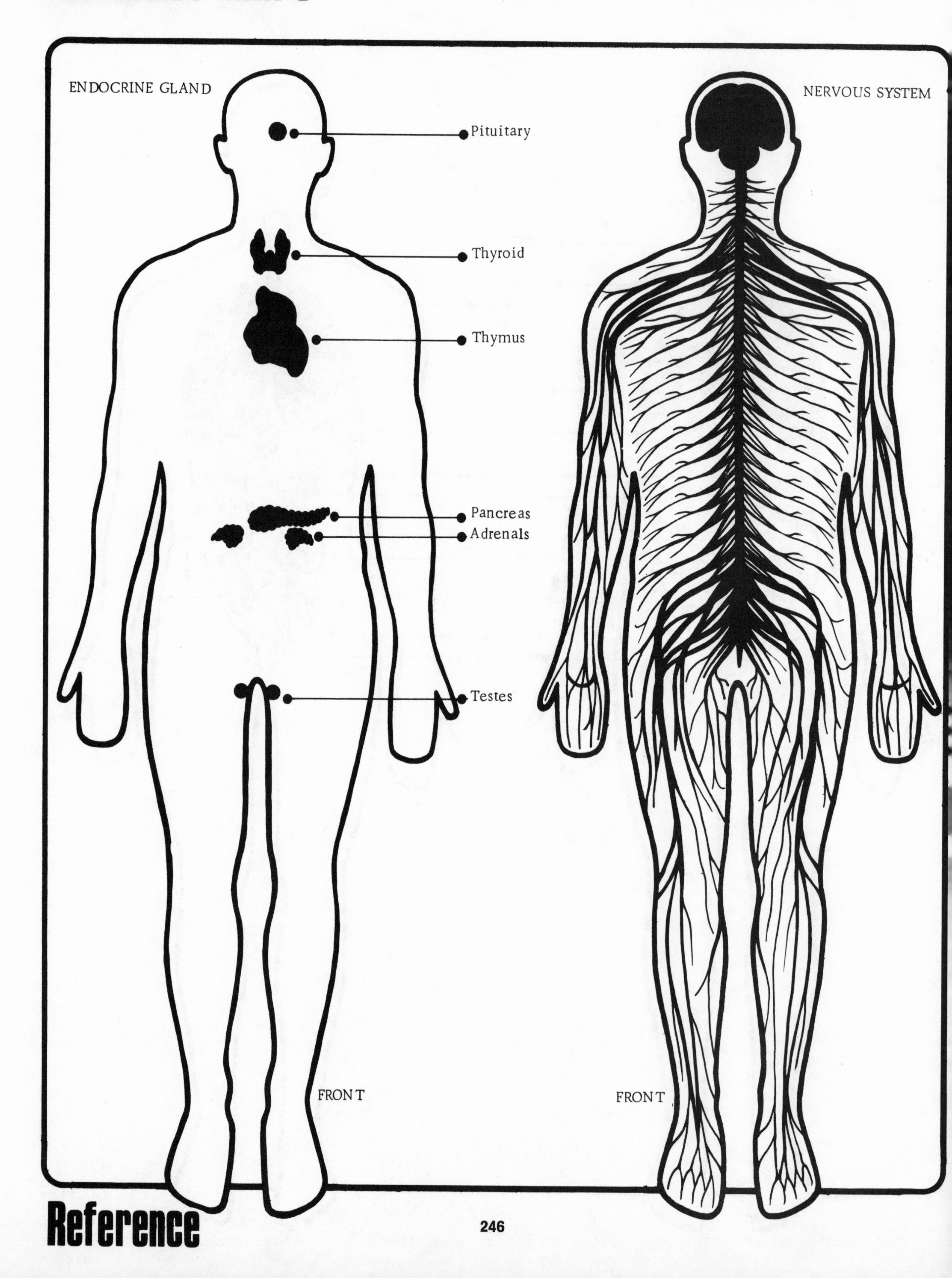

REPLACEABLE MAN

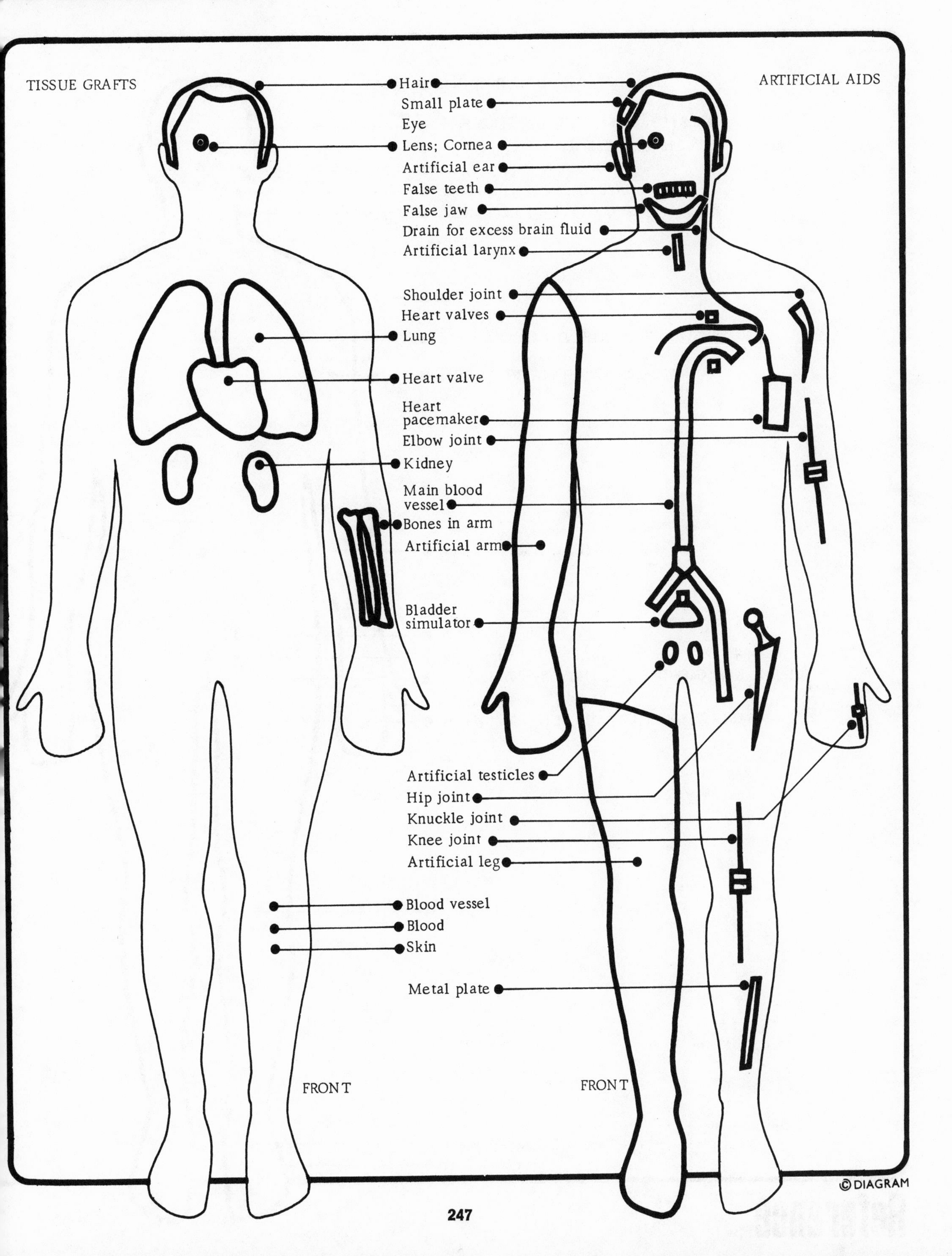

INDEX MAN

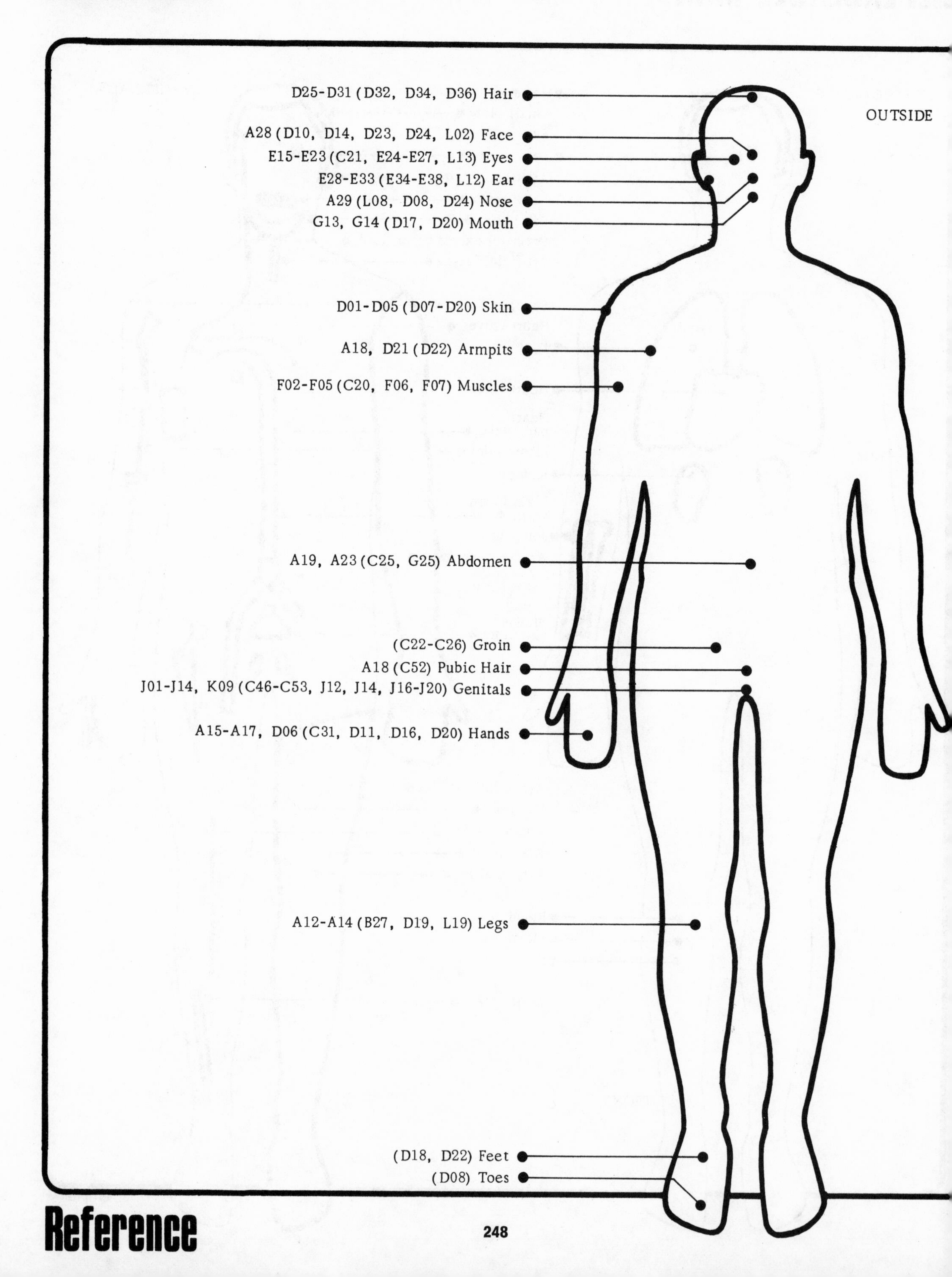

OUTSIDE
D25-D31 (D32, D34, D36) Hair
A28 (D10, D14, D23, D24, L02) Face
E15-E23 (C21, E24-E27, L13) Eyes
E28-E33 (E34-E38, L12) Ear
A29 (L08, D08, D24) Nose
G13, G14 (D17, D20) Mouth
D01-D05 (D07-D20) Skin
A18, D21 (D22) Armpits
F02-F05 (C20, F06, F07) Muscles
A19, A23 (C25, G25) Abdomen
(C22-C26) Groin
A18 (C52) Pubic Hair
J01-J14, K09 (C46-C53, J12, J14, J16-J20) Genitals
A15-A17, D06 (C31, D11, D16, D20) Hands
A12-A14 (B27, D19, L19) Legs
(D18, D22) Feet
(D08) Toes

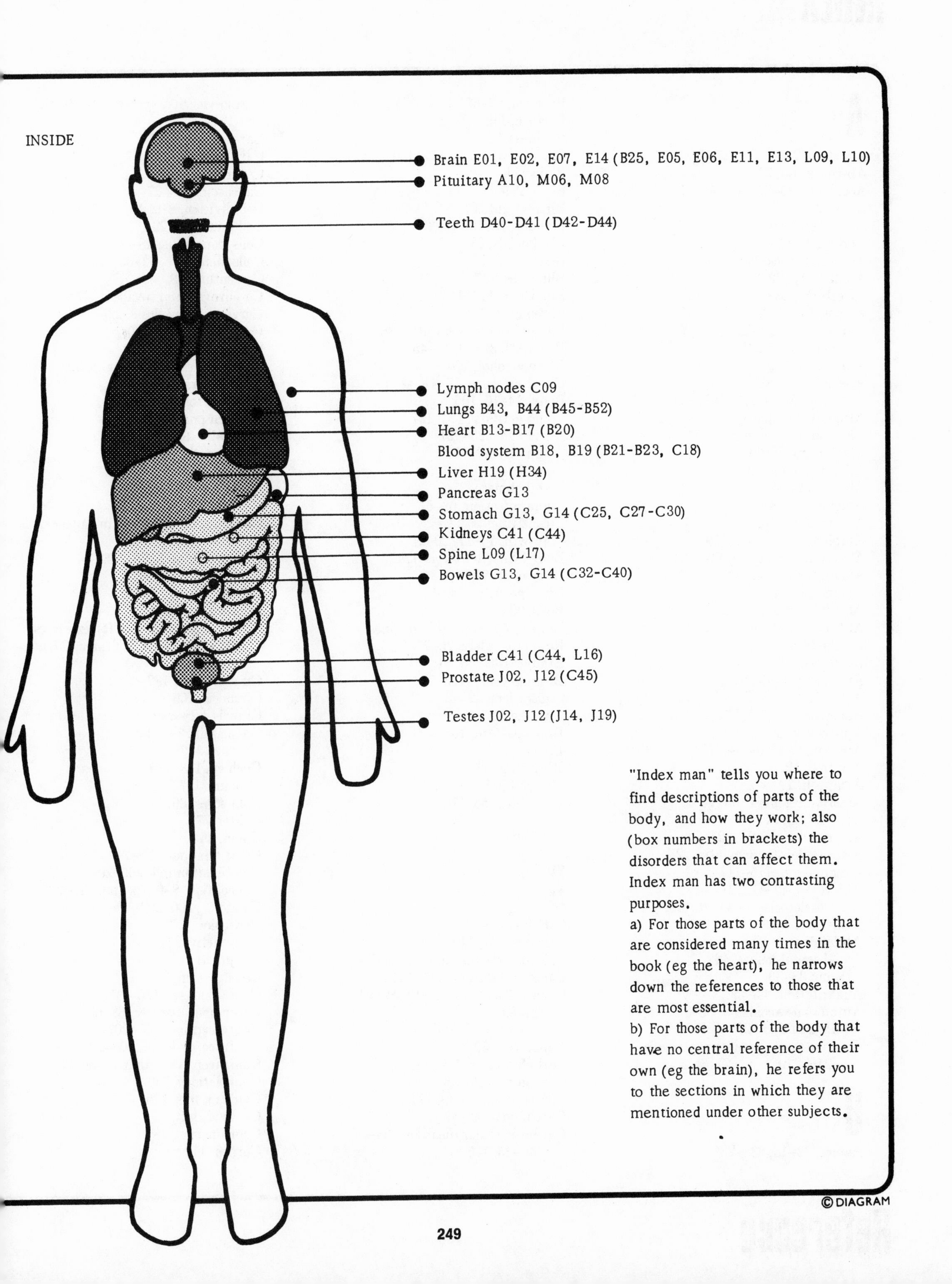

"Index man" tells you where to find descriptions of parts of the body, and how they work; also (box numbers in brackets) the disorders that can affect them. Index man has two contrasting purposes.

a) For those parts of the body that are considered many times in the book (eg the heart), he narrows down the references to those that are most essential.

b) For those parts of the body that have no central reference of their own (eg the brain), he refers you to the sections in which they are mentioned under other subjects.

INDEX

D

E

F

INDEX

N

O

P

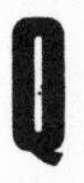

R

W

X

Y